MW00680908

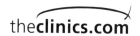

SURGICAL ONCOLOGY CLINICS OF NORTH AMERICA

Progress in Surgical Oncology:
A European Perspective

GUEST EDITOR
Bernard Nordlinger, MD

CONSULTING EDITOR
Nicholas J. Petrelli, MD

July 2008 • Volume 17 • Number 3

SAUNDERS

An Imprint of Elsevier, Inc.
PHILADELPHIA   LONDON   TORONTO   MONTREAL   SYDNEY   TOKYO

W.B. SAUNDERS COMPANY
A Division of Elsevier Inc.

1600 John F. Kennedy Boulevard, Suite 1800 • Philadelphia, PA 19103-2899

http://www.theclinics.com

SURGICAL ONCOLOGY CLINICS
OF NORTH AMERICA
July 2008
Editor: Catherine Bewick

Volume 17, Number 3
ISSN 1055-3207
ISBN-13: 978-1-4160-6359-9
ISBN-10: 1-4160-6359-5

The ideas and opinions expressed in the *Surgical Oncology Clinics of North America* do not necessarily reflect those of the Publisher. The Publisher does not assume any responsibility for any injury and/or damage to persons or property arising out of or related to any use of the material contained in this periodical. The reader is advised to check the appropriate medical literature and the product information currently provided by the manufacturer of each drug to be administered to verify the dosage, the method and duration of administration, or contra-indications. It is the responsibility of the treating physician or other health care professional, relying on independent experience and knowledge of the patient, to determine drug dosages and the best treatment for the patient. Mention of any product in this issue should not be construed as endorsement by the contributors, editors, or the Publisher of the product or manufacturers' claims.

Surgical Oncology Clinics of North America (ISSN 1055-3207) is published quarterly by Elsevier Inc., 360 Park Avenue South, New York, NY 10010-1710. Months of publication are January, April, July, and October. Business and editorial offices: 1600 John F. Kennedy Boulevard, Suite 1800, Philadelphia, PA 19103-2899. Customer service office: 6277 Sea Harbor Drive, Orlando, FL 32887–4800. Periodicals postage paid at New York, NY, and additional mailing offices. Subscription prices are $202.00 per year (US individuals), $308.00 (US institutions) $102.00 (US student/resident), $232.00 (Canadian individuals), $375.00 (Canadian institutions), $137.00 (Canadian student/resident), $272.00 (foreign individuals), $375.00 (foreign institutions), and $137.00 (foreign student/resident). Foreign air speed delivery is included in all *Clinics* subscription prices. All prices are subject to change without notice. POST-MASTER: Send address changes to *Surgical Oncology Clinics of North America,* Elsevier Journals Customer Service, 6277 Sea Harbor Drive, Orlando, FL 32887–4800. **Customer Service: 1-800-654-2452 (US). From outside the United States, call 1-407-563-6020. Fax: 1-407-363-9661. E-mail: JournalsCustomerService-usa@** elsevier.com.

Reprints. For copies of 100 or more, of articles in this publication, please contact the Commercial Reprints Department, Elsevier Inc., 360 Park Avenue South, New York, New York 10010-1710. Tel. (212) 633-3813 Fax: (212) 462-1935 email: reprints@elsevier.com.

Surgical Oncology Clinics of North America is covered in *Index Medicus and EMBASE/Excerpta Medica, Current Contents/Clinical Medicine, and ISI/BIOMED.*

Printed in the United States of America.

CONSULTING EDITOR

NICHOLAS J. PETRELLI, MD, Bank of America Endowed Medical Director, Helen F. Graham Cancer Center at Christiana Care Health System, Newark, Delaware; and Professor of Surgery, Thomas Jefferson University, Philadelphia, Pennsylvania

GUEST EDITOR

BERNARD NORDLINGER, MD, Hopital Ambroise–Paré, Service de Chirurgie Digestive, Boulogne–Billancourt, France

CONTRIBUTORS

MOSTAFA AMINI, MD, Director, Department of Pathology, San Giovanni–Addolorata Hospital, Rome, Italy

OMER AZIZ, MBBS, MRCS, Specialist Registrar and Honorary Research Fellow, Department of Bio Surgery and Surgical Technology, Imperial College London, St. Mary's Hospital, London, United Kingdom

FAUSTO BADELLINO, MD, Genova, Italy

RICHARD BRYANT, MD, Department of Gastrointestinal and Hepatobiliary Surgery, Hopital Henri Mondor–University of Paris, Creteil, France

OLIVIER R.C. BUSCH, MD, Department of Surgery, Academic Medical Center of the University of Amsterdam, Amsterdam, the Netherlands

DANIEL CHERQUI, MD, Professor of Surgery and Chief, Department of Gastrointestinal and Hepatobiliary Surgery, and Live Transplantation, Hopital Henri Mondor–University of Paris, Creteil, France

WILLY COOSEMANS, MD, PhD, Associate Professor of Surgery and Clinical Head, Department of Thoracic Surgery, University Hospitals Leuven, Leuven, Belgium

ARA W. DARZI, FRCS, FACS, FMedSci, KBE, Professor of Surgery, Department of Bio Surgery and Surgical Technology, Imperial College London, St. Mary's Hospital, London, United Kingdom

HERBERT DECALUWÉ, MD, Resident, Department of Thoracic Surgery, University Hospitals Leuven, Leuven, Belgium

GEORGES DECKER, MD, Consultant, Department of Thoracic Surgery, University Hospitals Leuven, Leuven, Belgium

PAUL De LEYN, MD, PhD, Associate Professor of Surgery and Clinical Head, Department of Thoracic Surgery, University Hospitals Leuven, Leuven, Belgium

ALEXANDER M.M. EGGERMONT, MD, PhD, Professor of Surgical Oncology, Erasmus University Medical Center–Daniel den Hoed Cancer Center, Rotterdam, the Netherlands

MASSIMO FARINA, MD, Surgeon, Department of Surgery, San Giovanni–Addolorata Hospital, Rome, Italy

LUCIO FORTUNATO, MD, Attending Surgeon, Department of Surgery, San Giovanni–Addolorata Hospital, Rome, Italy

DIRK J. GOUMA, MD, Department of Surgery, Academic Medical Center of the University of Amsterdam, Amsterdam, the Netherlands

DANIEL JAECK, MD, PhD, FRCS, Professor, Centre de Chirurgie Viscérale e de Transplantation, Hopital de Hautepierre, Hopitaux Universitaires de Strasbourg, Université Louis Pasteur, Strasbourg, France

ALEXIS LAURENT, MD, PhD, Department of Gastrointestinal and Hepatobiliary Surgery, Hopital Henri Mondor–University of Paris, Creteil, France

TONI LERUT, MD, PhD, FRCSI(Hon), FRCS, FACS, Professor of Surgery, The Huub and Imelda Spierings Chair in Thoracic and Esophageal Surgery, and Chairman, Department of Thoracic Surgery, University Hospitals Leuven, Leuven, Belgium

MARIO LISE, MD, Surgery Branch, Department on Oncological and Surgical Sciences, University of Padova, Padova, Italy

ALAIN LUCIANI, MD, PhD, Department of Radiology, Hopital Henri Mondor–University of Paris, Creteil, France

ALBERTO MARCHET, MD, Surgery Branch, Department on Oncological and Surgical Sciences, University of Padova, Padova, Italy

ALESSANDRA MASCARO, MD, Recipient of Fellowship of the American–Italian Cancer Foundation, Department of Surgery, San Giovanni–Addolorata Hospital, Rome, Italy

SIMONE MOCELLIN, MD, Surgery Branch, Department on Oncological and Surgical Sciences, University of Padova, Padova, Italy

JOHNNY MOONS, MScN, Department of Thoracic Surgery, University Hospitals Leuven, Leuven, Belgium

PHILIPPE NAFTEUX, MD, Joint Clinical Head, Department of Thoracic Surgery, University Hospitals Leuven, Leuven, Belgium

CONTRIBUTORS

R.J. NICHOLLS, MA, MChir, FRCS, Visiting Professor of Colorectal Surgery, Department of Biosurgery and Surgical Technology, St. Mary's Hospital, Imperial College; and Emeritus Consultant Surgeon, Department of Surgery, St. Mark's Hospital, London, United Kingdom

DONATO NITTI, MD, Professor, Surgery Branch, Department on Oncological and Surgical Sciences, University of Padova, Padova, Italy

PATRICK PESSAUX, MD, PhD, Professor, Centre de Chirurgie Viscérale e de Transplantation, Hopital de Hautepierre, Hopitaux Universitaires de Strasbourg, Université Louis Pasteur, Strasbourg, France

PIERLUIGI PILATI, MD, Surgery Branch, Department on Oncological and Surgical Sciences, University of Padova, Padova, Italy

GRAEME J. POSTON, MB, MS, FRCS(Ed), FRCS(Eng), Chairman of the Department of Surgery and Director, Division of Surgery, Digestive Diseases, Critical Care, and Anesthesia, Center for Digestive Diseases, University Hospital Aintree, Liverpool, United Kingdom

ALAIN SAUVANET, MD, Professor, Service de Chirurgie Digestive, Hopital Beaujon, Université Paris VII, AP–HP, Clichy-Cedex, France

CLAUDE TAYAR, MD, Department of Gastrointestinal and Hepatobiliary Surgery, Hopital Henri Mondor–University of Paris, Creteil, France

PARIS P. TEKKIS, MD, FRCS, Senior Lecturer and Consultant Surgeon, Department of Biosurgery and Surgical Technology, St. Mary's Hospital, Imperial College; and Honorary Consultant Surgeon, Department of Surgery, St. Mark's Hospital, London, United Kingdom

SALVATORE TOMA, MD, PhD, Professor of Medical Oncology, Dipartimento di Oncologia, Biologia e Genetica, Universitá di Genova, Genova, Italy

JEANNE TRAN van NHIEU, MD, Department of Pathology, Hopital Henri Mondor–University of Paris, Creteil, France

THOMAS M. van GULIK, MD, Department of Surgery, Academic Medical Center of the University of Amsterdam, Amsterdam, the Netherlands

DIRK van RAEMDONCK, MD, PhD, Associate Professor of Surgery and Clinical Head, Department of Thoracic Surgery, University Hospitals Leuven, Leuven, Belgium

CARLO EUGENIO VITELLI, MD, Director, Department of Surgery, San Giovanni–Addolorata Hospital, Rome, Italy

CHRISTIANE VOIT, MD, Department of Dermatology, Charité, Humboldt University, Berlin, Germany

CONTENTS

Despite radical surgery, the prognosis of patients who have gastric carcinoma remains unsatisfactory because of the intrinsic but unpredictable aggressiveness of this malignancy. During the past decade an ever-growing list of molecular prognostic factors has been proposed based on the discovery of the mechanisms underlying gastric cancer aggressiveness. Studies performed in larger and more homogeneous series of patients and adequate statistical analysis are warranted before any of the candidate biomarkers can be implemented in the routine clinical setting for the identification of patients at higher risk and thus for the selection of candidates for adjuvant or more aggressive therapies.

Tremendous progress has been made in surgery for cancer of the esophagus and gastroesophageal junction. After primary surgery, overall 5-year survival rates of 35% or more are obtained in high-volume units, and for advanced stage III cancer, 5-year survival reaches 25%. Multimodality therapy, in particular induction chemotherapy with or without radiotherapy, results in a complete response rate in up to 25% of the patients. Approximately 50% of the patients receiving such treatment do not respond, however, and their outcome is dismal. Therefore, further efforts are needed to elaborate more precise algorithms for selecting candidates for induction therapy versus primary surgery.

FORTHCOMING ISSUES

RECENT ISSUES

THE CLINICS ARE NOW ONLINE!

Access your subscription at:
http://www.theclinics.com

ELSEVIER
SAUNDERS

Surg Oncol Clin N Am
17 (2008) xiii–xiv

SURGICAL
ONCOLOGY CLINICS
OF NORTH AMERICA

Foreword

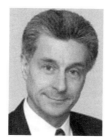

Nicholas J. Petrelli, MD
Consulting Editor

This issue of the *Surgical Oncology Clinics of North America* is entitled "Update on Surgical Oncology in Europe." The guest editor is Bernard Nordlinger, MD, from the Department of Digestive and Oncologic Surgery, Ambroise–Paré Hospital, Boulogne, France. Dr. Nordlinger is one of the world's experts in the field of hepatic resection for liver metastases.

This issue of the *Surgical Oncology Clinics of North America* contains an array of outstanding European investigators who have contributed to many of the advances in the surgical treatment of solid tumors over the last decade. The topics vary from the molecular prognostic factors in gastric cancer by Donato Nitti from Padova, Italy, to the laparoscopic resection for colorectal cancer. Dr. Alexander Eggermont from Rotterdam, The Netherlands, discusses the European approach to the management of melanoma, while Dr. Faust Badellino from Genova, Italy, discusses the European approach to the treatment of soft tissue sarcomas.

Our European surgical oncologists have made great contributions to the care of cancer patients. It is important that collaborative efforts between surgical oncologists in the United States and Europe become stronger. I congratulate Raphael Pollock, MD, past President of the Society of Surgical Oncology, who, during his tenure (2006–2007), formed the International Committee of the Society of Surgical Oncology. Joseph M. Klausner from Tel Aviv Sourasky Medical Center in Tel Aviv, Israel, is the appointed chair of this committee. Although the committee is young in existence, it is making efforts to potential new members in Europe and Israel in describing the advantages of joining the Society of Surgical Oncology. The committee is

doi:10.1016/j.soc.2008.04.017
surgonc.theclinics.com

also considering new representatives from France, Italy, Sweden, Holland, Switzerland, the United Kingdom, Argentina, Brazil, and Mexico for membership in the International Committee, with expectations of adding other surgeons from Japan and Russia; all of this to strengthen our collaborative efforts with our European colleagues.

I congratulate Dr. Nordlinger for bringing together a talented group of investigators to update readers about the present status of surgical oncology in Europe. In my opinion, this subject matter was long overdue for our readers.

Nicholas J. Petrelli, MD
Helen F. Graham Cancer Center
Christiana Care Health System
4701 Ogletown-Stanton Road
Suite 1233
Newark, DE 19713, USA

Department of Surgery
Thomas Jefferson University
College Building
1025 Walnut Street
Philadelphia, PA 19107, USA

E-mail address: npetrelli@christianacare.org

SURGICAL
ONCOLOGY CLINICS
OF NORTH AMERICA

ELSEVIER
SAUNDERS

Surg Oncol Clin N Am
17 (2008) xv–xvi

Preface

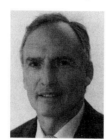

Bernard Nordlinger, MD
Guest Editor

The *Surgical Oncology Clinics of North America* dedicates this entire issue to European surgical oncology. Important advances have been made in recent years in surgical oncology— or rather in multimodality management of cancer that includes surgery.

When significant progress is made, reports are presented in major congresses and published in journals with worldwide distribution. The medical community finally does not care which part of the world the progress is coming from, as long as it is useful. And sometimes, the medical community does not even know where the author of an important report is working. So why an issue dedicated to European perspectives in surgical oncology?

Unlike North America, Europe is made of many countries that are very different from each other, from the north to the south and the west to the east. But there are some common ways of thinking and common strategies. They may differ from those of other continents.

European cooperative research groups, such as the European Organisation for Research and Treatment of Cancer (EORTC), have demonstrated their ability to address important questions concerning the treatment of cancer, and organize and conduct large clinical trials within and outside of Europe.

This issue includes contributions by leading experts from different European countries and is an opportunity to demonstrate the variety of fields in which European surgery has made major contributions to progress.

A broad spectrum of cancer-related topics are covered, including esophageal and gastric carcinoma, colorectal cancer, liver metastases, melanoma,

doi:10.1016/j.soc.2008.04.016

pancreatic neoplasm, hepatocellular cancer, soft tissue sarcoma, breast cancer, and laparoscopic surgery. I am grateful to all of the contributors for their efforts in providing state-of-the-art information. Of course, the information contained in these articles does not consider only progress coming from Europe but is a perspective as seen by recognized European experts.

As a whole, this issue provides a review of some of the most significant and clinically relevant advances in the field of surgical oncology in recent years. I hope the readers will find it informative and useful.

Bernard Nordlinger, MD
Hôpital Ambroise-Paré
Service de Chirurgie Digestive
9 avenue Charles De Gaulle
92100 Boulogne-Billancourt
France

E-mail address: bernard.nordlinger@apr.aphp.fr

ELSEVIER
SAUNDERS

Surg Oncol Clin N Am
17 (2008) 467–483

SURGICAL
ONCOLOGY CLINICS
OF NORTH AMERICA

Recent Advances in Conventional and Molecular Prognostic Factors for Gastric Carcinoma

Donato Nitti, MD*, Simone Mocellin, MD,
Alberto Marchet, MD, Pierluigi Pilati, MD,
Mario Lise, MD

*Surgery Branch, Department of Oncological and Surgical Sciences, University of Padova,
Via Giustiniani 2, 35128 Padova, Italy*

Despite its declining incidence, gastric cancer still ranks among the first 10 causes for cancer mortality worldwide, although significant geographic differences exist [1,2]. Currently, surgery represents the only potentially curative treatment [3–5]. Despite technical advances in surgery and the use of adjuvant therapies, the 5-year overall survival rates of patients who have resectable gastric cancer are unsatisfactory, ranging from 20% to 30% [3–5]. This low rate of survival is attributable, at least in part, to advanced disease at diagnosis. Indeed, only 30% to 60% of patients undergo surgical resections with curative intent in Western countries [3–6]. By contrast, early diagnosis based on mass screening programs has resulted in a significant decrease in mortality in some countries (eg, Japan) [7]. The other major determinant of poor gastric cancer prognosis is linked to the high biologic aggressiveness of this disease, which is characterized by the early development of metastatic potential and by significant resistance to conventional antineoplastic agents (eg, chemotherapeutic drugs and radiotherapy). In the absence of formal screening programs, most patients present with disease at an advanced pathologic stage and can expect a median survival of 24 months (5-year survival, 20%–30%) in tumors resected with curative intent and a median survival of 6 to 8 months after palliative procedures [3–5]. Currently, the most powerful prognostic factors are the TNM stage at diagnosis and the possibility of achieving an apparently

* Corresponding author.
E-mail address: donato.nitti@unipd.it (D. Nitti).

1055-3207/08/$ - see front matter © 2008 Elsevier Inc. All rights reserved.
doi:10.1016/j.soc.2008.02.010
surgonc.theclinics.com

radical surgery at laparotomy [3–5,8]. Besides the development of novel, more effective therapeutic strategies, efforts to improve the life expectancy of these patients are directed toward the identification of patients who have a higher risk of disease recurrence after radical surgery and the selection of patients who have a greater likelihood of responding to adjuvant treatments [9–11]. In a personalized cancer medicine approach [12], this identification would lead to the treatment of patients who most need adjuvant therapy (ie, those at high risk for the presence of minimal residual disease) and to the treatment of patients who are most likely to benefit from a given therapeutic regimen (ie, those who have a tumor sensitive to the anticancer agents administered). In this respect, the current version of the TNM staging system [8] is largely inappropriate, because the variability of prognosis within each stage does not allow the prediction of clinical outcome on a single-patient basis. Improvements in the current TNM system together with the identification of molecular markers of tumor aggressiveness are the pillars of the growing interest in the application of the principles of stratified medicine [13] to the management of patients who have gastric cancer. This article reviews the current knowledge of the latest developments regarding conventional prognostic factors that might lead to a novel version of the TNM system. Furthermore, recent progress in applying the insights of tumor biology for prediction of prognosis is reviewed and discussed.

Conventional prognostic factors

Tumor site

The tumor location has several important implications in the treatment and prognosis of gastric cancer. Although some studies showed no association between tumor site and clinical outcome [14,15], most investigators have reported that gastric carcinoma of the proximal third of the stomach represents a distinct clinical entity with specific prognostic implications [3,6,16–19]. In particular, proximal tumors have a higher frequency of larger size, extensive wall penetration, vessel invasion, lymph node metastasis, more advanced stage, and an overall worse survival than distal tumors. The clinical relevance of tumor location is underscored by the epidemiologic evidence that, despite the overall decrease in the incidence of gastric cancer, the incidence of tumors in the upper third of the stomach has risen significantly during the last few decades [20].

TNM staging system

The pathologic TNM stage consistently has been reported to be an independent prognostic factor for both disease-free and overall survival [2,3,8,21–23]. In particular, the depth of gastric wall invasion by the tumor (T category) allows a distinction to be made between cases that have a favorable prognosis (T1 tumors limited to the submucosa layer, also called "early gastric cancer") and those that have a poorer prognosis (T2–T4 tumors extending through the muscular layer, the visceral peritoneum, and through neighbor organs, also called "advanced gastric cancer"). On the other hand, the status of regional lymph nodes (N category, defined as the absolute number of positive lymph nodes at pathologic examination of the surgical specimen) predicts clinical outcome independently of the T category. Almost 10 years ago Siewert and colleagues [23] reported that the ratio between metastatic and removed lymph nodes (the N ratio) was the single most important independent prognostic factor, followed by residual tumor status and T category (n = 1654). Since then, many other investigators have confirmed that the N ratio might be a better way of classifying the lymph node status than the conventional N category [22,24–31]. With this regard, the present authors [21] have demonstrated in a large series (n = 1851) that using the N ratio in the staging system (which then should be called the "TRM" classification) in place of the N category provides more accurate prognostic than information can be achieved using the current TNM system. In fact, the overlapping of survival curves observed with the TNM classification is abolished completely with the TRM system, so better patient stratification can be obtained by using the N ratio.

Grading

Tumor grading refers to the degree of differentiation of malignant cells and classifies cancers into three categories: well, moderately, and poorly differentiated (or anaplastic). Although tumor grading has been associated with prognosis and is reported routinely in pathologic reports of gastric cancer specimens, the prognostic impact of this parameter remains to be proven. In fact, several retrospective studies have failed to identify grading as an independent prognostic factor [14,19,32].

Lymphatic and vascular invasion

The presence of malignant cells within tumor-associated vessels and lymphatics has been associated classically with a worse prognosis. Several histopathologic studies have demonstrated that lymphatic involvement is a statistically significant predictor of survival and that the presence of tumor emboli significantly influences tumor recurrence and death after curative resection [18,33,34]. For instance, Yokota and colleagues [18] found that lymphatic invasion retained its significance (relative risk, 11.4; 95% confidence interval, 2.6–49.5) in a multivariate analysis model (n = 266). These findings were supported recently in a report by Hyung and colleagues [34], who reported a poor prognosis associated with advanced T category and the presence of vascular invasion (n = 280). Analogously, Kooby and colleagues [35] demonstrated in adequately staged node-negative patients (n = 507) that vascular invasion is an independent negative prognostic factor and may be a predictor of biologic aggressiveness.

Type of surgery

The extent of surgical dissection at the time of primary tumor resection might influence both patient survival (therapeutic effect) and accurate staging (prognostic value), with the latter being particularly relevant for the assessment of nodal status. For instance, the type of gastric resection (total versus subtotal) in cases of gastric cancer of the distal stomach was found to be irrelevant in terms of patient survival [3]. Even worse, the use of splenectomy associated with gastric resection was demonstrated to affect patient clinical outcome negatively, at least in the absence of malignant infiltration of the spleen [36].

In contrast with this evidence, about which most investigators involved in gastric cancer management agree, a still open issue remains the extent of regional lymphadenectomy. In particular, a more limited node dissection (referred as to "D1 type lymphadenectomy") might be associated with shorter survival than a more extensive dissection (D2 type lymphadenectomy) [3,37]. The discrepancy in overall survival rates reported by Japanese (shorter survival) and Western centers led to the conduction of two large, multicentric, randomized prospective trials [38,39] that could not demonstrate a significant difference in overall survival. These results, however, may be confounded by surgical learning curves and poor surgeon compliance, and thus available data cannot rule out a survival benefit for patients who have intermediate TNM stage disease undergoing D2 type dissection [40]. While waiting for definitive evidence about the impact of lymph node dissection on survival in the only study addressing the impact of lymph node dissection on the prognostic value of the N ratio [21], the present authors have found that the accuracy of this prognostic factor is not influenced by the type of lymphadenectomy (D1 versus D2 lymphadenectomy). Because of the relatively limited number of patients analyzed, they could not establish a minimum number of lymph nodes to be removed to maintain the prognostic power of the N ratio. Nevertheless, given the linear positive correlation between the number of nodes excised and the likelihood of finding positive nodes [37], a minimum of 15 lymph nodes removed at the time of gastrectomy (as recommended by the American Joint Committee on Cancer in the TNM staging system) should be considered the standard approach for achieving adequate N staging.

Gastric cancer biology and molecular prognostic factors

During the metastatic process malignant cells must progress through a series of sequential and selective events consisting of tumor cell detachment, local invasion, motility, angiogenesis, vessel invasion, survival in the circulation, adhesion to endothelial cells, extravasation, and growth in different organs/tissues. Candidate molecules playing a key role in each of these steps have been identified and include cell-adhesion molecules, growth factors and their receptors, matrix degradation enzymes, and motility factors. As the cascade of molecular events leading to gastric cancer progression is elucidated [41–44], a growing number of biomarkers is being proposed to improve the ability to predict patients' clinical outcome and thus optimize their therapeutic management in terms of

1. Better risk stratification, which allows personalized adjuvant treatments by identifying patients who have the highest likelihood of harboring minimal residual disease and thus of experiencing disease recurrence
2. Identification of tumors with the highest sensitivity to the available therapeutic regimens (both in the metastatic and adjuvant setting), which would spare as many as 50% of patients useless treatments
3. Identification of novel molecular targets for the development of more tumor-specific (and thus more effective) therapeutic agents

Many of these molecules/factors have been investigated as prognostic factors that might improve the ability of conventional parameters to predict patients' clinical outcome, as described in the following sections.

Microsatellite instability

Microsatellite instability (MSI) is defined as the presence of replication errors resulting in insertions/deletions of bases within nucleotide repeats known as "microsatellite regions." MSI may occur in a subset of sporadic gastric cancers ranging from 25% to 50% [42,45]. Three levels of MSI can be identified: high-level MSI (MSI-H), generally defined as MSI in more than 30% of the standard markers; low-level MSI (MSI-L), when changes are exhibited in less than 30% of the markers, and microsatellite stable (MSS) in the absence of microsatellite alterations. Recently, mononucleotide repeat markers have been shown to be highly sensitive in detecting MSI-H tumors, and revised criteria have been proposed to define MSI-H as instability at mononucleotide loci and MSI-L as instability limited only to dinucleotide loci [46]. By adopting these criteria, Ottini and colleagues [47] reported a frequency of 17% for MSI-H, 14% for MSI-L, and 69% for MSS disease in a series of gastric cancer cases from a high-risk population in central Italy. These frequencies are consistent with frequencies observed in other gastric cancer series from Western populations [48]. In colon cancer, MSI is caused more often by mutations of the DNA mismatch repair genes *hMLH1* and *hMSH2* and less frequently by mutations in *hMSH6*, *hPMS1*, and *hPMS2* genes [49]. By contrast, in gastric cancer *hMLH1* and *hMSH2* mutations are relatively rare (12%–15% of MSI-H cases) [42,45]. *hMLH1* epigenetic silencing (caused by promoter hypermethylation), however, has been found to be responsible for the development of more than 50% of gastric cancers exhibiting MSI-H phenotype [42,45]. Simple genetic and/or epigenetic inactivation of DNA mismatch repair genes is not, by itself, a transforming event, and therefore additional genetic changes are believed to be necessary for tumor development and progression [41–44]. In particular, MSI-H gastric cancer is believed to progress through mutations in coding repetitive sequences in genes involved in cell growth regulation (*TGFbRII*, *IGFIIR*, and *TCF4*), in apoptosis (*Bax*, *Fas*, *Caspase-5*, *APAF-1*), and in DNA repair genes (*hMSH6*, *hMSH3*, *MED1*, *RAD50*, and *ATR*). Interestingly, the occurrence of mutations in specific cancer-related genes confers unique clinicopathologic features to MSI-H tumors as compared with MSS and MSI-L tumors. For instance, intestinal histotype, antral location, and lower prevalence of lymph node metastases have been associated with MSI-H gastric cancers [10,50,51]. This evidence is in line with reports showing that MSI-H gastric tumors have a better long-term survival than MSS/MSI-L counterparts [10,51–55]. Some investigators, however, have not found MSI to be an independent prognostic factor [56,57], and others have reported that MSI is associated with clinical outcome only in subsets of patients [58], a finding that leads to questions about the applicability of MSI as a prognostic marker in routine clinical practice.

Tumor invasiveness

A balance of activities between matrix metalloproteinases (MMPs) and their inhibitors plays a pivotal role in determining tumor invasiveness and metastasis [59]; as a corollary, measures of this imbalance represent a potential prognostic index [60]. Among different MMPs studied in gastric cancer, some investigators have reported that the expression of MMP-7 (also known as "matrilysin") is correlated with vessel invasion, lymph node status, and distant metastases [61,62]. Analogously, others have observed that the prognosis of patients who have MMP-1–positive gastric carcinomas (n = 76) is significantly worse than that of patients who have MMP-1–negative tumors (n = 27) [63]. Furthermore, the expression of membrane-type 1 MMP, an activator of MMP-2, is associated with poorer prognosis (n = 25), although its prognostic value is not independent when a multivariable model is applied to the data [64]. Finally, tissue inhibitors of MMP (TIMP) can inhibit tumor invasion through the inactivation of MMP: in a multivariate survival analysis (n = 50), Mimori and colleagues [65] reported that a high tumor/normal ratio of TIMP-1 correlates with traditional pathologic features and is an independent factor influencing patients' prognosis. Despite these positive findings, some caution is warranted to avoid overestimating the prognostic power of MMP expression. In fact, the series thus far reported are small, and some negative reports have been published [66,67].

Vascular endothelial growth factor

Vascular endothelial growth factor (VEGF) is a master promoter of angiogenesis and plays a fundamental role in many types of tumor [41], including gastric carcinoma [41]. Besides the evidence from many preclinical models, the importance of this molecule in favoring tumor growth is underscored by the positive results obtained in the clinical setting by neutralizing VEGF with specific monoclonal antibodies in patients who have some types of solid tumors [41], including gastric carcinoma [68]. Many investigators have reported on the negative correlation between VEGF expression in primary gastric tumors and patient survival [69–74], even after adjustment for the effect of both traditional and molecular factors [75]. Accordingly, the use of VEGF expression as a prognostic biomarker in the clinical setting has been advocated [76]. Also, VEGF plasma levels have been found to predict an unfavorable clinical outcome [77], although the experience in this field is much more limited.

Cell cycle, apoptosis, and p53

Cell-cycle checkpoints are regulatory pathways that control cell-cycle transitions, DNA replication, and chromosome segregation. Abnormalities in cell-cycle regulators are involved in stomach carcinogenesis through genomic instability and unbridled cell proliferation [41–44]. The *cyclin-E* gene is amplified in 15% to 20% of gastric cancers, and the overexpression of *cyclin-E* correlates with the aggressiveness of the cancer (n = 89) [78]. Reduction in the expression of *p27/Kip1*, a cyclin-dependent kinase inhibitor, frequently is associated with advanced gastric cancers, and the reduced expression of *p27/Kip1* also correlates significantly with deep invasion and lymph node metastasis. In fact, it has been shown that reduced *p27* expression is a negative prognostic factor for patients who have a *cyclin-E*–positive tumor (n = 241) [79]. An important regulator at the G1/S checkpoint is retinoblastoma (RB) protein. RB expression is lower in lymph node metastases than in the corresponding primary tumors [80]; furthermore, univariate and multivariate survival analyses have revealed that reduced expression of RB is associated with worse overall survival (n = 67). The product of the tumor suppressor gene, *p53*, is multifunctional and participates in cell-cycle regulation partly through *p21* induction, which promotes cell-cycle arrest by inhibiting the phosphorylation of the cyclin-dependent kinase complexes. Although more than 100 articles have been published concerning *p53* abnormalities in gastric cancer in relation to patients' prognosis, the prognostic impact remains controversial [11]. Recent reports indicate that abnormal expression of *p53* significantly affects cumulative survival and that *p53* status also may influence response to chemotherapy [81,82]. Okuyama and colleagues [83] suggested that the *p53/p21* status could represent a prognostic marker for survival in patients who have surgically resected gastric cancer (n = 195). In fact, the median survival time was significantly longer in the *p53*-negative/*p21*-positive group of patients. Recent studies indicate that inducible nitric oxide synthase (iNOS), VEGF, and *p53* are fundamental in the angiogenic process. In fact, it has been shown that iNOS and

VEGF overexpression can induce tumor-associated angiogenesis, whereas *p53* suppresses angiogenesis by down-regulating VEGF and iNOS, thus eventually influencing prognosis. In particular, in a series of 55 patients, Feng and colleagues [84] reported that a positive immunostaining reaction for the iNOS protein was correlated significantly with lymph node metastases, whereas *p53* expression was higher in poorly differentiated gastric carcinomas than in well-differentiated ones. Moreover, no positive immunostaining was observed for *p53*, iNOS, and VEGF in the histologically normal tissue and in chronic superficial gastritis; by contrast, *p53*-, iNOS-, and VEGF-positive immunostaining was observed in tissues of lesions ranging in severity from chronic atrophic gastritis, intestinal metaplasia, and dysplasia, with the positive rate increasing with lesion progression. These findings may indicate that p53 protein accumulation and increased expression of iNOS and VEGF might be responsible for gastric carcinogenesis and tumor aggressiveness, supporting their prognostic potential.

Cell adhesion

Among the cell adhesion factors that can influence gastric carcinoma, E-cadherin is the best characterized. E-cadherin, which is essential for cell–cell adhesion of epithelial cells, is encoded by the *CDH1* gene. Loss of expression of E-cadherin has been found in many sporadic cases, and germline *CDH1* mutations are believed to play a key role in the development of familial gastric cancer [85]. Moreover, *CDH1* promoter methylation or polymorphism can lead to the transcriptional down-regulation of the gene [86,87]. An inverse correlation has been detected between normal E-cadherin and *MUC1* expression, and it has been suggested that patients who have early gastric carcinoma (n = 209) presenting with a combination of normal E-cadherin and *MUC1*-negative expression possess a more favorable prognosis [88]. Similarly, Mingchao and colleagues [89] found an abnormal expression of E-cadherin and beta-catenin in 46% and 44% of gastric carcinomas (n = 13), respectively; these alterations occurred more frequently in diffuse than in intestinal-type gastric tumors, but other authors also have suggested that loss of E-cadherin could represent an early event in intestinal-type gastric carcinogenesis. Moreover, a significant correlation between abnormal beta-catenin expression and lymph node metastases was demonstrated, and 36% and 16% of gastric dysplasia stained abnormally for E-cadherin and beta-catenin, respectively, thus suggesting that an abnormal expression of the E-cadherin/beta-catenin complex in gastric dysplasia may be an early event in the tumorigenesis process as well as a useful prognostic marker if the results are validated in larger series.

Gene expression profiles

Because cancer is a polygenic disease, it seems logical to expect that high-throughput technologies such as gene microarray [90] and proteomics [91] will improve significantly the ability of obtain an overall picture of the molecular events governing gastric cancer progression. As a corollary, new sets of prognostic factors should be identified that overcome the intrinsic limit of single-molecule–based prediction of prognosis. Although the use of proteomics in this field is still in its infancy, several groups have tested gene microarray technology to find gene expression signatures specifically related to metastatic potential and prognosis. Hippo and colleagues [92] studied the expression profiles of 6800 genes and reported that overexpression of *RBP4, OCT2, IGF2, PFN2, KIAA1093, PCOLCE*, and *FN1* was associated with lymph node metastasis (n = 22). Hasegawa and colleagues [93] performed a genome-wide analysis of gene expression in well-differentiated gastric cancers (n = 20), using a cDNA microarray representing 23,040 genes and found that the altered expression of 12 genes (*DDOST, GNS, NEDD8, LOC51096, CCT3, CCT5, PPP2R1B, UBQLN1, AIM2, USP9X,* and two expressed sequence tags) was associated with lymph node metastasis. In line with these findings, in the authors' experience (n = 32), the combined expression of three genes by primary tumors (namely *BIK, Aurora Kinase B*, and *eIF5A2*) correctly predicted lymph node status in 30 cases (accuracy, 93%) [94]. Inoue and colleagues [95] developed a prognostic scoring system using a cDNA microarray. Seventy-eight genes were expressed differentially in patients who had aggressive or nonaggressive gastric cancers (n = 43). The prognostic score, calculated by summing up the value of a coefficient for each gene, can predict the stage of disease and the patient's prognosis. Finally, Yasui and colleagues [96] developed a custom-made oligo-DNA microarray with known genes related to the development and progression of cancer and marker genes for chemosensitivity. These investigators were able to identify clusters of genes that could be used to classify patients (n = 5) in different TNM stages correctly. Although these reported examples indicate that gene microarray analysis may be useful to search for novel prognostic factors, it also underscores heterogeneity of the results obtained so far in gastric cancer (as already reported for other malignancies [97]). This heterogeneity prevents researchers from implementing these findings in the clinical setting before larger and more homogeneous series of patients are analyzed and meta-analysis of comparable studies is performed.

Circulating tumor cells

Minimal residual disease is represented by single disseminated tumor cells detected by cytologic examination, immunohistochemical analysis, or polymerase chain reaction (PCR) in bone marrow, blood (circulating tumor cells, CTC), and lymph nodes in patients who have different tumor types, including gastric cancer [98]. Although conventional cytology-based methods detect one epithelial cell per 10^3 to 10^4 cells, PCR allows the detection of one epithelial cell per 10^6 to 10^7 cells. Although this 3- to 4-log gain in sensitivity is accompanied by a loss in specificity, PCR is the most popular method for studying minimal residual disease in oncology, and it represents the standard of care in the management of some hematologic malignancies [99]. In gastric carcinoma, the largest experience in the search for minimal residual disease has involved the detection of CTC. The presence of CTC in the peripheral blood of patients who have solid tumors has been widely proven and most often is based on the expression of epithelial (eg, cytokeratins) or tissue-specific antigens (eg, melanin synthesis enzymes for melanoma) by means of PCR or cytology methods [100]. The biologic significance of CTC in the determinism of cancer metastasis is openly debated, however. In fact, although the detection of CTC has been reported repeatedly to be associated with a worse prognosis in patients who have cutaneous melanoma [101], the findings are more controversial in epithelial cancers (eg, breast, colon carcinoma) [100]. In gastric carcinoma some investigators have described a significant negative association between CTC detection and patient survival [102–106], but others have not [107–109]. These conflicting results probably reflect the fact that most CTC have no metastatic potential, and their detection acts as a confounding factor in survival analysis. Accordingly, efforts should be made to characterize CTC to identify those playing a significant role in cancer progression. To this aim, molecular factors influencing the ability of CTC to survive in the peripheral blood, to migrate through the vessel wall, and to grow in the metastatic site should be tested, as already reported in pioneer studies. Shin and colleagues [110] reported that the expression of telomerase (an antiapoptotic factor) and *c-Met* (an oncogene playing a key role in the determinism of cancer metastatic potential) in the peripheral blood of patients who have gastric cancer does correlate with prognosis. Although these two molecules are expressed preferentially by malignant cells as compared with normal cells, these investigators, like many other researchers involved in this field, did not sort epithelial CTC from peripheral blood mononuclear cells before performing PCR analyses, therefore leading to questions about the assumption that the observed gene expression is linked necessarily to CTC.

Concluding remarks

It is increasingly evident that personalized treatment of cancer no longer can rely on the commonly used histopathologic factors, which are only gross indicators of the metastatic potential of tumors. Although the need for novel prognostic factors able to overcome the intrinsic limits of conventional parameters is widely acknowledged by researchers, no innovative indicator of cancer aggressiveness has been implemented in the routine prognostic evaluation of gastric cancer during the past 2 decades. As regards the conventional histopathologic parameters, the evidence based on data from thousands of patients that the N ratio is an independent prognostic factor has not led to an update of the TNM staging system, the most widely accepted and used prognostic scoring system. Clearly, the lack of an international coordinated effort in this direction is undermining the opportunity to improve the standard management of patients who have gastric cancer with a very simple adjustment of the pathologic report. This reluctance seems even less justified because the N ratio is being reported more and more frequently as an independent prognostic factor in other epithelial (eg, breast carcinoma [111]) and nonepithelial (eg, melanoma [112]) tumors. This experience in other cancers strengthens the results obtained in patients who have gastric carcinoma and suggests that the proportion of positive nodes might represent a generally applicable method to interpret better the prognostic significance of the presence of metastatic disease in the locoregional lymphatic basin. Even though the N ratio actually can improve the performance of current TNM staging system, one must acknowledge that the prognostic potential of conventional prognostic factors has reached a plateau of effectiveness that can be overcome only by implementing insights into the molecular processes in gastric cancer progression. During the past decade an ever-growing list of molecular prognostic factors has been proposed, based on the discovery of the mechanisms underlying gastric cancer aggressiveness. Despite this promise, virtually all biomarkers have been tested in small series (n < 100), often the clinicopathologic features of cases enrolled are heterogeneous, and often the effect of the new prognostic factor is not adjusted by means of a multivariable analysis (which takes into account the influence of the distribution of conventional prognostic factors between the groups of patients identified by the candidate prognostic factor). Accordingly, studies performed in larger and more homogeneous series are warranted before any of these biomarkers can be used in the routine clinical setting to identify patients at higher risk and thus to select patients for adjuvant or more aggressive therapies. In the meantime, meta-analyses might be performed to make the most of available data and to suggest which biomarker is more promising. No such study has ever been performed for gastric carcinoma, unlike other tumor types [113–115]. Finally, as advocated by the principles of stratified medicine [13], it is recommended strongly that clinical trials testing any therapeutic regimen always be coupled with ancillary studies addressing the potential of biomarkers as predictors of patients' clinical outcomes. If systematically applied, this approach will increase rapidly the number of cases needed for sound statistical analysis and thus will speed the pace of discovery of clinically relevant (ie, characterized by high accuracy) prognostic factors.

Summary

The most powerful prognostic factors for gastric carcinoma are the TNM stage at diagnosis and the possibility of achieving an apparently radical tumor resection at laparotomy. Despite radical surgery, the prognosis of patients who have gastric carcinoma remains unsatisfactory because of the intrinsic and substantially unpredictable aggressiveness of this malignancy.

Although the current TNM staging system probably can be improved by using the ratio between positive and resected lymph nodes, the prognostic potential of conventional prognostic factors has reached a plateau of effectiveness that can be overcome only by the implementation of insights into the molecular processes of the progression of gastric cancer. During the past decade an ever-growing list of molecular prognostic factors has been proposed based on the discovery of the mechanisms underlying gastric cancer aggressiveness. Moreover, the implementation of high-throughput technologies such as gene microarray is speeding the pace of discovery of novel and more effective prognostic biomarkers. Studies performed in larger and more homogeneous series of patients and adequate statistical analysis are warranted before any of the candidate biomarkers can be implemented in the routine clinical setting to identify patients at higher risk and thus to select patients to undergo adjuvant or more aggressive therapies.

References

[1] Jemal A, Siegel R, Ward E, et al. Cancer statistics, 2006. CA Cancer J Clin 2006;56:106–30.
[2] Hohenberger P, Gretschel S. Gastric cancer. Lancet 2003;362:305–15.
[3] Dicken BJ, Bigam DL, Cass C, et al. Gastric adenocarcinoma: review and considerations for future directions. Ann Surg 2005;241:27–39.
[4] Foukakis T, Lundell L, Gubanski M, et al. Advances in the treatment of patients with gastric adenocarcinoma. Acta Oncol 2007;46:277–85.
[5] Clark CJ, Thirlby RC, Picozzi V Jr, et al. Current problems in surgery: gastric cancer. Curr Probl Surg 2006;43:566–670.
[6] Hundahl SA, Phillips JL, Menck HR. The National Cancer Data Base report on poor survival of U.S. gastric carcinoma patients treated with gastrectomy: fifth edition. American Joint Committee on Cancer staging, proximal disease, and the "different disease" hypothesis. Cancer 2000;88:921–32.
[7] Inoue M, Tsugane S. Epidemiology of gastric cancer in Japan. Postgrad Med J 2005;81: 419–24.
[8] Greene FL. TNM staging for malignancies of the digestive tract: 2003 changes and beyond. Semin Surg Oncol 2003;21:23–9.
[9] Yasui W, Oue N, Aung PP, et al. Molecular-pathological prognostic factors of gastric cancer: a review. Gastric Cancer 2005;8:86–94.
[10] Scartozzi M, Galizia E, Freddari F, et al. Molecular biology of sporadic gastric cancer: prognostic indicators and novel therapeutic approaches. Cancer Treat Rev 2004;30:451–9.
[11] Anderson C, Nijagal A, Kim J. Molecular markers for gastric adenocarcinoma: an update. Mol Diagn Ther 2006;10:345–52.
[12] Sikora K. Personalized medicine for cancer: from molecular signature to therapeutic choice. Adv Cancer Res 2007;96:345–69.
[13] Trusheim MR, Berndt ER, Douglas FL. Stratified medicine: strategic and economic implications of combining drugs and clinical biomarkers. Nat Rev Drug Discov 2007;6:287–93.
[14] Takahashi I, Matsusaka T, Onohara T, et al. Clinicopathological features of long-term survivors of scirrhous gastric cancer. Hepatogastroenterology 2000;47:1485–8.
[15] Kikuchi S, Sato M, Katada N, et al. Surgical outcome of node-positive early gastric cancer with particular reference to nodal status. Anticancer Res 2000;20:3695–700.
[16] Borch K, Jonsson B, Tarpila E, et al. Changing pattern of histological type, location, stage and outcome of surgical treatment of gastric carcinoma. Br J Surg 2000;87:618–26.

[17] Msika S, Benhamiche AM, Jouve JL, et al. Prognostic factors after curative resection for gastric cancer. A population-based study. Eur J Cancer 2000;36:390–6.

[18] Yokota T, Kunii Y, Teshima S, et al. Significant prognostic factors in patients with early gastric cancer. Int Surg 2000;85:286–90.

[19] Adachi Y, Shiraishi N, Suematsu T, et al. Most important lymph node information in gastric cancer: multivariate prognostic study. Ann Surg Oncol 2000;7:503–7.

[20] Crew KD, Neugut AI. Epidemiology of upper gastrointestinal malignancies. Semin Oncol 2004;31:450–64.

[21] Marchet A, Mocellin S, Ambrosi A, et al. The ratio between metastatic and examined lymph nodes (N ratio) is an independent prognostic factor in gastric cancer regardless of the type of lymphadenectomy: results from an Italian multicentric study in 1853 patients. Ann Surg 2007;245:543–52.

[22] Kim JP, Lee JH, Kim SJ, et al. Clinicopathologic characteristics and prognostic factors in 10 783 patients with gastric cancer. Gastric Cancer 1998;1:125–33.

[23] Siewert JR, Bottcher K, Stein HJ, et al. Relevant prognostic factors in gastric cancer: ten-year results of the German Gastric Cancer Study. Ann Surg 1998;228:449–61.

[24] Liu C, Lu P, Lu Y, et al. Clinical implications of metastatic lymph node ratio in gastric cancer. BMC Cancer 2007;7:200.

[25] Kunisaki C, Makino H, Akiyama H, et al. Clinical significance of the metastatic lymph-node ratio in early gastric cancer. J Gastrointest Surg 2008;12:542–9.

[26] Celen O, Yildirim E, Berberoglu U. Prognostic impact of positive lymph node ratio in gastric carcinoma. J Surg Oncol 2007;96:95–101.

[27] Cheong JH, Hyung WJ, Shen JG, et al. The N ratio predicts recurrence and poor prognosis in patients with node-positive early gastric cancer. Ann Surg Oncol 2006;13:377–85.

[28] Kunisaki C, Shimada H, Nomura M, et al. Clinical impact of metastatic lymph node ratio in advanced gastric cancer. Anticancer Res 2005;25:1369–75.

[29] Rodriguez-Santiago JM, Munoz E, Marti M, et al. Metastatic lymph node ratio as a prognostic factor in gastric cancer. Eur J Surg Oncol 2005;31:59–66.

[30] Nitti D, Marchet A, Olivieri M, et al. Ratio between metastatic and examined lymph nodes is an independent prognostic factor after D2 resection for gastric cancer: analysis of a large European monoinstitutional experience. Ann Surg Oncol 2003;10:1077–85.

[31] Takagane A, Terashima M, Abe K, et al. Evaluation of the ratio of lymph node metastasis as a prognostic factor in patients with gastric cancer. Gastric Cancer 1999;2:122–8.

[32] Inoue K, Nakane Y, Michiura T, et al. Histopathological grading does not affect survival after R0 surgery for gastric cancer. Eur J Surg Oncol 2002;28:633–6.

[33] Scartozzi M, Galizia E, Verdecchia L, et al. Lymphatic, blood vessel and perineural invasion identifies early-stage high-risk radically resected gastric cancer patients. Br J Cancer 2006;95:445–9.

[34] Hyung WJ, Lee JH, Choi SH, et al. Prognostic impact of lymphatic and/or blood vessel invasion in patients with node-negative advanced gastric cancer. Ann Surg Oncol 2002;9: 562–7.

[35] Kooby DA, Suriawinata A, Klimstra DS, et al. Biologic predictors of survival in node-negative gastric cancer. Ann Surg 2003;237:828–35 [discussion: 835–7].

[36] Wanebo HJ, Kennedy BJ, Winchester DP, et al. Role of splenectomy in gastric cancer surgery: adverse effect of elective splenectomy on longterm survival. J Am Coll Surg 1997;185:177–84.

[37] Nitti D, Marchet A, Mammano E, et al. Extended lymphadenectomy (D2) in patients with early gastric cancer. Eur J Surg Oncol 2005;31:875–81.

[38] Bonenkamp JJ, Hermans J, Sasako M, et al. Extended lymph-node dissection for gastric cancer. N Engl J Med 1999;340:908–14.

[39] Cuschieri A, Weeden S, Fielding J, et al. Patient survival after D1 and D2 resections for gastric cancer: long-term results of the MRC randomized surgical trial. Surgical Co-operative Group. Br J Cancer 1999;79:1522–30.

[40] McCulloch P, Nita ME, Kazi H, et al. Extended versus limited lymph nodes dissection technique for adenocarcinoma of the stomach. Cochrane Database Syst Rev 2004; CD001964.

[41] Cervantes A, Rodriguez Braun E, Perez Fidalgo A, et al. Molecular biology of gastric cancer. Clin Transl Oncol 2007;9:208–15.

[42] Hamilton JP, Meltzer SJ. A review of the genomics of gastric cancer. Clin Gastroenterol Hepatol 2006;4:416–25.

[43] Stock M, Otto F. Gene deregulation in gastric cancer. Gene 2005;360:1–19.

[44] Kountouras J, Zavos C, Chatzopoulos D. New concepts of molecular biology on gastric carcinogenesis. Hepatogastroenterology 2005;52:1305–12.

[45] Ottini L, Falchetti M, Lupi R, et al. Patterns of genomic instability in gastric cancer: clinical implications and perspectives. Ann Oncol 2006;17:97–102.

[46] Umar A, Boland CR, Terdiman JP, et al. Revised Bethesda guidelines for hereditary nonpolyposis colorectal cancer (Lynch syndrome) and microsatellite instability. J Natl Cancer Inst 2004;96:261–8.

[47] Ottini L, Falchetti M, Saieva C, et al. MRE11 expression is impaired in gastric cancer with microsatellite instability. Carcinogenesis 2004;25:2337–43.

[48] Bacani J, Zwingerman R, Di Nicola N, et al. Tumor microsatellite instability in early onset gastric cancer. J Mol Diagn 2005;7:465–77.

[49] Gologan A, Krasinskas A, Hunt J, et al. Performance of the revised Bethesda guidelines for identification of colorectal carcinomas with a high level of microsatellite instability. Arch Pathol Lab Med 2005;129:1390–7.

[50] Ottini L, Palli D, Falchetti M, et al. Microsatellite instability in gastric cancer is associated with tumor location and family history in a high-risk population from Tuscany. Cancer Res 1997;57:4523–9.

[51] Simpson AJ, Caballero OL, Pena SD. Microsatellite instability as a tool for the classification of gastric cancer. Trends Mol Med 2001;7:76–80.

[52] Schneider BG, Bravo JC, Roa JC, et al. Microsatellite instability, prognosis and metastasis in gastric cancers from a low-risk population. Int J Cancer 2000;89:444–52.

[53] Choi SW, Choi JR, Chung YJ, et al. Prognostic implications of microsatellite genotypes in gastric carcinoma. Int J Cancer 2000;89:378–83.

[54] Artunedo Pe P, Moreno Azcoita M, Alonso A, et al. Prognostic significance of high microsatellite instability in a Spanish series of gastric adenocarcinomas. Anticancer Res 2000;20: 4009–14.

[55] Azmy IA, Balasubramanian SP, Wilson AG, et al. Role of tumour necrosis factor gene polymorphisms (-308 and -238) in breast cancer susceptibility and severity. Breast Cancer Res 2004;6:R395–400.

[56] Wirtz HC, Muller W, Noguchi T, et al. Prognostic value and clinicopathological profile of microsatellite instability in gastric cancer. Clin Cancer Res 1998;4:1749–54.

[57] Hayden JD, Cawkwell L, Quirke P, et al. Prognostic significance of microsatellite instability in patients with gastric carcinoma. Eur J Cancer 1997;33:2342–6.

[58] Beghelli S, de Manzoni G, Barbi S, et al. Microsatellite instability in gastric cancer is associated with better prognosis in only stage II cancers. Surgery 2006;139:347–56.

[59] Noel A, Jost M, Maquoi E. Matrix metalloproteinases at cancer tumor-host interface. Semin Cell Dev Biol 2008;19:52–60.

[60] de Mingo M, Moran A, Sanchez-Pernaute A, et al. Expression of MMP-9 and TIMP-1 as prognostic markers in gastric carcinoma. Hepatogastroenterology 2007;54:315–9.

[61] Liu XP, Kawauchi S, Oga A, et al. Prognostic significance of matrix metalloproteinase-7 (MMP-7) expression at the invasive front in gastric carcinoma. Jpn J Cancer Res 2002; 93:291–5.

[62] Lee KH, Shin SJ, Kim KO, et al. Relationship between E-cadherin, matrix metalloproteinase-7 gene expression and clinicopathological features in gastric carcinoma. Oncol Rep 2006;16:823–30.

[63] Inoue T, Yashiro M, Nishimura S, et al. Matrix metalloproteinase-1 expression is a prognostic factor for patients with advanced gastric cancer. Int J Mol Med 1999;4: 73–7.

[64] Caenazzo C, Onisto M, Sartor L, et al. Augmented membrane type 1 matrix metalloproteinase (MT1-MMP):MMP-2 messenger RNA ratio in gastric carcinomas with poor prognosis. Clin Cancer Res 1998;4:2179–86.

[65] Mimori K, Mori M, Shiraishi T, et al. Clinical significance of tissue inhibitor of metalloproteinase expression in gastric carcinoma. Br J Cancer 1997;76:531–6.

[66] Mrena J, Wiksten JP, Nordling S, et al. MMP-2 but not MMP-9 associated with COX-2 and survival in gastric cancer. J Clin Pathol 2006;59:618–23.

[67] Joo YE, Seo KS, Kim HS, et al. Expression of tissue inhibitors of metalloproteinases (TIMPs) in gastric cancer. Dig Dis Sci 2000;45:114–21.

[68] Shah MA, Ramanathan RK, Ilson DH, et al. Multicenter phase II study of irinotecan, cisplatin, and bevacizumab in patients with metastatic gastric or gastroesophageal junction adenocarcinoma. J Clin Oncol 2006;24:5201–6.

[69] Lieto E, Ferraraccio F, Orditura M, et al. Expression of vascular endothelial growth factor (VEGF) and epidermal growth factor receptor (EGFR) is an independent prognostic indicator of worse outcome in gastric cancer patients. Ann Surg Oncol 2008;15:69–79.

[70] Kolev Y, Uetake H, Iida S, et al. Prognostic significance of VEGF expression in correlation with COX-2, microvessel density, and clinicopathological characteristics in human gastric carcinoma. Ann Surg Oncol 2007;14:2738–47.

[71] Kondo K, Kaneko T, Baba M, et al. VEGF-C and VEGF-A synergistically enhance lymph node metastasis of gastric cancer. Biol Pharm Bull 2007;30:633–7.

[72] Nikiteas NI, Tzanakis N, Theodoropoulos G, et al. Vascular endothelial growth factor and endoglin (CD-105) in gastric cancer. Gastric Cancer 2007;10:12–7.

[73] Juttner S, Wissmann C, Jons T, et al. Vascular endothelial growth factor-D and its receptor VEGFR-3: two novel independent prognostic markers in gastric adenocarcinoma. J Clin Oncol 2006;24:228–40.

[74] Shida A, Fujioka S, Ishibashi Y, et al. Prognostic significance of vascular endothelial growth factor D in gastric carcinoma. World J Surg 2005;29:1600–7.

[75] Vidal O, Soriano-Izquierdo A, Pera M, et al. Positive VEGF immunostaining independently predicts poor prognosis in curatively resected gastric cancer patients: results of a study assessing a panel of angiogenic markers. J Gastrointest Surg 2007; [epub ahead of print].

[76] Roukos DH, Liakakos T, Karatzas G, et al. Can VEGF-D and VEGFR-3 be used as biomarkers for therapeutic decisions in patients with gastric cancer? Nat Clin Pract Oncol 2006;3:418–9.

[77] Wang TB, Deng MH, Qiu WS, et al. Association of serum vascular endothelial growth factor-C and lymphatic vessel density with lymph node metastasis and prognosis of patients with gastric cancer. World J Gastroenterol 2007;13:1794–7 [discussion: 179–8].

[78] Bani-Hani KE, Almasri NM, Khader YS, et al. Combined evaluation of expressions of cyclin E and p53 proteins as prognostic factors for patients with gastric cancer. Clin Cancer Res 2005;11:1447–53.

[79] Xiangming C, Natsugoe S, Takao S, et al. The cooperative role of p27 with cyclin E in the prognosis of advanced gastric carcinoma. Cancer 2000;89:1214–9.

[80] Feakins RM, Nickols CD, Bidd H, et al. Abnormal expression of pRb, p16, and cyclin D1 in gastric adenocarcinoma and its lymph node metastases: relationship with pathological features and survival. Hum Pathol 2003;34:1276–82.

[81] Fondevila C, Metges JP, Fuster J, et al. p53 And VEGF expression are independent predictors of tumour recurrence and survival following curative resection of gastric cancer. Br J Cancer 2004;90:206–15.

[82] Pinto-de-Sousa J, Silva F, David L, et al. Clinicopathological significance and survival influence of p53 protein expression in gastric carcinoma. Histopathology 2004;44: 323–31.

[83] Okuyama T, Maehara Y, Kabashima A, et al. Combined evaluation of expressions of p53 and p21 proteins as prognostic factors for patients with gastric carcinoma. Oncology 2002; 63:353–61.

[84] Feng CW, Wang LD, Jiao LH, et al. Expression of p53, inducible nitric oxide synthase and vascular endothelial growth factor in gastric precancerous and cancerous lesions: correlation with clinical features. BMC Cancer 2002;2:8.

[85] Carneiro F, Oliveira C, Suriano G, et al. Molecular pathology of familial gastric cancer. J Clin Pathol 2008;61:25–30.

[86] Machado JC, Oliveira C, Carvalho R, et al. E-cadherin gene (CDH1) promoter methylation as the second hit in sporadic diffuse gastric carcinoma. Oncogene 2001;20:1525–8.

[87] Humar B, Graziano F, Cascinu S, et al. Association of CDH1 haplotypes with susceptibility to sporadic diffuse gastric cancer. Oncogene 2002;21:8192–5.

[88] Tanaka M, Kitajima Y, Sato S, et al. Combined evaluation of mucin antigen and E-cadherin expression may help select patients with gastric cancer suitable for minimally invasive therapy. Br J Surg 2003;90:95–101.

[89] Mingchao, Stockton P, Sun K, et al. Loss of E-cadherin expression in gastric intestinal metaplasia and later stage p53 altered expression in gastric carcinogenesis. Exp Toxicol Pathol 2001;53:237–46.

[90] Mocellin S, Provenzano M, Rossi CR, et al. DNA array-based gene profiling: from surgical specimen to the molecular portrait of cancer. Ann Surg 2005;241:16–26.

[91] Mocellin S, Rossi CR, Traldi P, et al. Molecular oncology in the post-genomic era: the challenge of proteomics. Trends Mol Med 2004;10:24–32.

[92] Hippo Y, Taniguchi H, Tsutsumi S, et al. Global gene expression analysis of gastric cancer by oligonucleotide microarrays. Cancer Res 2002;62:233–40.

[93] Hasegawa S, Furukawa Y, Li M, et al. Genome-wide analysis of gene expression in intestinal-type gastric cancers using a complementary DNA microarray representing 23,040 genes. Cancer Res 2002;62:7012–7.

[94] Marchet A, Mocellin S, Belluco C, et al. Gene expression profile of primary gastric cancer: towards the prediction of lymph node status. Ann Surg Oncol 2007;14:1058–64.

[95] Inoue H, Matsuyama A, Mimori K, et al. Prognostic score of gastric cancer determined by cDNA microarray. Clin Cancer Res 2002;8:3475–9.

[96] Yasui W, Oue N, Ito R, et al. Search for new biomarkers of gastric cancer through serial analysis of gene expression and its clinical implications. Cancer Sci 2004;95:385–92.

[97] Gyorffy B, Lage H. A Web-based data warehouse on gene expression in human malignant melanoma. J Invest Dermatol 2007;127:394–9.

[98] Wolfrum F, Vogel I, Fandrich F, et al. Detection and clinical implications of minimal residual disease in gastro-intestinal cancer. Langenbecks Arch Surg 2005;390:430–41.

[99] Cazzaniga G, Gaipa G, Rossi V, et al. Monitoring of minimal residual disease in leukemia, advantages and pitfalls. Ann Med 2006;38:512–21.

[100] Mocellin S, Keilholz U, Rossi CR, et al. Circulating tumor cells: the 'leukemic phase' of solid cancers. Trends Mol Med 2006;12:130–9.

[101] Mocellin S, Hoon D, Ambrosi A, et al. The prognostic value of circulating tumor cells in patients with melanoma: a systematic review and meta-analysis. Clin Cancer Res 2006; 12:4605–13.

[102] Ishigami S, Sakamoto A, Uenosono Y, et al. Carcinoembryonic antigen messenger RNA expression in blood can predict relapse in gastric cancer. J Surg Res 2007; [epub ahead of print].

[103] Uen YH, Lin SR, Wu CH, et al. Clinical significance of MUC1 and c-Met RT-PCR detection of circulating tumor cells in patients with gastric carcinoma. Clin Chim Acta 2006;367:55–61.

[104] Wu CH, Lin SR, Yu FJ, et al. Development of a high-throughput membrane-array method for molecular diagnosis of circulating tumor cells in patients with gastric cancers. Int J Cancer 2006;119:373–9.

[105] Illert B, Fein M, Otto C, et al. Disseminated tumor cells in the blood of patients with gastric cancer are an independent predictive marker of poor prognosis. Scand J Gastroenterol 2005;40:843–9.

[106] Yeh KH, Chen YC, Yeh SH, et al. Detection of circulating cancer cells by nested reverse transcription-polymerase chain reaction of cytokeratin-19 (K19)—possible clinical significance in advanced gastric cancer. Anticancer Res 1998;18:1283–6.

[107] Pituch-Noworolska A, Kolodziejczyk P, Kulig J, et al. Circulating tumour cells and survival of patients with gastric cancer. Anticancer Res 2007;27:635–40.

[108] Ikeguchi M, Kaibara N. Detection of circulating cancer cells after a gastrectomy for gastric cancer. Surg Today 2005;35:436–41.

[109] Piva MG, Navaglia F, Basso D, et al. CEA mRNA identification in peripheral blood is feasible for colorectal, but not for gastric or pancreatic cancer staging. Oncology 2000; 59:323–8.

[110] Shin JH, Chung J, Kim HO, et al. Detection of cancer cells in peripheral blood of stomach cancer patients using RT-PCR amplification of tumour-specific mRNAs. Aliment Pharmacol Ther 2002;16(Suppl 2):137–44.

[111] Woodward WA, Vinh-Hung V, Ueno NT, et al. Prognostic value of nodal ratios in node-positive breast cancer. J Clin Oncol 2006;24:2910–6.

[112] Rossi CR, Mocellin S, Pasquali S, et al. N-ratio: a novel independent prognostic factor for patients with stage-III cutaneous melanoma. Ann Surg Oncol 2008;15:310–5.

[113] Malats N, Bustos A, Nascimento CM, et al. p53 As a prognostic marker for bladder cancer: a meta-analysis and review. Lancet Oncol 2005;6:678–86.

[114] Zhu CQ, Shih W, Ling CH, et al. Immunohistochemical markers of prognosis in non-small cell lung cancer: a review and proposal for a multiphase approach to marker evaluation. J Clin Pathol 2006;59:790–800.

[115] Mocellin S, Hoon DS, Pilati P, et al. Sentinel lymph node molecular ultrastaging in patients with melanoma: a systematic review and meta-analysis of prognosis. J Clin Oncol 2007;25: 1588–95.

ELSEVIER
SAUNDERS

Surg Oncol Clin N Am
17 (2008) 485–502

SURGICAL
ONCOLOGY CLINICS
OF NORTH AMERICA

Multidisciplinary Treatment of Advanced Cancer of the Esophagus and Gastroesophageal Junction: A European Center's Approach

Toni Lerut, MD, PhD, FRCSI(Hon), FRCS, FACS*,
Johnny Moons, MScN, Willy Coosemans, MD, PhD,
Herbert Decaluwé, MD, Georges Decker, MD,
Paul De Leyn, MD, PhD, Philippe Nafteux, MD,
Dirk van Raemdonck, MD, PhD

*Department of Thoracic Surgery, University Hospitals Leuven,
Herestraat 49, 3000 Leuven, Belgium*

Cancer of the esophagus and gastroesophageal junction (GEJ) is estimated to be among the 10 most common malignancies worldwide and the sixth most common cause of cancer-related mortality. Cancer of the esophagus is diagnosed in approximately 450.000 patients per year [1–3]. These cases exhibit remarkable geographic variation in incidence (eg, the incidence of adenocarcinoma of the esophagus), and GEJ, in particular Barrett's adenocarcinoma, has risen substantially during the past 2 decades [4]. Particularly in the United States and Europe (eg, Denmark and Scotland), the incidence of adenocarcinoma is now higher than that of squamous cell carcinoma [5].

The vast majority of the patients suffering from a cancer of the esophagus and GEJ present with symptoms of dysphagia and weight loss because of an obstructive tumor [6]. About three of four patients present with an advanced-stage carcinoma because of the tumor depth (T3–T4, a transmural tumor extending into surrounding structures) and/or because of lymph node involvement. In this subset of patients, about half have distant metastatic disease at the time of diagnosis.

* Corresponding author.
 E-mail address: toni.lerut@uzleuven.be (T. Lerut).

1055-3207/08/$ - see front matter © 2008 Elsevier Inc. All rights reserved.
doi:10.1016/j.soc.2008.02.007
surgonc.theclinics.com

During the last 3 decades diagnostic modalities, surgical techniques, and perioperative management have improved substantially, resulting in a decrease in postoperative mortality and in an increase in disease-free survival and overall cancer-specific long-term survival.

Despite these efforts, however, the majority of patients die from metastatic disease. This mortality has resulted in an intense search for other therapeutic modalities (ie, chemotherapy or chemoradiotherapy in combination with surgery) in an effort to improve the outcome.

This article focuses on the treatment of advanced carcinoma of the esophagus and GEJ.

Primary surgery

According to data from literature, up to 80% of patients may have positive nodes at the time of surgery [7]. Indeed, lymphatic dissemination occurs as an early event, lymph nodes being involved in as many as 50% of patients presenting with a T1b tumor [8]. Moreover, the esophageal wall is characterized by an extensive submucosal lymphatic plexus favoring a rather chaotic pattern of metastatic dissemination, as shown, in particular, by the meticulous studies coming mainly from Japanese publications. According to the location of the tumor (upper, middle, or distal third of the esophagus), cervical lymph nodes are involved in 46.3%, 29.7%, and 27% of the patients, respectively, whereas abdominal nodes are involved in 12.2%, 39.9%, and 74% of patients, respectively [7]. Furthermore, regardless of tumor location, involvement of distant lymph nodes is unpredictable because of the high incidence of skip metastases [8].

Finally, because of the absence of a serosa, particularly in the upper and middle third of the esophagus, there is a higher tendency to spread into surrounding vital structures (eg, pars membranacea of the trachea, aortic adventitia) by the time the diagnosis is made. As a result R0 resection, the prerequisite for a curative surgery, may be impeded in a substantial number of patients suffering from a carcinoma of the esophagus and GEJ.

The patient's general condition (eg, weight loss, regurgitation, and underlying cardiopulmonary disease related to tobacco use, together with alcohol abuse, particularly in squamous cell carcinoma [9]) may limit the surgical possibilities. In patients who have Barrett's adenocarcinoma, on the other hand, an excessive body mass index often complicates surgical therapy [9,10]. The increasing age of the population, particularly in Western countries, and related comorbidities also add to the overall risk for candidates for surgical resection. Today more than 25% of patients undergoing operation are classified as having an American Society of Anesthesiologists score of III or IV.

During the recent decades three literature reviews have evaluated postoperative mortality and long-term outcome, each basically covering one of the 3 decades (ie, the 1970s, the 1980s, and the 1990s).

The first review, published in 1980 by Earlam and Cunha-Melo [11], reported postoperative mortality as high as 29% and 5-year survival as low as 4% after resection for esophageal cancer.

The second review by Müller and colleagues [12] in 1990 highlighted a substantial decrease in postoperative mortality to 13% and an increase in 5-year survival to 20%.

Finally, the most recent review by Jamieson and colleagues [13] in 2004 involving 70,756 patients reported an overall postoperative mortality of 6.7% and a 5-year survival of 27.9%.

The trends depicted in these three reviews are well reflected by the authors' own experience, in which 5-year survival reached 40% during the last decade, twice the rate in the authors' experience before 1990 (Fig. 1).

It generally is accepted today that, in centers of postoperative excellence, the mortality factor can be kept below 5%, despite the limiting comorbidity. An increasing number of publications indicate that there is a clear volume–outcome relationship between low- and high-volume surgeons as well as between low- and high-volume centers dealing with the treatment of complex surgical procedures such as esophagectomy [14–16].

Some studies suggested that a significant reduction in postoperative mortality to less than 5% can be achieved only with an experience of more than 20 esophagectomies per year [17–19].

Despite the substantial reduction of postoperative mortality, systemic and locoregional recurrence remains a challenging problem after esophagectomy. Much controversy persists as to the extent of lymphadenectomy that should be performed and its potential impact on the outcome.

In essence there are two attitudes toward this issue. Some authors believe that the presence of positive nodes, even a single node, equals systemic disease, and that in the presence of such a poor prognostic factor, surgery will not change the outcome, whatever the extent of resection. Systematic removal of lymph nodes therefore is considered of no benefit at all, and it

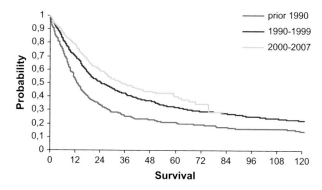

Fig. 1. Overall outcome after resectional surgery for cancer of the esophagus and gastroesophageal junction in 2000 patients according to different time periods. Survival is stated in months. University of Leuven data, 1975–2007.

is argued that surgical trauma should be kept as minimal as possible. This goal can be achieved by performing a transhiatal esophagectomy, as advocated by Orringer [20], or, as advocated more recently by Luketich [21], using a totally thoracoscopic and laparoscopic approach.

Others believe that the natural disease can be influenced positively by more aggressive surgery even in the presence of positive lymph nodes. Skinner [22] introduced the concept of en bloc resection in 1969. The operation consists of an excision of the tumor within a wide envelope of surrounding tissue containing both pleural spaces laterally, the pericardium anteriorly, the thoracic duct posteriorly, and including lymphatic tissue in the posterior mediastinum as well as in the upper abdominal compartment. In his initial experience, 5-year survival increased by as much as 18% in a series of 111 patients.

Mainly under the Japanese influence, much attention has been paid to a meticulous extensive lymphadenectomy in the management of esophageal cancer. In the chest this lymphadenectomy includes the upper mediastinal lymph nodes (eg, the aortopulmonary nodes), the nodes along the left recurrent nerves, and the brachiocephalic nodes [7]. At the consensus meeting if the International Society for Diseases of the Esophagus in Milan, this type of thoracic lymphadenectomy was labeled "total extended lymphadenectomy," as opposed to the standard lymphadenectomy, in which the upper border is limited to the level of the subcarinal lymph nodes [23].

In an effort to maximize the extent of lymphadenectomy the so-called "third field" (ie, bilateral cervical lymphadenectomy) has been added to the dissection [24].

Over the years a number of authors have claimed that more aggressive surgery has resulted in a substantial improvement in accuracy of pathologic staging, disease-free survival, and long-term survival (cure rate).

It is easy to understand that a more extensive lymphadenectomy can improve the accuracy of the pathologic lymph node staging. The chances of identifying involved nodes increases with the number of resected and labeled lymph nodes. It has been suggested that at least 15 nodes should be resected [24]. Factors that have proven to have prognostic significance are the number and ratio of positive nodes, extracapsular lymph node involvement, location of positive nodes, grade of differentiation, lymphatic vessel invasion, blood vessel invasion, and perineural invasion, and completeness (R status) of resection [25,26].

More controversial is the impact of radical surgery on disease-free survival and cure rate. Data from literature seem to indicate that en bloc esophagectomy and more extensive lymphadenectomy result in better locoregional tumor control than obtained with standard esophagectomy, which usually is performed through a transhiatal approach. In general, there is locoregional recurrence without the presence of distant metastasis in less than 10% of patients undergoing the radical surgery, versus 20% to 45% of patients after standard esophagectomy (Table 1).

Table 1
Impact of extent of surgery on local control

Author [reference]	No. of subjects	Local recurrence (%)
En bloc esophagectomy		1–10
Matsubara et al [27]	171	10
Altorki and Skinner [28]	111	8
Hagen et al [29]	100	1
Collard et al [30]	324	4
Swanson et al [31]	250	5.6
Lerut et al [32]	174	5.2
Transhiatal esophagectomy		23–47
Hulscher et al [33]	137	23
Becker et al [34]	35	31
Gignoux et al [35]		47
Nygaard et al [36]	186	35

Data from The University of Leuven, Leuven, Belgium.

Only one randomized, controlled trial has been performed to date. This trial, the Dutch trial, published by Hulscher and colleagues [37] compared an extended resection including two-field lymphadenectomy with a limited resection for adenocarcinoma of the esophagus and GEJ. A mean of 16 ± 9 nodes were identified in the resection specimen after limited resection, versus 31 ± 4 after extended resection. Although the difference was not significant, there was a strong trend favoring extended resection with a disease-free survival at 8 years of 39% after extended resection versus 27% after limited resection. For long-term, 8-year survival, the figures were 39% for extended resection versus 29% for limited resection. A subsequent subset analysis indicated a 17% survival benefit at 5 years in favor of the extended resection for distal-third adenocarcinoma [38].

Beside the single randomized, controlled trial, a growing number of retrospective and prospective observational studies seem to endorse the trend reflected by the Dutch trial that radical surgery favors both disease-free survival and local control as well as in overall 5-year survival (Table 2) [7–41].

More importantly, in many reports 5-year survival in stage III (T3–4N1) disease after radical surgery with two-field lymphadenectomy exceeds the threshold of 25% (Table 3) [7–42]. These figures are in sharp contrast with the results after limited resection: Orringer and colleagues [20], for example, reported a 5-year survival of 12% with similar-staged disease treated by transhiatal standard resection, and Killinger and colleagues [43] reported a 5-year survival of 10% for stage III disease, again reported after limited esophagectomy.

In the authors' experience, it seems that when fewer than six lymph nodes are involved, and they are located in the peritumoral area, a 5-year survival of 38% could be obtained (Fig. 2).

Table 2
Overall survival after radical surgery

Author [reference]	No. of patients	Survival (%)	
		3-year	5-year
Akiyama et al [7]	913	52.6	42.4
Ando et al [39]	419	52	40
Isono et al [40]	1740	42	34.3
Altorki and Skinner [28]	111	52	40
Hagen et al [29]	100	60	52
Collard [30]	235 R0	65	49
	324 R0–2	50	35
Lerut et al [32]	195	55	39
Hulscher et al [37]	114	42	40

Data from The University of Leuven, Leuven, Belgium.

Induction neoadjuvant therapy

Despite all efforts to refine the indications for surgery and improve the outcome after primary surgery, a majority of patients die from systemic and locoregional metastasis. This outcome has generated an interest in the use of a combined multimodality approach. During the recent decades neo-adjuvant (induction) protocols aiming at downstaging of the cancer have been widely tested. Unfortunately, however, different trials have yielded conflicting results. Several literature reviews and meta-analyses have been published on this subject.

Preoperative radiotherapy

Five randomized trials have compared preoperative radiotherapy plus surgery versus surgery alone. None of these trials could show an improvement in resectability or outcome. A meta-analysis of these trials including an update of individual patient data failed to show a significant survival benefit with the use of preoperative radiotherapy [44].

Table 3
Survival after radical surgery stage III $(T_{3-4}N_1)$

Author [reference]	No. of patients	5-year survival (%)
Akiyama et al [7]	175	27 (2F)/56 (3F)
Ando et al [39]	201	37.6
Baba et al [42]	22	30
Altorki and Skinner [28]	33	34.5 (4-year)
Hagen et al [29]	32	26
Collard et al [30]	98	30
Lerut et al [32]	162	26

Abbreviations: 2F, 2 field lymphadenectomy; 3F, 3 field lymphadenectomy.
Data from The University of Leuven, Leuven, Belgium.

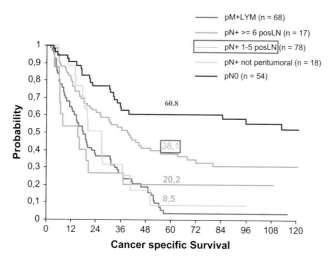

Fig. 2. Five-year survival in 235 patients presenting with cT3N0–1 according to the pathologic classification in subsets of pN0 and pN1–5 positive peritumoral nodes (pN) plus non-peritumoral nodes (pM + LYM). Survival is stated in months. University of Leuven data, 1991–1999.

Induction chemotherapy

Pilot studies and phase II trials using preoperative chemotherapy, either as monotherapy or combining several chemotherapeutic drugs, mostly based on 5-fluorouracil and cisplatinum, have shown clinical response rates varying between 40% and 70%. None of these studies, however, has shown evidence of improvement in overall survival as compared with surgery alone.

Similarly, randomized, controlled trials (Table 4) failed to indicate a clear survival benefit in favor of the combined arm [36–40,42–51].

The two largest trials showed conflicting results. The intergroup trial from the United States [49] that enrolled 467 patients who had resectable esophageal squamous cell carcinoma and adenocarcinoma did not show a difference in resection rate or in 3-year survival (23% versus 26% respectively) between the surgery-alone arm and the induction-plus-surgery arm.

In contrast, the United Kingdom Medical Research Council (UK MRC) trial [51] that enrolled 802 patients who had resectable esophageal squamous cell carcinoma and adenocarcinoma indicated a significant survival benefit at 2 years (48% versus 35%, respectively) in favor of the induction arm.

The Cochrane meta-analysis by Malthaner and colleagues [52] analyzed 11 randomized, controlled trials and concluded that there was no significant survival benefit for induction chemotherapy plus surgery versus surgery alone, although a nonsignificant reduction in local recurrence of 19% was noticed with preoperative chemotherapy. A second and more recent meta-analysis by Gebski and colleagues [53] indicated no survival benefit for

Table 4
Randomized, controlled trials of induction chemotherapy

Author [reference]	Chemotherapy (N)	Chemotherapy plus surgery (N)	Hazard ratio
Roth et al [45]	19	20	0.71
Nygaard et al [36]	56	25	1.22
Schlag [46]	22	24	0.97
Maipang et al [47]	24	22	1.66
Law et al [48]	74	73	0.73
Kelsen et al [49]	33	234	1.07
Ancona et al [50]	48	48	0.85
Medical Research Council Oesophageal Cancer Research Working Group [51]	400	403	0.79

squamous cell carcinoma but a possible significant benefit for all-cause mortality in adenocarcinomas (hazard ratio, 0.78; $P = .014$) in the UK MRC trial.

Induction chemoradiotherapy

The goal of combining chemotherapy and radiation therapy is to take advantage of the radiosensitizing effects of chemotherapy to reduce the tumor size and maximize local control along with its systemic effect on circulating tumor cells.

As a result, much attention has been given to the use of neoadjuvant chemoradiotherapy, as reflected by numerous published trials. At this point seven randomized, controlled trials [36–40,42–59] have been published in peer-reviewed journals (Table 5), and four more trials have been published in abstract form [60–63]. Of the fully published trials, only one was able to demonstrate a clear survival benefit in favor of the combined chemoradiotherapy-plus-surgery arm (32% at 3 years) versus the surgery-alone arm (6% at 3 years). This trial, however, was widely criticized, particularly in the surgical community, because the substandard survival at 3 years in the surgical arm (6%) probably resulted from a major selection bias.

Of concern are the considerable variations in different aspects of these trials (eg, location of tumor, histologic type, clinical stage, variation in the drug, dose, volume, schedules, and number of cycles of chemotherapy and radiotherapy administered). These variations may cause differences in response to the treatment and differences in outcome [64].

Moreover, most of these randomized trials lack sufficient power to indicate significant differences.

To remediate this limitation, a number of meta-analyses have been reported (Box 1). Three of these meta-analyses concluded that induction chemoradiotherapy improves 2- or 3-year survival with an increased R0 resection rate and a lower recurrence rate [52–65].

Table 5
Randomized, controlled trials of induction chemoradiation therapy

Author [reference]/ study arm	No. of patients	Resection (%)	PCR (%)	Operative mortality	3-year survival (%)
Nygaard et al [36]					
CRT + surgery	47	66	ns	24	17
Surgery alone	41	68		13	9
Le Prise et al [54]					
CRT + surgery	41	85	10	8	19
Surgery alone	45	84		7	14
Apinop et al [55]					
CRT + surgery	35	74	20	12	26
Surgery alone	34	100		15	20
Walsh et al [56]					
CRT + surgery	58	90	22	10	32
Surgery alone	55	100		4	6
Bosset et al [57]					
CRT + surgery	143	78	20	12	36
Surgery alone	139	68		4	34
Urba et al [58]					
CRT + surgery	50	ns	28	ns	30
					15 (8 years)
Surgery alone	50	ns		ns	15
					10 (8 years)
Burmeister et al [59]					
CRT + surgery	129	82	16	5	25 (5 years)
Surgery alone	128	86		5	22

Abbreviations: CRT, chemoradiation therapy; ns, not significant; PCR, pathological complete response.

The meta-analysis by Greer and colleagues [66] indicated a small, non–statistically significant improvement in overall survival. In the meta-analysis by Fiorica and colleagues [67], however, the surgical arm was favored because of the negative impact of postoperative mortality in the induction arm.

Several comments should be made about the results of these randomized trials and meta-analyses.

Box 1. Meta-analyses of induction chemoradiation therapy

Malthaner and colleagues [52]: Improved 2/3- year survival
Urschel and colleagues [65]: Improved R0 resection
Gebski and colleagues [53]: Lower recurrence rate
Greer and colleagues [66]: Small, non–statistically significant improvement in overall survival
Fiorica and colleagues [67]: Impact of postoperative mortality favors surgery-alone arm

Even in a meta-analysis, the strength of a chain is determined by its weakest link. In all the trials there is a notorious lack in defining the quality criteria for the surgical arm because of a lack of standardization and a lack of instruments for quality control [68]. Overall 3-year survival figures for surgery alone seem to be below 25% in all but one trial. Given that in the different trials all patients had stage T0-3N0-1 disease, these figures compare poorly with today's results of primary surgery, which achieves 5-year survival figures above 35% overall and over 25% for stage III (T3N1) disease in many high-volume centers.

As a result the validity of the meta-analysis must be questioned. It is well known that the quality of meta-analysis may become a more important source of bias than the reporting and dissemination of trials themselves [69].

A second comment relates to the exclusion criteria in these trials. In general, patients older than 70 years and/or presenting with renal, cardiac, or pulmonary complications were excluded. This subset of patients, however, represents approximately 25% of the candidates for a treatment with curative option. A majority of this subset nevertheless may undergo successful primary surgery. The results in the group of very old patients (> 75 years) in the authors' institution have been rewarding, as shown in Fig. 3, with a survival rate of 43.2% after R0 resection. Postoperative hospital mortality was 7.2%. The incidence of isolated locoregional recurrences in that group was 5.6%, and the combined incidence of locoregional plus distant metastases was 6.5%, the incidence of generalized distant metastases being 25%. All patients were followed for at least 3 years. These figures show that, with careful selection, advanced age (a population constantly increasing in Western societies) is no longer a contraindication for therapies with curative options, including major surgery.

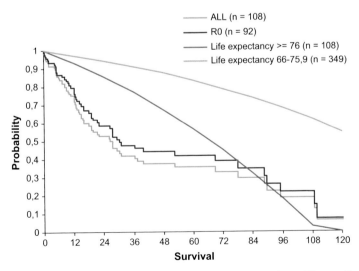

Fig. 3. Cancer-specific outcome after primary surgery in patients aged over 75 years. Survival is stated in months. University of Leuven data, 1991–2006.

Whether combined modality treatment is feasible in this subset of elderly patients without a too high a risk of morbidity and mortality requires further study, as does the final outcome of such therapeutic regimens.

A third comment on the randomized trials relates to the problem of mismatch of clinical staging even in the era of positron emission tomograph (PET) scanning and refinement by echoendoscopic techniques. A recent analysis performed on a series of 296 de novo cancers of the esophagus and GEJ at the authors' institution revealed both understaging of node involvement and, more importantly, overstaging (ie, false-positive nodes) in 21.6% of the cases. After radical primary surgery, node-negative patients, even those who have T3 tumors, have a good prognosis, with 5-year survival reaching 60% in the authors' experience (see Fig. 2). As a result, one can hypothesize that patients who are clinically staged as node positive but in fact are false positive will be a cause of artificial upgrading. This upgrading is calculated as affecting at least 5% of the results presented in the induction-plus-surgery arm, because in reality they were N0.

Finally, in addition to a higher postoperative morbidity, there is at least a trend for higher postoperative mortality in the induction-plus-surgery group, as also shown by the authors' own experience [70].

In particular, the combination of induction chemoradiotherapy and aggressive lymphadenectomy results in increased postoperative morbidity and mortality. There seems to be a direct correlation with the increase of the applied doses and extent of radiotherapy.

Primary surgery versus induction therapy: how to select candidates

Thus, candidates for primary surgery versus combined treatment modality should be selected carefully, with consideration of the pros and cons of both primary surgery and induction therapy. A first prerequisite is that all physicians involved in the selection process should be aware that today the reference standard of primary surgery is an overall 5-year survival rate higher than 35%, and many centers in both the East and the West exceed this figure, attaining rates as high as 50%. For advanced stage III (T3–4N1) disease the 5-year survival figures today are between 25% and 35% (see Table 3).

It seems that, if only a limited number of nodes are involved, primary surgery can attain 5-year survival rates exceeding 35%. In the authors' own experience in patients who had a cT3N0-1 staging and who had fewer than six involved nodes located in the peritumoral region on final pathologic examination, a 5-year survival rate as high as 38% was attained (see Fig. 2). This subset of patients is a substantial group, representing 33% of all cT3N0–1 patients analyzed in the authors' study.

In patients who had six or more involved nodes and distant lymph node metastases on pathologic staging, the 5-year survival rate dropped significantly below 10%.

On the other hand, approximately 20% to 25% of patients receiving induction chemoradiotherapy show a complete response on final pathologic examination with a 5-year survival rate exceeding the results expected from primary surgery [36–40,42–59].

At least 50% of patients, however, do not respond to induction chemo-radiotherapy. In their study of the value of induction chemotherapy, Ancona and colleagues [50] showed that the patients who did not respond had a dismal 5-year survival rate of 12%. Unfortunately, at this point there are no markers that make it possible to distinguish between patients who will respond and those who will not respond. One reason, among others, why nonresponders have a survival lower than expected is thought to be related to the loss of precious time between the start of induction and the point at which surgery is performed, usually approximately 3 to 4 months after initiation of the induction therapy. Efforts are made to assess possible early response by performing a PET scan shortly after the first cycle of chemotherapy. It has been suggested that such a PET scan is a good prognostic indicator [71] and may become a more precise clinical tool to distinguish responders from nonresponders [72,73]. Nonresponders then could go either immediately to surgery or to a palliative setting, according the findings at the time of initial clinical staging and the early postinduction PET assessment.

Obviously, given the difficulties in detecting early responders, the search for a more precise algorithm becomes mandatory. It must take into account the results obtained with primary surgery, particularly in cases with limited peritumoral node involvement, and the likelihood that these results will be superior to the overall results obtained after induction therapy.

In this respect, PET scanning again may become an important tool. Choi and colleagues [74] found that there were no long-term survivors when three or more separate positive nodes were detected on PET scan. Pathologic stage III patients who had one or two positive nodes on PET scan had 5-year survival rates of 50% and 25%, respectively.

No substantial data are available on the value of adjuvant chemotherapy plus radiotherapy. In addition to some observational studies, two randomized trials have been performed and failed to show a benefit of postoperative chemotherapy [52]. One nonrandomized study, however, indicated that postoperative chemoradiotherapy may prolong survival in patients who have positive lymph nodes [75].

Definitive chemoradiotherapy

The first attempts to treat patients who had cancer of the esophagus with definitive chemoradiotherapy without surgery were published by Cooper and colleagues [76] in 1999.

Although a 5-year survival rate of 32% was obtained, the final outcome was burdened by the high incidence of local recurrence in nearly 50% of the patients. As a result there seemed to be no further incentive to explore this therapeutic option on a broader, multicentric basis.

With the recent introduction of PET scanning and with its ability to assess response to chemotherapy making it a prognostic predictor [70–72], renewed interest has been directed toward the nonsurgical treatment of cancer of the esophagus, mainly for squamous cell carcinoma. Three aspects are important: survival, disease-free survival, and quality of life.

In a trial performed in France and published by Bedenne and colleagues [77], 444 cT3N0–1M0 patients were entered in the study. Only the 259 patients who responded to initial chemoradiotherapy were included for randomization.

Survival at 4 years showed no difference between chemoradiation plus surgery versus definitive chemoradiotherapy. In the surgical arm, however, early postoperative and 6-month mortality was high, 9% and 16%, respectively. The main issue not discussed in the original publication is what happened to the 144 (40%) nonresponders.

An assumption on this issue can be made from the publication on salvage surgery by Piessen and colleagues [78], whose center included a substantial number of patients in the French trial. In that publication salvage surgery seemed to result in a R0 resection in 61% of the cases, with a 5-year survival of 13%, versus 0% in the remaining 37 R1–2 resections. Combining R0 and R1–2 resections, the overall 5-year survival after salvage surgery is estimated to be below 10%. If these patients are added to the results obtained in the 259 responders in the publication by Bedenne [77], the overall 5-year survival in the whole series can be estimated at approximately 18%, well inferior to the results obtained today in centers of excellence with primary surgery in stage III disease (see Table 3).

In the German trial published by Stahl and colleagues [79] dealing with 172 cT3–4N0–1M0 patients randomly assigned to chemoradiation plus surgery or to definitive chemoradiation, the 3-year survival rates are 24.4% and 31.3%, respectively. Again, postsurgery mortality was high, 11.3%, which may be related to the participation of as many as much as 11 centers, not all of which were high-volume centers.

Furthermore, cancer-related death was 46.5% in the surgery arm versus 72% in the definitive chemoradiotherapy arm. Overall, 5-year survival was 29% in the surgical arm versus 17% in the definitive chemoradiotherapy arm. Another important issue is disease-free survival, in particular locoregional disease–free survival. Locoregional recurrence is a major source of impaired quality of life, which is increasingly becoming a focus of attention. Disease-free survival at 2 years in the Stahl [79] publication was 64.3% in the surgical arm and 40.7% in the definitive chemoradiotherapy arm. In the publication by Bedenne [77], the local recurrence rate at 2 years was 33.6% in the surgery arm versus 43% in the chemoradiation-only arm. Of these patients, 32.3% required stent placement, indicating an inferior quality of life. These figures can be compared with the authors' own results, with a disease-free survival rate of 46% at 5 years and a rate of locoregional recurrence with or without distant metastasis at 5 years of only 15% [32]. This experience also was reflected by the Dutch trial on extent of surgery, which showed a disease-free survival rate of 39% at 8 years after more radical primary surgery [37].

Clearly, at this point, the available results should be interpreted with caution before they are disseminated more broadly.

Summary

The treatment of cancer of the esophagus and GEJ remains a complex and challenging issue. During the last 2 decades tremendous progress has been made, resulting in a doubling of the 5-year survival rate after primary surgery. Today more than one in three patients is a long-term survivor after treatment with curative intent.

This progress is the result of better diagnosis that allows better distinction between curative versus palliative setting. Better surgical techniques and perioperative management also have contributed substantially to decreasing postoperative mortality and to better overall long-term survival, with 5-year survival rates, including including advanced stage III disease, better than 25%. These figures are the modern reference standard to which all other therapeutic modalities should be compared. Some new nonsurgical technologies are promising, in particular endomucosal resection in high-grade dysplasia and early T1a cancer (not discussed in this article). This procedure functions as a precise staging procedure and as a valid therapeutic modality as well.

In advanced carcinoma, however, controversy remains concerning the real value of multimodality treatment. Although meta-analyses seem to favor the combination of induction chemoradiotherapy plus surgery, the results should be analyzed with great care, and these therapeutic regimens still are considered as investigational.

At this point only complete responders seem to benefit from these induction regimens. Furthermore, given the more favorable result obtained with primary surgery in patients who have a limited number of peritumoral positive nodes, further efforts should be made to elaborate a more precise algorithm along this line.

In this respect the promising prognostic value of PET scans assessing lymph node involvement and the significance of the number of PET-positive nodes and their location in relation to the primary tumor requires further validation. Of equal importance, when using induction therapy, is the need for further validation of the prognostic value of early response observed by PET scan in the early phase of induction therapy.

At this point definitive chemoradiotherapy is far from being a valid therapeutic option, given the inferior results when incorporating the poor results of salvage surgery as and the high incidence of locoregional recurrence jeopardizing the quality of life in at least one of three patients treated with such a regimen. Multidisciplinary tumor boards evaluating the value of each of the different diagnostic and therapeutic options and modalities therefore are of paramount importance, and the leadership of the experienced surgeon is an essential element.

References

[1] Devesa SS, Blot WJ, Fraumen JF Jr. Changing patterns in the incidence of esophageal and gastric carcinoma in the United States. Cancer 1998;83(10):2049–53.

[2] Ward EM, Thun MJ, Hannan LM, et al. Interpreting cancer trends. Ann N Y Acad Sci 2006; 1076:29–53.

[3] Parkin DM, Pisarie P, Ferlay J. Global cancer statistics. CA Cancer J Clin 1999;49(1):33–64.

[4] Pera M, Manterola C, Vidal O, et al. Epidemiology of esophageal adenocarcinoma. J Surg Oncol 2005;92(3):151–9.

[5] Bossetti C, Levi F, Ferlay J, et al. Trends in oesophageal cancer incidence and mortality in Europe. Int J Cancer 2007;122:1118–29.

[6] Watt E, Whyte F. The experience of dysphagia and its effect on the quality of life of patients with oesophageal cancer. Eur J Cancer Care (Engl) 2003;12(2):183–93.

[7] Akiyama H, Tsurumaru M, Udagawa H, et al. Radical lymph node dissection for cancer of the thoracic esophagus. Ann Surg 1994;220(3):364–72.

[8] Nishimaki T, Suzuki T, Kanda T, et al. Extended radical esophagectomy for superficially invasive carcinoma of the esophagus. Surgery 1999;125(2):142–7.

[9] Vaughan TL, Davis S, Kristal A, et al. Obesity, alcohol, and tobacco as risk factors for cancers of the esophagus and gastric cardia: adenocarcinoma versus squamous cell carcinoma. Cancer Epidemiol Biomarkers Prev 1995;4(2):85–92.

[10] Chow WH, Blot WJ, Vaughan TL, et al. Body mass index and risk of adenocarcinoma of the esophagus and gastric cardia. J Natl Cancer Inst 1998;90(2):150–5.

[11] Earlam R, Cunha-Melo JR. Oesophageal squamous cell carcinoma: I. A critical review of surgery. Br J Surg 1980;67(6):381–90.

[12] Müller JM, Erasmi H, Stelzner M, et al. Surgical therapy of esophageal carcinoma. Br J Surg 1990;77(8):845–57.

[13] Jamieson GG, Mathew G, Ludemann R, et al. Postoperative mortality following esophagectomy and problems in reporting its rate. Br J Surg 2004;91(8):943–7.

[14] van Lanschot JJ, Hulscher JB, Buskens CJ, et al. Hospital volume and hospital mortality for esophagectomy. Cancer 2001;91(8):1574–8.

[15] Dimick JB, Goodney PP, Orringer MB, et al. Specialty training and mortality after esophageal cancer resection. Ann Thorac Surg 2005;80(1):282–6.

[16] Birkmeyer JD, Dimick JB, Staiger DO. Operative mortality and procedure volume as predictors of subsequent hospital performance. Ann Surg 2006;243(3):411–7.

[17] Christian CK, Gustafson ML, Betensky RA, et al. The Leapfrog volume criteria may fall short in identifying high-quality surgical centres. Ann Surg 2003;238(4):447–55 [discussion: 455–7].

[18] Metzger R, Bollschweiler E, Vallböhmer D, et al. High volume centres for esophagectomy: what is the number needed to achieve low postoperative mortality? Dis Esophagus 2004; 17(4):310–4.

[19] Killeen SD, O'Sullivan MJ, Coffey JC, et al. Provider volume and outcomes for oncological procedures. Br J Surg 2005;92(4):389–402.

[20] Orringer MB, Marshall B, Iannettoni MD. Transhiatal esophagectomy: clinical experience and refinements. Ann Surg 1999;230(3):392–400.

[21] Luketich JD, Alvelo-Rivera M, Buenaventura PO, et al. Minimally invasive esophagectomy: outcomes in 222 patients. Ann Surg 2003;238(4):486–94.

[22] Skinner DB. En bloc resection for neoplasms of the esophagus and cardia. J Thorac Cardiovasc Surg 1983;85(1):59–71.

[23] Fumagalli U, Panel of experts. Resective surgery for cancer of the thoracic esophagus. Results of a consensus conference held at the VIth World Congress of the International Society for Diseases of the Esophagus. Dis Esophagus 1996;9:30–8.

[24] Fujita H, Sueyoshi S, Tanaka T, et al. Optimal lymphadenectomy for squamous cell carcinoma in the thoracic esophagus: comparing the short and long-term outcome among the four types of lymphadenectomy. World J Surg 2003;27(5):571–9.

[25] Lagarde S, ten Kate F, Reitsma J, et al. Prognostic factors in adenocarcinoma of the esophagus or gastroesophageal junction. J Clin Oncol 2006;24:4347–55.

[26] Lerut T, Coosemans W, Decker G, et al. Leuven Collaborative Workgroup for Esophageal Carcinoma. Extracapsular lymph node involvement is a negative prognostic factor in T3 adenocarcinoma of the distal esophagus and gastroesophageal junction. J Thorac Cardiovasc Surg 2003;126(4):1121–8.

[27] Matsubara T, Ueda M, Yanagida O, et al. How extensive should lymph node dissection be for cancer of the thoracic esophagus? J Thorac Cardiovasc Surg 1994;107(4):1073–8.

[28] Altorki N, Skinner D. Should en bloc esophagectomy be the standard of care for esophageal carcinoma? Ann Surg 2001;234(5):581–7.

[29] Hagen JA, DeMeester SR, Peters JH, et al. Curative resection for esophageal adenocarcinoma: analysis of 100 en bloc esophagectomies. Ann Surg 2001;234(4):520–30.

[30] Collard JM, Otte JB, Fiasse R, et al. Skeletonizing en bloc esophagectomy for cancer. Ann Surg 2001;234(1):25–32.

[31] Swanson SJ, Batirel HF, Bueno R, et al. Transthoracic esophagectomy with radical mediastinal and abdominal lymph node dissection and cervical esophagogastrostomy for esophageal carcinoma. Ann Thorac Surg 2001;72(6):1918–24.

[32] Lerut T, Nafteux P, Moons J, et al. Three-field lymphadenectomy for carcinoma of the esophagus and gastroesophageal junction in 174 R0 resections: impact on staging, disease-free survival, and outcome: a plea for adaptation of TNM classification in upper-half esophageal carcinoma. Ann Surg 2004;240(6):962–72.

[33] Hulscher JB, van Sandick JW, Tijssen JG, et al. The recurrence pattern of esophageal carcinoma after transhiatal resection. J Am Coll Surg 2000;191(2):143–8.

[34] Becker CD, Barbier PA, Terrier F, et al. Patterns of recurrence of esophageal carcinoma after transhiatal esophagectomy and gastric interposition. AJR Am J Roentgenol 1987;148(2): 273–7.

[35] Gignoux M, Roussel A, Paillot B, et al. The value of preoperative radiotherapy in esophageal cancer: Results of a study of the E.O.R.T.C. World J Surg 2005;11(4):426–32.

[36] Nygaard K, Hagen S, Hansen HS, et al. Preoperative radiotherapy prolongs survival in operable esophageal carcinoma: a randomized, multicenter study of preoperative radiotherapy and chemotherapy. The second Scandinavian trial in esophageal cancer. World J Surg 1992;16(6):1104–9.

[37] Hulscher JB, van Sandick JW, de Boer AG, et al. Extended transthoracic resection compared with limited transhiatal resection for adenocarcinoma of the esophagus. N Engl J Med 2002; 347(21):1662–9.

[38] Hulscher JB, van Lanschot JJ. Individualised surgical treatment of patients with an adenocarcinoma of the distal esophagus or gastro-esophageal junction. Dig Surg 2005; 22(3):130–4 [epub 2005 May 16].

[39] Ando N, Ozawa S, Kitagawa Y, et al. Improvement in the results of surgical treatment of advanced squamous esophageal carcinoma during 15 consecutive years. Ann Surg 2000; 232(2):225–32.

[40] Isono K, Sato H, Nakayama K. Results of a nationwide study on the three-field lymph node dissection of esophageal cancer. Oncology 1991;48(5):411–20.

[41] Roder JD, Busch R, Stein HJ, et al. Ratio of invaded to removed lymph nodes as a predictor of survival in squamous cell carcinoma of the oesophagus. Br J Surg 1994;81(3):410–3.

[42] Baba M, Aikou T, Yoshinaka H, et al. Long-term results of subtotal esophagectomy with three-field lymphadenectomy for carcinoma of the thoracic esophagus. Ann Surg 1994; 219:310–6.

[43] Killinger WA, Rice TW, Adelstein DJ, et al. Stage II esophageal carcinoma: the significance of T and N. J Thorac Cardiovasc Surg 1996;111(5):935–40.

[44] Arnott SJ, Duncan W, Gignoux M, et al. Oesophageal cancer collaborative group. Preoperative radiotherapy for esophageal carcinoma. Cochrane Database Syst Rev 2005;19(4): CD001799.

[45] Roth J, Pass H, Flanagan M, et al. Randomized clinical trial of preoperative and postoperative adjuvant chemotherapy with cisplatin, vindesine, and bleomycin for carcinoma of the esophagus. J Thorac Cardiovasc Surg 1998;96:242–8.

[46] Schlag P. Randomized trial of preoperative chemotherapy for squamous cell carcinoma of the esophagus. Arch Surg 1992;127:1446–50.

[47] Maipang T, Vasinnanukorn P, Petpichetchian C, et al. Induction chemotherapy in the treatment of patients with carcinoma of the esophagus. J Surg Oncol 1994;56:191–7.

[48] Law S, Fok M, Chow S, et al. Preoperative chemotherapy versus surgical therapy alone for squamous cell carcinoma of the esophagus: a prospective randomized trial. J Thorac Cardiovasc Surg 1997;114:210–7.

[49] Kelsen D, Ginsberg R, Pajak T, et al. Chemotherapy followed by surgery compared with surgery alone for localized esophageal cancer. N Engl J Med 1998;339:1979–84.

[50] Ancona E, Ruol A, Santi S, et al. Only pathologic complete response to neoadjuvant chemotherapy improves significantly the long term survival of patients with resectable esophageal squamous cell carcinoma. Cancer 2001;91:2165–74.

[51] Medical research council Oesophageal cancer working group. Surgical resection with or without preoperative chemotherapy in esophageal cancer: a randomised controlled trial. Lancet 2002;359:1727–34.

[52] Malthaner R, Wong R, Rumble R, et al. Neoadjuvant or adjuvant therapy for respectable esophageal cancer: a systematic review and meta-analysis. BMC Med 2004;2:35.

[53] Gebski V, Burmeister B, SMithers BM, et al, Australian Gastro-Intestinal Trials Group. Survival benefits from neoadjuvant chemoradiotherapy or chemotherapy in oesophageal carcinoma: a meta-analysis. Lancet Oncol 2007;8(3):226–34.

[54] Le Prise E, Etienne P, Meunier B, et al. A randomized study of chemotherapy, radiation therapy, and surgery versus surgery for localized squamous cell carcinoma of the esophagus. Cancer 1994;73:1779–84.

[55] Apinop C, Puttisak P, Preecha N. A prospective study of combined therapy in esophageal cancer. Hepatogastroenterology 1994;41:391–3.

[56] Walsh T, Noonan N, Hollywood D, et al. A comparison of multimodal therapy and surgery for esophageal adenocarcinoma. N Engl J Med 1996;335:462–7.

[57] Bosset J, Gignoux M, Triboulet J, et al. Chemoradiotherapy followed by surgery compared with surgery alone in squamous cell cancer of the esophagus. N Engl J Med 1997;337:161–7.

[58] Urba S, Orringer M, Turrisi A, et al. Randomized trial of preoperative chemoradiation versus surgery alone in patients with locoregional esophageal carcinoma. J Clin Oncol 2001;19:305–13.

[59] Burmeister B, SMithers M, Gebski V, et al. A randomized phase III study comparing surgery alone with chemoradiation therapy followed by surgery for resectable carcinoma of the esophagus: an intergroup study of the Trans-Tasman Radiation Oncology Group (TROG) and the Australian Gastro-Intestinal Trials Group (AGITG). Lancet Oncol 2005;6:659–68.

[60] Lee JL, Park SI, Kim SB, et al. A single institutional phase III trial of preoperative chemotherapy with hyperfractionation radiotherapy plus surgery versus surgery alone for respectable esophageal squamous cell carcinoma. Ann Oncol 2004;15(6):947–54.

[61] Walsh T. The role of multimodality therapy in improving survival: a prospective randomised trial. In: Predicting, defining and improving outcomes for esophageal carcinoma [MD thesis]. Dublin: Trinity College, University of Dublin; 1995. p. 124–50.

[62] Tepper J, Krasna M, Niedzwiecki D, et al. Superiority of trimodality therapy to surgery alone in esophageal cancer: results of CALGB 9781. J Clin Oncol 2006;24(Suppl 18S): 4012 [abstract].

[63] Carstens H, Albertsson M, Friesland S, et al. A randomized trial of chemoradiotherapy versus surgery alone in patients with resectable esophageal cancer. J Clin Oncol 2007; 25(18S):4530.

[64] Geh JI, Bond SJ, Bentzen SM, et al. Systematic overview of preoperative (neoadjuvant) chemoradiotherapy trials in oesophageal cancer: evidence of a radiation and chemotherapy dose response. Radiother Oncol 2006;78(3):236–44 [epub 2006 Mar 20].

[65] Urschel J, Vasan H. A meta-analysis of randomized controlled trials that compared neoadjuvant chemoradiation and surgery to surgery alone for resectable esophageal cancer. Am J Surg 2003;185:538–43.

[66] Greer S, Goodney P, Sutton J, et al. Neoadjuvant chemoradiotherapy for esophageal carcinoma: a meta-analysis. Surgery 2005;137:172–7.

[67] Fiorica F, Di Bona D, Schepis F, et al. Preoperative chemoradiotherapy for esophageal cancer: a systematic review and meta-analysis. Gut 2004;53:925–30.

[68] Jadad AR, Moore RA, Carroll D, et al. Assessing the quality of reports of randomized clinical trials: is blinding necessary? Control Clin Trials 1996;17(1):1–12.

[69] Egger M, Ebrahim S, Smith GD. Where now for meta-analysis? Int J Epidemiol 2002;31:1–5.

[70] Hagry O, Coosemans W, De Leyn P, et al. Effect of preoperative chemoradiotherapy on postsurgical morbidity and mortality in cT3-4+/-cM1lymph cancer of the oesophagus and gastroesophageal junction. Eur J Cardiothorac Surg 2003;24(2):179–86.

[71] Flamen P, Van Cutsem E, Lerut A, et al. Positron emission tomography for assessment of the response to induction radiochemotherapy in locally advanced oesophageal cancer. Ann Oncol 2002;13(3):361–8.

[72] Lordick F, Ott K, Krause BJ, et al. PET to assess early metabolic response and to guide treatment of adenocarcinoma of the oesophagogastric junction: the MUNICON phase II trial. Lancet Oncol 2007;8(9):797–805.

[73] Kim LK, Ryu JS, Kim SB, et al. Value of complete metabolic response by (18)F-fluorodeoxyglucose-positron emission tomography in oesophageal cancer for prediction of pathologic response and survival after preoperative chemoradiotherapy. Eur J Cancer 2007;43(9): 1385–91.

[74] Choi JY, Jang HJ, Shim YM, et al. 18F-FDG PET in patients with esophageal squamous cell carcinoma undergoing curative surgery: prognostic implications. J Nucl Med 2004;45(11): 1843–50.

[75] Bédard EL, Inculet RI, Malthaner RA, et al. The role of surgery and postoperative chemoradiation therapy in patients with lymph node positive esophageal carcinoma. Cancer 2001;91(12):2423–30.

[76] Cooper JS, Guo MD, Herskovic A, et al. Chemoradiotherapy of locally advanced esophageal cancer: long-term follow-up of a prospective randomized trial (RTOG 85-01). Radiation Therapy Oncology Group. JAMA 1999;281(17):1623–7.

[77] Bedenne L, Michel P, Bouché O, et al. Chemoradiation followed by surgery compared with chemoradiation alone in squamous cancer of the esophagus: FFCD 9102. J Clin Oncol 2007; 25(10):1160–8.

[78] Piessen G, Briez N, Triboulet JP, et al. Patients with locally advanced esophageal carcinoma non responder to radiochemotherapy: who will benefit from surgery? Ann Surg Oncol 2007; 14(7):2036–44.

[79] Stahl M, Stuschke M, Lehmann N, et al. Chemoradiation with and without surgery in patients with locally advanced squamous cell carcinoma of the esophagus. J Clin Oncol 2005;23(10):2310–7.

ELSEVIER
SAUNDERS

Surg Oncol Clin N Am
17 (2008) 503–517

SURGICAL
ONCOLOGY CLINICS
OF NORTH AMERICA

Staging of Advanced Colorectal Cancer

Graeme J. Poston, MB, MS, FRCS(Ed), FRCS(Eng)*

*Division of Digestive Diseases, Critical Care and Anesthesia, Center for Digestive Diseases,
University Hospital Aintree, Lower Lane, Liverpool L9 7AL, UK*

Only 10 years ago the management of advanced colorectal cancer was relatively straightforward. A few patients (accounting for less than 10%) who had limited liver-only disease meeting the stringent criteria of the day (1–3 unilobar metastases, preferably presenting metachronously, and resectable with a generous margin of healthy liver tissue) were offered the chance of surgery with curative intent [1]. If they survived the surgery, they had a 30% to 40% chance of being alive 5 years later [2]. For all others, the chance of remaining alive 5 years after diagnosis was less than 1% [3,4]. The American Joint Committee on Cancer (AJCC) staging system for advanced colorectal cancer was equally straightforward: all patients who had metastatic disease beyond the immediate lymph node basin of the primary tumor fell into stage IV, for whom the prognosis was grim.

The situation in 2008 has changed completely for both "resectable" and "unresectable" patients. The definition of resectability with curative intent is now the ability to clear (with negative margins) all measurable disease from the liver while leaving a future remnant liver (FRL) with a volume equaling 20% to 30% of the total healthy liver at presentation [5–7]. Factors determining the extent of safe liver resection include performance status, age, patient fitness, and concurrent parenchymal liver disease [5–7]. Limited resectable extrahepatic disease, hilar lymph node metastases, lung, ovarian, adrenal metastases, and local or regional recurrence are no longer considered formal contraindications [8,9]. Nonresectable extrahepatic disease (including positive celiac axis lymph nodes), significant parenchymal liver disease (Child class B and C), and lack of fitness to undergo the procedure [5] remain barriers to hepatectomy.

These advances are not reflected in the present approach to staging advanced colorectal cancer. Dukes, in his seminal paper on the staging of

* Department of Surgery, Liverpool Supra-Regional Hepatobiliary Centre, University Hospital Aintree, Lower Lane, Liverpool L9 7AL, United Kingdom.
E-mail address: graeme.poston@aintree.nhs.uk

1055-3207/08/$ - see front matter © 2008 Elsevier Inc. All rights reserved.
doi:10.1016/j.soc.2008.02.009

primary rectal cancer in 1932, deliberately excluded patients whose cancer had already spread to the liver at the time of diagnosis [10]. Including these patients was pointless, because they had incurable disease and inevitably would die soon [11]; therefore there was no Dukes' stage D. Even when Dukes [12] updated his findings 15 years later, it was only to reinforce the observations of the original paper. The first successful liver resection for metastatic colorectal cancer was performed in 1943 [13]. Despite this achievement, and the modifications to the Duke's classification made by Astler and Coller [14] in 1954, clinicians continue to group all patients who have colorectal cancer with distant metastases within an all-encompassing group, D/stage IV.

Historically, relative contraindications to liver resection have included synchronous presentation of primary colorectal cancer and liver metastasis, especially with a rectal primary tumor; a stage III primary colorectal tumor; multiple diffusely distributed liver metastases; multiple metastases; a metastasis larger than 5 cm; the presence of extrahepatic disease; a disease-free interval of less than 1 year from the diagnosis of the primary tumor; a high serum carcinoembryonic antigen level (> 200 ng/mL); and advanced age [15,16]. None of these factors individually (Box 1) precludes the offer of surgery, and only when more than three factors coincide does the postsurgical prognosis appear poorer [15,16]. These scoring systems, however, were derived before the modern use of effective chemotherapy became widely adopted.

Novel surgical strategies to bring more patients to liver surgery include preoperative portal vein embolization to increase the FRL to an acceptably safe volume and two-stage hepatectomy to allow compensatory hepatic hyperplasia to occur before completion of an R0 resection [5–7]. These recent changes in the definition of resectability mean that more than 20% of patients who have liver metastases now can be considered

---

Box 1. Predictive factors for poorer outcome after hepatectomy for colorectal liver metastases

- Synchronous detection
- Rectal primary tumor
- Stage III primary disease
- More than three metastases
- Largest metastasis > 5 cm in diameter
- Bilobar disease
- High serum carcinoembryonic antigen levels (> 200 ng/mL)
- Extrahepatic disease

Data from Nordlinger B, Guiguet M, Vaillant J-C, et al. Surgical resection of colorectal carcinoma metastases to the liver. Cancer 1996;77:1254–62; and Fong Y, Fortner J, Sun R, et al. Clinical score for predicting recurrence after hepatic resection for metastatic colorectal cancer: analysis of 1001 consecutive cases. Ann Surg 1999;230:309–16.

for surgery with curative intent at the outset, and 5-year and 10-year over-all survival exceeds 50% and 25%, respectively, in single [17–19] and multicenter series [8,20].

The 2003 French guidelines on the management of colorectal liver metastases recognize an important subcategory of patients being considered for liver resection [21]. These guidelines stratify operable patients into those who are "easily" resectable (involvement of up to four of the eight anatomic liver segments; noninvolvement of the vena cava; at least one hepatic vein and the contralateral portal pedicle clear of disease) as Class 1. Those whose disease is "potentially" resectable but involves five to six liver segments and/or specific major contralateral vascular structures within the liver are defined as Class 2 [21]. These guidelines recommend that whereas Class 1 resections should be within the ability of most hepatobiliary surgeons, Class 2 resections should be performed by very experienced liver surgeons working within recognized major liver units [21]. The benefit of destructive therapies using radiofrequency and microwave ablation techniques remains to be proven [19,22,23].

In the light of these advances [8], the staging of advanced colorectal cancer must discriminate between patients whose extrahepatic metastatic disease is potentially curable (with surgical resection) and those whose disease is not potentially curable. The lungs are the most common site of metastatic disease in patients who have extra-abdominal metastatic colorectal cancer [24–27], and lung resection for colorectal metastases has been performed successfully for more than 50 years [28]. The reported long-term survival very closely mirrors that seen after hepatectomy (5-year median survival rate of 41% after lung resection), with similar low operative morbidity and mortality [26,29–75]. It also has been argued, however, that favorable outcome after pulmonary resection in these highly selected patients is predetermined by the biology of their disease and is not actually a consequence of the surgical intervention [76]. The prognostic factors linked to better outcome following resection of pulmonary colorectal metastases are listed in Box 2.

Today, chemotherapy alone can extend the median survival of patients who have nonresectable disease by as much as 2 years [77–80]. The addition of monoclonal biologic agents offers a prospect of median survival extending beyond 2 years, and 20% of these patients will be alive 4 years after the detection of nonoperable liver disease [81–84]. The biggest breakthrough in the management of advanced colorectal cancer during the last decade has been the ability of medical oncologists, using modern cytotoxic agents, to convert inoperable liver disease to resectability [85–118].

Resectability rates after chemotherapy vary widely, from 6% to 60%. These wide discrepancies probably reflect patient selection, study design, and variations in institutional definitions of resectability [85–118]. It now is clear that resection rates directly reflect response rates to chemotherapy [119], and 5-year survival rates after subsequent liver resection often approach those seen after primary liver resection in initially resectable disease [87,88]. Although there are anecdotal reports of complete pathologic

Box 2. Prognostic factors repeatedly identified as being linked to better outcome after resection of pulmonary colorectal metastases

- Normal pre-thoracotomy carcinoembryonic antigen levels
- Solitary lung metastasis (If there is more than one metastasis, survival after surgery for unilateral disease is better than that seen after surgery for bilateral disease).
- Size of metastasis < 3 cm
- Prolonged disease-free interval/metachronous detection of lung disease
- Hilar/mediastinal lymphadenopathy
- Presence of extrathoracic disease
- Grade/stage of the primary colorectal tumor

Data from Refs. [30–75].

responses to modern combination cytotoxic chemotherapy [120,121], such observations have not been reported in any of the large-scale studies. The rate of radiologic complete response in single-institution reports is approximately 7% [122], and mapping of resection should continue to rely on prechemotherapy (baseline) imaging studies to minimize the rate of hepatic recurrence following liver resection after preoperative chemotherapy [107,121,123].

Furthermore, the response to chemotherapy may well be a surrogate marker for the subsequent success of liver surgery. Few patients whose disease progresses during chemotherapy, while remaining resectable, are alive 5 years after hepatectomy [122]. Combining the advances in surgical resection (redefinition of resectability and conversion of inoperable disease to resectability using chemotherapy) with modern chemotherapy regimens, the overall 5-year survival in advanced colorectal cancer now exceeds 20% in specialist centers [85–87,98,100,104,109,110,113,114].

Patients whose disease has metastasized beyond the lymph node basin of the primary tumor remain collectively grouped by the 2002 sixth edition of the AJCC *Cancer Staging Manual* as stage IV, with no differentiation reflecting a difference in prognosis based on the site and extent of metastatic disease [124]. This restriction probably reflects a continuing reliance on the TNM system of cancer staging introduced by the Union International Contre le Cancer in 1958, at a time when patients who had advanced colorectal cancer had little prospect of surviving more than 6 months from the time of diagnosis.

The present stage IV covers a range of patients whose outlook varies from incurable, with a prognosis of perhaps only 6 months, to potentially curable, clearly not matching the other current stage-based treatment strategies and outcomes in stages I, II, and III. Furthermore, the new approach of converting incurable nonresectable metastatic disease to resectability with potentially curative intent (changing a prognosis of 0% at 5 years to in excess of 35%, and probable cure) represents a paradigm shift in therapeutic strategy for which there currently is no appropriate terminology. Such a strategy is not "downstaging" within the current terminology, because these patients presently remain within a globally encompassing stage IV. The concept of "downsizing" remains something people do with their homes in later middle age, after the children leave home, and has no oncologic equivalent.

Further considerations

This argument could be developed further by dividing the group of patients initially considered to have unresectable disease into those who, in the opinion of an experienced multidisciplinary team (MDT) comprising surgeons, oncologists, radiologists, and pathologists, could become resectable after a course of chemotherapy and those whose disease would remain incurable even after an apparent complete radiologic response to treatment. Also, consideration must be given to distinguishing between patients who have liver-only disease, those who have disease involving both the liver and extrahepatic sites, and those who have metastatic disease exclusively outside the liver (eg, peritoneal carcinomatosis or disease involving the aortic lymph node chain). The standard of care that now is obligatory by law in several European countries (including the United Kingdom and France) is that all patients diagnosed as having cancer must be discussed within the setting of an MDT, and the management decisions made by that team must be documented in the patient's case record.

In addition to identifying clinically meaningful subgroups based on metastatic location and resectability, a distinction also must be made based on the rationale for the administration of chemotherapy. Thus one could distinguish chemotherapy given in the true neoadjuvant setting, to a patient determined to be resectable with curative intent, from chemotherapy given to patients who are borderline resectable or whose disease might become resectable if they achieved a sufficient response to chemotherapy. Some have previously termed the latter approach as "neotherapeutic" chemotherapy to distinguish it from true neoadjuvant chemotherapy [125]. Another view is that this strategy could be termed "induction" chemotherapy.

Last, clinicians should remember that patients deemed to be hopelessly incurable at detection of their advanced disease are with increasing frequency achieving such dramatic responses to chemotherapy, even in second- and third-line regimens, that they can be offered resection of the hepatic metastases with potentially curative intent. These are the fortuitous patients who are brought "accidentally" to hepatectomy [126].

Staging advanced colorectal cancer: possible ways forward?

A recent proposal for staging colorectal cancer spread beyond the N2 lymph node basin of the primary tumor [127] limits stage IV to liver-only disease and is further stratified by the MDT on intention to treat and prognosis into

- IVA: Easily resectable with curative intent at detection (French classification I [21])
- IVB: Technically difficult/borderline resectability at detection (French classification II [21])
- IVC: Potentially resectable after neotherapeutic chemotherapy in the opinion of an experienced MDT
- IVD: Little or no hope of being rendered resectable with curative intent after conventional chemotherapy (involvement of more than six anatomic segments, less than 25% FRL predicted after surgery, involvement of all three hepatic veins and/or both portal pedicles, significant coexisting parenchymal liver disease)

Based on this system, the spread of tumor beyond the liver would be classified as stage V disease and then must be considered by the MDT as either potentially curable or beyond cure but amenable to palliative therapy with a survival benefit. Therefore there would be two further subcategories:

- VA: Resectable (including hepatic with extrahepatic disease). This group would include lung metastases, positive hepatic hilar lymph nodes, adrenal and splenic metastases, direct extension from the liver into adjacent organs including diaphragm, and low-volume peritoneal disease.
- VB: Extrahepatic disease that is not resectable with curative intent

An alternative, less rigorous, approach would be to stratify advanced disease according to resectability for cure, regardless of anatomic site. Stage IV then would include all metastatic disease that is considered resectable with curative intent by an experienced anatomic site-specific MDT and might be subdivided into

- IVA: Liver resectable
- IVB: Extrahepatic (± liver) resectable

With this approach, stage V would include patients who have metastatic disease that is considered unresectable with curative intent by an experienced site-specific MDT at detection. Stage V could be further substratified into

- VA: Disease that in the opinion of an experienced MDT might become resectable with curative intent after neotherapeutic chemotherapy
- VB: Disease that has little or no prospect of ever becoming resectable after chemotherapy, whatever the intention of the chemotherapy administration

Another alternative proposal groups all distant disease within stage IV. The MDT would subclassify such disease into the categories of resectable with curative intent (IVR) and unresectable with curative intent

(IVU) [125]. The IVR and IVU categories could be stratified further into hepatic only (a), extrahepatic only (b), and both hepatic and extrahepatic (c) (Table 1).

Because the overall 5-year survival for both resectable hepatic and extra-hepatic disease is now equivalent to that for stage III disease, another way of looking at staging would be to equate such disease to stage III. Presently, stage III includes metastatic disease that is resectable with curative intent en bloc with the primary tumor (ie, the draining lymph nodes already infil-trated by carcinoma are resected with the primary tumor). The 5-year sur-vival for patients who have C1 (involving the muscularis propria, with nodal metastases, Astler-Coller system) and C2 (penetrating muscularis propria, with nodal metastases, Astler-Coller system) stage disease is similar to that seen after resection of French class I liver metastases [21] and other easily resectable distant disease (lung, adrenal, portal lymph nodes, and low-volume peritoneal). Stage IV then would apply to all disease for which sur-gical resection does not offer potential long-term survival benefit. With the growing knowledge of tumor biology, stage IV might be stratified further according to predicted response (by the MDT) to chemotherapy and tar-geted biologic therapies.

A novel approach, still under discussion, is a grid-based staging system (Table 2). Although more complicated, this approach might lead to a better system for the classification of patients at the outset. Patients then would be treated according to their position on the grid. Those classified as A1 and A2 would receive surgery only, those classified as B1, B2, B3, and A3 would receive neoadjuvant therapy, and those classified as C1–4, B4, and A4 would receive palliative chemotherapy.

Discussions among experts in the field suggest that, in its present form, the grid staging system probably is too complicated for everyday use, but it probably is appropriate for clinical trials in which some standardized form of patient stratification would allow more meaningful cross-trial com-parisons. This discussion is particularly important in view of the paucity of randomized trial data and the ethical dilemmas that preclude randomized trials going forward. The general consensus in Europe is that by replacing the more traditional two-part classification of resectable or unresectable

Table 1
Staging classification based on resectability with curative intent and unresectability with cura-tive intent

Category	Disease stage
IVRa	Resectable liver-only disease
IVRb	Resectable extrahepatic (but no liver) disease
IVRc	Resectable hepatic and extrahepatic disease
IVUa	Unresectable liver-only disease
IVUb	Unresectable extrahepatic (no liver) disease
IVUc	Hepatic and extrahepatic disease unresectable at one or more sites

Table 2
A proposed grid staging system

	Extrahepatic metastases			
Hepatic metastases	None	Resectable	Initially unresectable	Unresectable
None	NA			
Resectable	A1 (M1a)	A2 (M2a)	A3 (M3a)	A4 (M4a)
Initially unresectable	B1 (M1b)	B2 (M2b)	B3 (M3b)	B4 (M4b)
Unresectable	C1 (M1c)	C2 (M2c)	C3 (M3c)	C4 (M4c)

with three stratification groups, namely, resectable, unresectable, and unlikely to become resectable, patients who are classified as having initially unresectable disease will be followed more carefully and will have a better
chance of a good, long-term clinical outcome (see Table 2) [126].

If the ABC grid classification risks confusion with Dukes' system, desig-
nations such as M1–4 (or M0, M1a, M1b, and M1c) could be used, as proposed by the European Colorectal Metastases Treatment Group in their
recent paper [127], to describe the degree of extrahepatic disease involvement, and the designators "a," "b," and "c" could be used to describe
whether the hepatic metastases are resectable, initially unresectable, or unlikely to become resectable.

Summary

The treatment of advanced metastatic colorectal cancer is now multimodal, and long-term survival, with or without disease, is increasingly the
norm [127]. This situation is not reflected in the current staging system beyond the present stage III. Whatever the solution, it is evident that the current staging system (AJCC version 6, 2002) [125] for advanced colorectal
cancer is flawed, is out of date, and does not reflect current treatment strategies or prognoses for patients who have metastatic disease. A new staging
system is long overdue.

Such restratification would encourage improved patient work-up and
would bring the possibility of using curative treatment strategies for patients
who have advanced disease to the attention of physicians at an early stage. It
also would encourage high-quality patient follow-up and greater and more
careful monitoring of patients initially assigned to palliative therapy who
may, despite an initially unfavorable assessment, achieve a sufficiently
good response to be brought accidentally to further surgery with potentially
curative intent.

A new staging system should enable more direct comparison of results
from different institutions and would allow further stratification for subset
analyses within future trials of new treatment strategies. Advanced colorectal cancer is rapidly evolving from an acute terminal illness into a chronic
and manageable condition. Last, the increasing evidence of chemotherapy

response sufficient to render previously nonresectable disease resectable with curative intent opens the possibility that achieving resectability could become a recognized secondary end point for future clinical trials in medical oncology.

References

[1] Hughes KS, (On behalf of the Registry of Hepatic Metastases). Resection of the liver for colorectal carcinoma metastases: a multi-institutional study of indications for resection. Surgery 1988;103:278–88.

[2] Scheele J, Stang R, Altendorf-Hofmann A, et al. Resection of colorectal liver metastases. World J Surg 1995;19:59–71.

[3] Rougier P, Milan C, Lazorthes F, et al. Prospective study of prognostic factors in patients with unresected hepatic metastases from colorectal cancer. Br J Surg 1995;82: 1397–400.

[4] Scheithauer W, Rosen H, Kornek G-V. Randomised comparison of combination chemotherapy plus supportive care with supportive care alone in patients with metastatic colorectal cancer. Br Med J 1993;306:752–5.

[5] Poston GJ, Adam R, Alberts S, et al. Oncosurge: a strategy for improving resectability with curative intent in metastatic colorectal cancer. J Clin Oncol 2005;23:7125–34.

[6] Abdalla E, Barnett CC, Doherty D, et al. Extended hepatectomy in patients with hepatobiliary malignancies with and without preoperative portal vein embolization. Arch Surg 2002;137:675–80.

[7] Vauthey JN, Chaoui A, Do KA, et al. Standardized measurement of the future liver remnant prior to extended liver resection: methodology and clinical associations. Surgery 2000; 127:512–9.

[8] Elias D, Liberale G, Vernerey D, et al. Hepatic and extrahepatic colorectal metastases: when resectable, their localization does not matter, but their total number has a prognostic effect. Ann Surg Oncol 2005;12:900–9.

[9] Jaeck D. The significance of hepatic pedicle lymph node metastases in surgical management of colorectal liver metastases and of other liver malignancies. Ann Surg Oncol 2003;10: 1007–11.

[10] Dukes CE. The classification of cancer of the rectum. J Pathol Bacteriol 1932;35:323–32.

[11] Rolleston H, McNee JW. Malignant tumours, diseases of the liver, gallbladder and bile ducts. London: Macmillan & Co; 1927. p. 489–551.

[12] Dukes CE. The surgical pathology of rectal cancer. J Clin Pathol 1949;2:95–8.

[13] Poston GJ. Standing on the shoulders of giants. Eur J Surg Oncol 2008;34:253–5.

[14] Astler VB, Coller FA. The prognostic significance of direct extension of carcinoma of the colon and rectum. Ann Surg 1954;139:846–52.

[15] Nordlinger B, Guiguet M, Vaillant J-C, et al. Surgical resection of colorectal carcinoma metastases to the liver. Cancer 1996;77:1254–62.

[16] Fong Y, Fortner J, Sun R, et al. Clinical score for predicting recurrence after hepatic resection for metastatic colorectal cancer: analysis of 1001 consecutive cases. Ann Surg 1999;230: 309–16.

[17] Figueras J, Valls C, Rafecas J, et al. Resection rates and effect of postoperative chemotherapy on survival after colorectal liver metastases. Br J Surg 2001;88:980–5.

[18] Choti MA, Sitzmann JV, Tiburi MF, et al. Trends in long-term survival following liver resection for hepatic colorectal metastases. Ann Surg 2002;235:759–66.

[19] Abdalla E, Vauthey JN, Ellis LM, et al. Recurrence and outcomes following hepatic resection, radiofrequency ablation, and combined resection/ablation for colorectal liver metastases. Ann Surg 2004;239:818–25.

[20] Pawlik TM, Scoggins CR, Zorzi D, et al. Effect of surgical margin status on survival and site of recurrence after hepatic resection for colorectal metastases. Ann Surg 2005;241: 715–22.

[21] Chiche L. When is first-line resection of hepatic metastases indicated? Gastroenterol Clin Biol 2003;27(S2):B11–3, B41–61.

[22] Poston GJ. Radiofrequency ablation of colorectal liver metastases: where are we really going? J Clin Oncol 2005;23:1342–4.

[23] Higgins H, Berger DL. RFA for liver tumors: does it really work? Oncologist 2006;11: 801–8.

[24] Kanemitsu Y, Kato T, Hirai T, et al. Preoperative probability model for predicting overall survival after resection of pulmonary metastases from colorectal cancer. Br J Surg 2004;91: 112–20.

[25] Yoshidome H, Ito H, Kimura F, et al. Surgical treatment for extrahepatic recurrence after hepatectomy for colorectal metastases. Hepatogastroenterology 2004;51:1805–9.

[26] Inoue M, Ohta M, Iuchi K, et al. Benefits of surgery for patients with pulmonary metastases from colorectal cancer. Ann Thorac Surg 2004;78:238–44.

[27] Pihl E, Hughes ES, McDermott FT, et al. Lung recurrence after curative surgery for colorectal cancer. Dis Colon Rectum 1987;30:417–9.

[28] Okumura S, Kondo H, Tsuboi M, et al. Pulmonary resection for metastatic colorectal cancer: experiences with 159 patients. J Thorac Cardiovasc Surg 1996;112:867–74.

[29] Elias D, Sideris L, Pocard M, et al. Results of R0 resection for colorectal liver metastases associated with extrahepatic disease. Ann Surg Oncol 2004;11:274–80.

[30] Ambiru S, Miyazaki M, Ito H, et al. Resection of hepatic and pulmonary metastases in patients with colorectal carcinoma. Cancer 1998;82:274–8.

[31] Baron O, Amini M, Duveau D, et al. Surgical resection of pulmonary metastases from colorectal carcinoma. Five-year survival and main prognostic factors. Eur J Cardiothorac Surg 1996;10:347–51.

[32] Brister SJ, de Varennes B, Gordon PH, et al. Contemporary operative management of pulmonary metastases of colorectal origin. Dis Colon Rectum 1988;31:786–92.

[33] Gough DB, Donohue JH, Trastek VA, et al. Resection of hepatic and pulmonary metastases in patients with colorectal cancer. Br J Surg 1994;81:94–6.

[34] Goya T, Miyazawa N, Kondo H, et al. Surgical resection of pulmonary metastases from colorectal cancer. 10-year follow-up. Cancer 1989;64:1418–21.

[35] Lehnert T, Knaebel HP, Duck M, et al. Sequential hepatic and pulmonary resections for metastatic colorectal cancer. Br J Surg 1999;86:241–3.

[36] Mansel JK, Zinsmeister AR, Pairolero PC, et al. Pulmonary resection of metastatic colorectal adenocarcinoma. A ten year experience. Chest 1986;89:109–12.

[37] McAfee MK, Allen MS, Trastek VF, et al. Colorectal lung metastases: results of surgical excision. Ann Thorac Surg 1992;53:780–5 [discussion: 785–6].

[38] McCormack PM, Burt ME, Bains MS, et al. Lung resection for colorectal metastases. 10-year results. Arch Surg 1992;127:1403–6.

[39] Mori M, Tomoda H, Ishida T, et al. Surgical resection of pulmonary metastases from colorectal adenocarcinoma. Special reference to repeated pulmonary resections. Arch Surg 1991;126:1297–301 [discussion: 1302].

[40] Murata S, Moriya Y, Akasu T, et al. Resection of both hepatic and pulmonary metastases in patients with colorectal carcinoma. Cancer 1998;83:1086–93.

[41] Regnard JF, Grunenwald D, Spaggiari L, et al. Surgical treatment of hepatic and pulmonary metastases from colorectal cancers. Ann Thorac Surg 1998;66:214–8 [discussion: 218–9].

[42] Sauter ER, Bolton JS, Willis GW, et al. Improved survival after pulmonary resection of metastatic colorectal carcinoma. J Surg Oncol 1990;43:135–8.

[43] Scheele J, Altendorf-Hofmann A, Stangl R, et al. Pulmonary resection for metastatic colon and upper rectum cancer. Is it useful? Dis Colon Rectum 1990;33:745–52.

[44] Shirouzu K, Isomoto H, Hayashi A, et al. Surgical treatment for patients with pulmonary metastases after resection of primary colorectal carcinoma. Cancer 1995;76:393–8.
[45] Smith JW, Fortner JG, Burt M. Resection of hepatic and pulmonary metastases from colorectal cancer. Surg Oncol 1992;1:399–404.
[46] van Halteren HK, van Geel AN, Hart AA, et al. Pulmonary resection for metastases of colorectal origin. Chest 1995;107:1526–31.
[47] Wilking N, Petrelli NJ, Herrera L, et al. Surgical resection of pulmonary metastases from colorectal adenocarcinoma. Dis Colon Rectum 1985;28:562–4.
[48] Yano T, Hara N, Ichinose Y, et al. Results of pulmonary resection of metastatic colorectal cancer and its application. J Thorac Cardiovasc Surg 1993;106:875–9.
[49] Zanella A, Marchet A, Mainente P, et al. Resection of pulmonary metastases from colorectal carcinoma. Eur J Surg Oncol 1997;23:424–7.
[50] Ashley AC, Deschamps C, Alberts SR. Impact of prognostic factors on clinical outcome after resection of colorectal pulmonary metastases. Clin Colorectal Cancer 2006;6:32–7.
[51] Headrick JR, Miller DL, Nagorney DM, et al. Surgical treatment of hepatic and pulmonary metastases from colon cancer. Ann Thorac Surg 2001;71:975–9 [discussion: 979–80].
[52] Iizasa T, Suzuki M, Yoshida S, et al. Prediction of prognosis and surgical indications for pulmonary metastasectomy from colorectal cancer. Ann Thorac Surg 2006;82: 254–60.
[53] Ike H, Shimada H, Ohki S, et al. Results of aggressive resection of lung metastases from colorectal carcinoma detected by intensive follow-up. Dis Colon Rectum 2002;45:468–73 [discussion: 473–5].
[54] Ike H, Shimada H, Togo S, et al. Sequential resection of lung metastasis following partial hepatectomy for colorectal cancer. Br J Surg 2002;89:1164–8.
[55] Irshad K, Ahmad F, Morin JE, et al. Pulmonary metastases from colorectal cancer: 25 years of experience. Can J Surg 2001;44:217–21.
[56] Kobayashi K, Kawamura M, Ishihara T. Surgical treatment for both pulmonary and hepatic metastases from colorectal cancer. J Thorac Cardiovasc Surg 1999;118:1090–6.
[57] Koga R, Yamamoto J, Saiura A, et al. Surgical resection of pulmonary metastases from colorectal cancer: four favourable prognostic factors. Jpn J Clin Oncol 2006;36:643–8.
[58] Lee WS, Yun SH, Chun HK, et al. Pulmonary resection for metastases from colorectal cancer: prognostic factors and survival. Int J Colorectal Dis 2007;22:699–704.
[59] Moore KH, McCaughan BC. Surgical resection for pulmonary metastases from colorectal cancer. ANZ J Surg 2001;71:143–6.
[60] Nagakura S, Shirai Y, Nomura T, et al. Long-term survival after resection of colonic adenocarcinoma with synchronous metastases to the liver, adrenal gland, and aortic-caval lymph nodes: report of a case. Dis Colon Rectum 2002;45:1679–80.
[61] Negri F, Musolino A, Cunningham D, et al. Retrospective study of resection of pulmonary metastases in patients with advanced colorectal cancer: the development of a preoperative chemotherapy strategy. Clin Colorectal Cancer 2004;4:101–6.
[62] Ogata Y, Matono K, Hayashi A, et al. Repeat pulmonary resection for isolated recurrent lung metastases yields results comparable to those after first pulmonary resection in colorectal cancer. World J Surg 2005;29:363–8.
[63] Patel NA, Keenan RJ, Medich DS, et al. The presence of colorectal hepatic metastases does not preclude pulmonary metastasectomy. Am Surg 2003;69:1047–53 [discussion: 1053].
[64] Pfannschmidt J, Muley T, Hoffmann H, et al. Prognostic factors and survival after complete resection of pulmonary metastases from colorectal carcinoma: experiences in 167 patients. J Thorac Cardiovasc Surg 2003;126:732–9.
[65] Rena O, Casadio C, Viano F, et al. Pulmonary resection for metastases from colorectal cancer: factors influencing prognosis. Twenty-year experience. Eur J Cardiothorac Surg 2002; 21:906–12.
[66] Rizk NP, Downey RJ. Resection of pulmonary metastases from colorectal cancer. Semin Thorac Cardiovasc Surg 2002;14:29–34.

[67] Saito Y, Omiya H, Kohno K, et al. Pulmonary metastasectomy for 165 patients with colorectal carcinoma: a prognostic assessment. J Thorac Cardiovasc Surg 2002;124:1007–13.

[68] Sakamoto T, Tsubota N, Iwanaga K, et al. Pulmonary resection for metastases from colorectal cancer. Chest 2001;119:1069–72.

[69] Shah SA, Haddad R, Al-Sukhni W, et al. Surgical resection of hepatic and pulmonary metastases from colorectal carcinoma. J Am Coll Surg 2006;202:468–75.

[70] Shiono S, Ishii G, Nagai K, et al. Predictive factors for local recurrence of resected colorectal lung metastases. Ann Thorac Surg 2005;80:1040–5.

[71] Vogelsang H, Haas S, Hierholzer C, et al. Factors influencing survival after resection of pulmonary metastases from colorectal cancer. Br J Surg 2004;91:1066–71.

[72] Watanabe I, Arai T, Ono M, et al. Prognostic factors in resection of pulmonary metastasis from colorectal cancer. Br J Surg 2003;90:1436–40.

[73] Yamada H, Katoh H, Kondo S, et al. Surgical treatment of pulmonary recurrence after hepatectomy for colorectal liver metastases. Hepatogastroenterology 2002;49:976–9.

[74] Yedibela S, Klein P, Feuchter K, et al. Surgical management of pulmonary metastases from colorectal cancer in 153 patients. Ann Surg Oncol 2006;13:1538–44.

[75] Zink S, Kayser G, Gabius HJ, et al. Survival, disease-free interval, and associated tumor features in patients with colon/rectal carcinomas and their resected intra-pulmonary metastases. Eur J Cardiothorac Surg 2001;19:908–13.

[76] Treasure T, Utley M, Hunt I. When professional opinion is not enough. BMJ 2007;334:831–2.

[77] Tournigand C, Andre T, Achille E, et al. FOLFIRI followed by FOLFOX6 or the reverse sequence in advanced colorectal cancer: a randomized GERCOR study. J Clin Oncol 2004;22:229–37.

[78] Goldberg RM, Sargent DJ, Morton RF, et al. A randomized controlled trial of fluorouracil plus leucovorin, irinotecan, and oxaliplatin combinations in patients with previously untreated metastatic colorectal cancer. J Clin Oncol 2004;22:23–30.

[79] Grothey A, Sargent D, Goldberg RM, et al. Survival of patients with advanced colorectal cancer improves with the availability of fluorouracil-leucovorin, irinotecan, and oxaliplatin in the course of treatment. J Clin Oncol 2004;22:1209–14.

[80] Cals L, Rixe O, Francois E, et al. Dose-finding study of weekly 24-h continuous infusion of 5-fluorouracil associated with alternating oxaliplatin or irinotecan in advanced colorectal cancer patients. Ann Oncol 2004;15:1018–24.

[81] Saltz LB, Meropol NJ, Loehrer PJ, et al. Phase II trial of cetuximab in patients with refractory colorectal cancer that expresses the epidermal growth factor receptor. J Clin Oncol 2004;22:1201–8.

[82] Cunningham D, Humblet Y, Siena S, et al. Cetuximab monotherapy and cetuximab plus irinotecan in irinotecan-refractory metastatic colorectal cancer. N Engl J Med 2004;351:337–45.

[83] Hurwitz H, Fehrenbacher L, Novotny W, et al. Bevacizumab plus irinotecan, fluorouracil, and leucovorin for metastatic colorectal cancer. N Engl J Med 2004;350:2335–42.

[84] Ardalan B, Livingstone A, Franceschi D, et al. A phase II study of irinotecan, fluoroxuridine and leucovorin (IFLUX) as a first-line chemotherapy in advanced colorectal cancer. J Clin Oncol 2005;23(16s):270s.

[85] Bismuth H, Adam R, Levi F, et al. Resection of nonresectable liver metastases from colorectal cancer after neoadjuvant chemotherapy. Ann Surg 1996;224:509–20 [discussion: 520–2].

[86] Akasu T, Moriya Y, Takayama T. A pilot study of multimodality therapy for initially unresectable liver metastases from colorectal carcinoma: hepatic resection after hepatic arterial infusion chemotherapy and portal embolization. Jpn J Clin Oncol 1997;27:331–5.

[87] Adam R, Avisar E, Ariche A, et al. Five-year survival following hepatic resection after neoadjuvant therapy for nonresectable colorectal cancer. Ann Surg Oncol 2001;8:347–53.

[88] Giacchetti S, Itzuki M, Gruia G, et al. Long-term survival of patients with unresectable co-lorectal cancer liver metastases following infusional chemotherapy with 5-fluorouracil, leu-covorin, oxaliplatin and surgery. Ann Oncol 1999;10:663–9.

[89] Meric F, Patt YZ, Curley SA, et al. Surgery after downstaging of unresectable hepatic tu-mors with intra-arterial chemotherapy. Ann Surg Oncol 2000;7:490–5.

[90] Shankar A, Leonard P, Renaut AJ, et al. Neo-adjuvant therapy improves respectability rates for colorectal liver metastases. Ann R Coll Surg Engl 2001;83:85–8.

[91] Gil-Delgado MA, Guinet F, Castaing D, et al. Prospective phase II trial of irinotecan, 5-fluorouracil, and leucovorin in combination as salvage therapy for advanced colorectal can-cer. Am J Clin Oncol 2001;24:101–5.

[92] Wein A, Reidel C, Kockerling F, et al. Impact of surgery on survival in palliative patients with metastatic colorectal cancer after first line treatment with weekly 24-hour infusion of high-dose 5-fluotouracil and folinic acid. Ann Oncol 2001;12:1721–7.

[93] Rivoire M, de Cian F, Meeus P, et al. Combination of neoadjuvant chemotherapy with cryotherapy and surgical resection for the treatment of unresectable liver metastases from colorectal carcinoma. Cancer 2002;95:2283–92.

[94] Miyanari N, Mori T, Takahashi K, et al. Evaluation of aggressively treated patients with unresectable multiple liver metastases from colorectal cancer. Dis Colon Rectum 2002; 45:1503–9.

[95] Falcone A, Masi G, Cupini S, et al. Biweekly chemotherapy with oxaliplatin, irinotecan, infusional fluorouracil, and leucovorin: a pilot study in patients with metastatic colorectal cancer. J Clin Oncol 2002;20:4006–14.

[96] Ho WM, Mok TS, Ma BB, et al. Liver resection after irinotecan (CPT-11), 5-fluorouracil (5FU) and folinic acid (FA) in patients (pts) with unresectable liver metastases (Mets) from colorectal cancer (CRC). Proceedings of the American Society of Clinical Oncology 2003;22:312.

[97] Alberts SR, Donohue JH, Mahoney MR, et al. Liver resection after 5-fluorouracil, leuco-vorin and oxaliplatin for patients with metastatic colorectal cancer (MCRC) limited to the liver. A North Central Cancer Treatment Group (NCCTG) phase II study. Proceedings of the American Society of Clinical Oncology 2003;22:263.

[98] Zelek L, Bugat R, Cherqui D, et al. Multimodal therapy with intravenous biweekly leuco-vorin, 5-fluorouracil and irinotecan combined with hepatic arterial infusion pirarubicin in non-resectable hepatic metastases from colorectal cancer (a European Association for Re-search in Oncology trial). Ann Oncol 2003;14:1537–42.

[99] Pozzo C, Basso M, Cassano A, et al. Neoadjuvant treatment of unresectable liver disease with irinotecan and 5-fluorouracil plus folinic acid in colorectal carcinoma patients. Ann Oncol 2004;15:933–9.

[100] Adam R, Delvart V, Pascal G, et al. Rescue surgery for unresectable colorectal liver metas-tases downstaged by chemotherapy: a model to predict long-term survival. Ann Surg 2004; 240:644–57.

[101] Rougier P, Raoul J-L, van Laethem J-L, et al. Cetuximab+FOLFIRI as first-line treatment for metastatic colorectal cancer. Proceedings of the American Society of Clinical Oncology 2004;22:248.

[102] Tabernero JM, van Cutsem E, Sastre J, et al. An international phase II study of cetuximab in combination with oxaliplatin/5-fluorouracil (5-FU)/folinic acid (FOLFOX-4) in the first-line treatment of patients with metastatic colorectal cancer expressing epidermal growth factor receptor (EGFR): preliminary results. Proceedings of the American Society of Clinical Oncology 2004;22:248.

[103] de la Camara J, Rodriguez J, Rotellar F, et al. Triplet therapy with oxaliplatin, irinotecan, 5-fluorouracil and folinic acid within a combined modality approach in patients with liver metastases from colorectal cancer. Proceedings of the American Society of Clinical Oncol-ogy 2004;23:268.

[104] Leonard GS, Fong Y, Jarnagin W, et al. Liver resection after hepatic infusion (HAI) plus systemic oxaliplatin (OXAL) combination in pretreated patients with extensive unresectable colorectal liver metastases. Proceedings of the American Society of Clinical Oncology 2004;23:256.

[105] Falcone A, Masi G, Cupini S, et al. Surgical resection of metastases (mts) after biweekly chemotherapy with irinotecan, oxaliplatin and 5-fluorouracil/leucovorin (FOLFOXIRI) in initially unresectable metastatic colorectal cancer (MCRC). Proceedings of the American Society of Clinical Oncology 2004;23:258.

[106] Fisher GA, Kuo T, Cho CD, et al. A phase II study of gefitinib in combination with FOL-FOX-4 (IFOX) in patients with metastatic colorectal cancer. Proceedings of the American Society of Clinical Oncology 2004;23:249.

[107] Gruenberger T, Schuell B, Kornek G, et al. Neoadjuvant chemotherapy for resectable colorectal cancer metastases: Impact on magnitude of liver resection and survival. Proceedings of the American Society of Clinical Oncology 2004;23:270.

[108] Alberts SR, Horvath WL, Sternfeld WC, et al. Oxaliplatin, fluorouracil, and leucovorin for patients with unresectable liver-only metastases from colorectal cancer: a North Central Cancer Treatment Group Phase II Study. J Clin Oncol 2005;23:published on-line October 17th.

[109] Diaz-Rubio E, Tabernero J, van Cutsem E, et al. Cetuximab in combination with oxaliplatin/5-fluorouracil (5-FU)/folinic acid (FA) (FOLFOX-4) in the first-line treatment of patients with epidermal growth factor receptor (EGFR)-expressing metastatic colorectal cancer: an international phase II study. J Clin Oncol 2005;23(16S):254s.

[110] Abad A, Anton A, Massuti B, et al. Resectability of liver metastases (LM) in patients with advanced colorectal cancer (ACRA) after treatment with the combination of oxaliplatin (OXA), irinotecan (IRI) and 5FU. Final results of a phase II study. J Clin Oncol 2005; 23(16S):275s.

[111] Bouchahda M, Tanaka K, Adam R, et al. Three-drug chemotherapy via hepatic artery as salvage treatment for patients with liver-only metastases from colorectal cancer. J Clin Oncol 2005;23(16s):175s.

[112] Martoni A, Pinto C, di Fabio F, et al. Phase II randomized trial on protracted 5-flururacil infusion plus oxaliplatin (FOX) versus capecitabine plus oxaliplatin (XELOX) as first-line treatment in advanced colorectal cancer (ACRC): preliminary results of the Italian FOCA study. J Clin Oncol 2005;23(16s):275s.

[113] Moosmann N, Kern W, Waggershausser T, et al. Hepatic artery infusion of 5-fluorouracil, folinic acid plus oxaliplatin for liver metastases from colorectal cancer. Final analysis of a phase I/II study. J Clin Oncol 2005;23(16s):278s.

[114] Folprecht G, Lutz MP, Seufferlein T, et al. Cetuximab and irinotecan/5-FU/FA (AIO) as first line treatment in metastatic colorectal cancer (mCRC): final results and pharmacokinetic data of a phase I/IIa study. J Clin Oncol 2005;23(16s):281s.

[115] Sufferlein T, Dittrich C, Riemann J, et al. A phase I/II study of cetuximab in combination with 5-fluorouracil (5-FU)/folinic acid (FA) plus weekly oxaliplatin (L-OHP)(FUFOX) in the first-line treatment of patients with metastatic colorectal cancer (mCRC) expressing epidermal growth factor receptor (EGFR). Preliminary results. J Clin Oncol 2005; 23(16s):281s.

[116] Garassino I, Carnaghi C, Rimassa L, et al. Definitive results of hybrid chemotherapy with intravenous (iv) oxaliplatin (OXA) and folinic acid (FA), and intra-hepatic infusion (HAI) of 5-fluorouracil (5-FU) in patients with colorectal liver metastases. J Clin Oncol 2005; 23(16s):288s.

[117] Shimonov M, Hayat H. Alternating hepatic artery chronotherapy with CPT-11 and systemic chronotherapy with 5-FU/FA+carboplatin for metastatic colorectal cancer confined to the liver: a phase II study. J Clin Oncol 2005;23(16s):297s.

[118] Seium Y, Stupp R, Ruhstaller T, et al. Oxaliplatin combined with irinotecan and 5-fluoro-uracil/leucovorin (OCFL) in metastatic colorectal cancer: a phase I-II study. Ann Oncol 2005;16:762–6.

[119] Folprecht G, Grothey A, Alberts S, et al. Neoadjuvant treatment of unresectable colorectal liver metastases: correlation between tumour response and resection rates. Ann Oncol 2005; 16:1311–9.

[120] Elias D, Youssef O, Sideris L, et al. Evolution of missing colorectal liver metastases following inductive chemotherapy and hepatectomy. J Surg Oncol 2004;86:4–9.

[121] Schrag D, Weiser M, Schattner M, et al. An increasingly common challenge: management of the complete responder with multi-focal metastatic colorectal cancer. J Clin Oncol 2005; 23:1799–802.

[122] Adam R, Pascal G, Castaing D, et al. Tumor progression while on chemotherapy: a contra-indication to liver resection for multiple colorectal metastases. Ann Surg 2004;240:1052–61.

[123] Vauthey J-N, Abdalla EK. Unresectable hepatic colorectal metastases: need for new surgical strategies. Ann Surg Oncol 2006;13:5–6.

[124] American Joint Committee on Cancer cancer staging manual. 6th edition. New York: Springer Verlag; 2002.

[125] Poston G, Adam R, Vauthey JN. Downstaging or downsizing: time for a new staging system in advanced colorectal cancer? J Clin Oncol 2006;24:2702–6.

[126] Van Cutsem E, Nordlinger B, Adam R, et al. Towards a pan-European consensus on the treatment of patients with colorectal liver metastases. Eur J Cancer 2006;42:2212–21.

[127] Nordlinger B, Van Cutsem E, Rougier P, et al. Does chemotherapy prior to liver resection increase the potential for cure in patients with metastatic colorectal cancer? A report from the European Colorectal Metastases Treatment Group. Eur J Cancer 2007 [E-pub ahead of print].

ELSEVIER
SAUNDERS

Surg Oncol Clin N Am
17 (2008) 519–531

SURGICAL
ONCOLOGY CLINICS
OF NORTH AMERICA

Laparoscopic Resection for Colorectal Cancer: Evidence to Date

Omer Aziz, MBBS, MRCS,
Ara W. Darzi, FRCS, FACS, FMedSci, KBE*

*Department of Bio Surgery and Surgical Technology, Imperial College London,
10th Floor QEQM Building, St Mary's Hospital, Praed St., London W2 1NY, UK*

It is estimated that every year 150,000 Europeans are affected by colorectal cancer [1]. Curative laparoscopic surgery for colorectal cancer aims to minimize postoperative morbidity and mortality while providing patients with a definitive resection. Many laparoscopic procedures for benign disease have been shown to reduce postoperative surgical recovery when compared with their open counterparts. The best example is the laparoscopic cholecystectomy, which now is used successfully throughout the world [2]. Although the general benefits of laparoscopy have driven its adoption, laparoscopy affords specific benefits to surgery for colorectal cancer. These benefits have come to light, particularly during the past 5 years, through the publication of a large number of high-quality randomized trials comparing laparoscopic with open surgery for colorectal resections. These trials, which are discussed later in this article, have helped establish and further define the specific benefits of laparoscopic surgery for colorectal cancer.

In providing curative surgery for colorectal cancer, laparoscopic procedures must fulfill a number of criteria. First, the oncologic quality of the resected specimen must be at least as good as in open surgery with high vessel ligation, lymph node dissection, and adequate resection margins. In laparoscopic surgery for mid and low rectal cancers (anterior and abdominoperineal resections), the adequacy of total mesorectal excision is particularly important, because it has been shown to be crucial in reducing local recurrence and in improving 5-year survival [3]. Second, laparoscopic port- and wound-site metastasis rates must not be higher than in open surgery, a subject that has been raised as a point of concern in the past [4,5]. Finally, the long-term results of laparoscopic surgery for colorectal cancer must be

* Corresponding author.
E-mail address: a.darzi@imperial.ac.uk (A.W. Darzi).

1055-3207/08/$ - see front matter © 2008 Elsevier Inc. All rights reserved.
doi:10.1016/j.soc.2008.02.003   *surgonc.theclinics.com*

equivalent to those for open surgery in terms of local recurrence, hepatic metastases, and 5-year disease-free survival. These results have become available recently through many the large-scale, randomized studies whose follow-up periods now have reached this stage.

Laparoscopic surgery for rectal cancers is an entity that requires special mention in this article. Intraoperative neurologic damage during pelvic surgery can impair urinary function, sexual function, and continence, significantly affecting a patient's quality of life [6–8]. In addition, neoadjuvant chemoradiotherapy (used preoperatively to downstage rectal cancers) may affect the difficulty of laparoscopic surgery for rectal cancer [9]. Finally, it is known that laparoscopic rectal surgery is technically more difficult than other colorectal resections because of the need for total mesorectal excision and lower anastomoses; therefore it is important to consider the surgical experience required to achieve good oncologic outcomes [10].

The use of laparoscopy brings with it additional costs for equipment, investment in infrastructure, and surgeons' training. With laparoscopic procedures being used in almost every hospital in Europe, the infrastructure costs have been reduced dramatically. It is still important, however, to understand the impact that the additional cost of instruments and training of laparoscopic surgeons has on a health care system as a whole. This article considers the evidence on the long-term cost effectiveness of laparoscopic versus open surgery as well as the guidelines of organizations such as the United Kingdom National Institute for Heath and Clinical Excellence (NICE), which uses cost-effectiveness thresholds to determine whether an intervention is suitable for widespread use across a health care system.

Important randomized trials of laparoscopic versus open surgery for colorectal cancer

To date, the largest and best-known randomized, controlled trials of laparoscopic versus open surgery for colorectal cancer are the Conventional versus Laparoscopic-Assisted Surgery in Patients with Colorectal Cancer (CLASICC) [11], Colon Cancer Laparoscopic or Open Resection (COLOR) [12], Clinical Outcomes of Surgical Therapy (COST) [10], and the Barcelona Group (Lacey and colleagues Ref. [13]) trials. The important characteristics and main findings of these studies are as summarized in Table 1.

The last 3 years have seen the publication of a number of meta-analytic studies that have combined data from these and other, smaller, randomized, controlled individual trials of laparoscopic versus open colorectal cancer resection. Meta-analysis is a technique that can be used to evaluate the existing literature in both a qualitative and quantitative way by comparing and integrating the results of different studies and taking into account variations in characteristics that can influence the overall estimate of the outcome of interest. Although some of these studies have focused on short-term outcomes (operative outcomes, early postoperative complications, and postoperative recovery) following laparoscopic versus open surgery [14,15], other, more recent meta-analyses have tried to compare oncologic outcomes, survival, and tumor recurrence [16–18]. Finally, one meta-analysis has focused specifically on results from laparoscopic versus open surgery for rectal cancer [19]. The key findings of these studies are discussed later in this article.

Early postoperative recovery following laparoscopic colorectal resection

In comparison with open surgery, laparoscopy, with its access to the peritoneal cavity through small incisions and reduced handing of abdominal viscera, offers significantly reduced abdominal wall and tissue trauma. Magnification of the laparoscopic image makes a meticulous dissection possible, avoiding unnecessary blood loss. Laparoscopically assisted colectomy, however, does require the removal of the specimen through a tailored abdominal incision, so a continuous abdominal wound is not avoided completely. Nonetheless, the reduced tissue trauma has been shown to translate into a benefit in postoperative recovery.

A Cochrane review of 25 randomized, controlled trials comparing the short-term benefits of laparoscopic and open colorectal resection surgery (for benign and malignant disease) has shown significantly reduced intraoperative blood loss with laparoscopic surgery than with open surgery, with a weighted mean difference (WMD) of -71.8 cm^3 (95% confidence interval [CI], -113.0 to -30.8; $P = .0006$). Results from a meta-analysis of the intensity of postoperative pain using a 0 to 100 visual analogue scale revealed that on day 1 the WMD between laparoscopic and open groups was -9.3 (95% CI , -13.2 to -5.4; $P = .0001$), significantly favoring laparoscopy. At day 2 this difference was no longer significant, but at day 3 patients who had undergone laparoscopic surgery experienced significantly less pain (WMD, -12.9; 95% CI, -19.8 to -6.0; $P = .0002$). The laparoscopic group also benefited from a shorter duration of postoperative ileus (time from surgery to passage of flatus) by 1 day when compared with open surgery (WMD, 1.03; 95% CI, -1.30 to -0.76; $P = .0001$) and had significantly improved postoperative pulmonary function (day 1 and 3 forced vital capacity) [15]. These findings have been confirmed by the meta-analyses by Abraham and colleagues [14] and by Reza and colleagues [20] focusing only on patients undergoing laparoscopic or open resections for colorectal cancers. All three studies found a significantly shorter length of hospital stay and reduced incidence of wound infection with laparoscopic surgery than with open surgery for colorectal cancer.

Postoperative mortality

The Cochrane review of 2394 participants from 17 trials comparing laparoscopic with open colorectal resections found no difference in mortality

Table 1
Large and multicenter trials of laparoscopic versus open colorectal surgery

Study	Recruitment period	Number of patients	Centers where surgery was performed	Colon cancers included	Exclusion criteria	Main outcomes of interest
COST	August 1994– August 2001	872 patients (intention to treat this number)	United States and Canada (48 centers)	Colonic adenocarcinomas (rectal and transverse colon cancers included)	Pregnancy, familial polyposis, inflammatory bowel disease, advanced local or metastatic disease, concurrent or previous malignant tumors, obstructing or perforating tumors	Time to tumor recurrence
CLASICC	July 1998– July 2002	794 patients (both intention to treat and actually treated)	United Kingdom (27 centers)	Cancer of colon or rectum (transverse colon cancers excluded)	Synchronous adenocarcinomas, obstructing tumors, previous malignancy in the past 5 years, absolute contraindications to pneumoperitoneum	Circumferential and longitudinal resection margin positivity; in-hospital mortality

COLOR	March 1997–March 2003	1248 patients (intention to treat this number)	The Netherlands, Sweden, Spain, France, Italy, Germany, and the United Kingdom (29 centers)	Cancer of left or right colon (transverse colon and splenic flexure tumors excluded)	Pregnancy, distant metastases, synchronous colon cancer, other malignancy, previous ipsilateral colon surgery, obstructing tumors, adjacent organ invasion, body mass index greater than 30	Cancer-free survival at 3 years after surgery
Barcelona Group	November 1993–July 1998	219 patients intention to treat this number	Spain (single center)	Colon cancers more than 15 cm from anal verge (rectal and transverse colon cancers excluded)	Previous colonic surgery, distant metastasis, obstructing tumors, adjacent organ invasion	Cancer-related survival

Abbreviations: CLASICC, Conventional versus Laparoscopic-Assisted Surgery in Patients with Colorectal Cancer; COLOR, Colon Cancer Laparoscopic or Open Resection; COST, Clinical Outcomes of Surgical Therapy.

between laparoscopic (0.8%) and conventional (1.1%) surgery (relative risk, 0.78; 95% CI, -0.34–1.8; $P = .55$) [15]. More recently, a meta-analysis by Bonjer and colleagues [16] has reported mortality to be 1.6% for open surgery versus 1.4% for laparoscopic surgery (odds ratio, 1.3; 95% CI, 0.5–3.4; $P = .63$).

Conversion rate

In 2004 Abraham's and colleagues' [14] meta-analysis of 12 randomized, controlled studies including 1130 patients reported a conversion rate of 15.1% across laparoscopic colorectal resections, with extent of disease, adhesions, poor visualization of important structures, inability to mobilize the left colon, and intraoperative complications of laparoscopy such as hypercapnia or surgical emphysema being the most common causes. The more recent review by Bonjer and colleagues [16] in 2007 reported the conversion rate of laparoscopic to open surgery as 19.0%. Results from the CLASICC study have shown patient factors that are important in conversion from laparoscopic to open surgery to be larger body mass index, male sex, patients who have rectal cancer, patients graded American Society of Anesthesiologists grade III, and the presence of greater local tumor spread [21]. The last factor is not surprising, because locally advanced cancers that involve adjacent pelvic viscera through direct spread or local perforation would prove a more challenging en bloc resection for the laparoscopic surgeon. The CLASICC study did not find age or previous surgery to be independent predictors of conversion, as might have been expected.

Oncologic quality of resection

The oncologic principles used in laparoscopic surgery for colorectal cancer are the same as in open surgery and include the use of a no-touch resection technique with en bloc removal of the primary tumor along with adherent or locally involved structures and high ligation of vascular and lymphatic structures [22]. As in all types of surgery, but especially in laparoscopy, where manual dexterity may be limited, surgeon inexperience may compromise the oncologic quality of resection. That consideration aside, views of the surgical planes such as the mesorectum are far superior with laparoscopy than with open surgery, potentially improving the quality of resection.

In their meta-analysis of 1536 patients (796 undergoing laparoscopic surgery and 740 undergoing open surgery), Bonjer and colleagues [16] found the mean number of lymph nodes to be 11.8 ± 7.4 in the laparoscopically resected specimens and 12.2 ± 7.8 in the open colectomy specimens, a difference that was not statistically different ($P = .40$). The same group found positive resection margins in 2.1% of open colectomy specimens versus

1.3% of laparoscopic specimens, a difference that was not significant (odds ratio, 1.8; 95% CI, 0.7–4.5; $P = .23$). These findings are mirrored in the study published by Jackson and colleagues [17].

Disease-free survival and recurrence

In their meta-analysis of the four largest and best-established randomized, controlled trials, Bonjer and colleagues [16] found 3-year disease-free survival to be 75.3% with laparoscopic resection versus 75.8% following open surgery (95% CI, −5%–4%). Overall survival was reported as 83.5% and 82.2%, respectively (95% CI, −3%–5%). The authors went on to use Cox proportional hazards regression model analyses for disease-free survival and overall survival stratified by trial, adjusting for sex and tumor stage, and found no difference between the treatments. The more recent meta-analysis by Jackson and colleagues [17] also found no difference in cancer-related survival and disease recurrence between the two groups.

Recently published 5-year outcomes data from the COST group trial, which followed 852 patients randomly assigned to either laparoscopic or open colorectal resections for cancer, showed an overall survival of 74.6% with laparoscopic resection versus 76.4% with open surgery ($P = .93$) [23]. Disease-free survival was 68.4% and 69.2% ($P = .94$), respectively. Local recurrence rates were 2.6% and 2.3% ($P = .79$), respectively, and overall rates of recurrence were 21.8% and 19.4% ($P = .25$), respectively. There was no significant difference in hepatic and pulmonary metastases between the groups in this study. These findings are mirrored by the recent publication of the 3-year results from the multicenter, randomized, controlled CLASICC trial, which did not find any differences in long-term outcomes between the laparoscopic and open surgery groups [24].

The COST study's 5-year follow-up data also did not show a significantly higher wound-site or laparoscopic port-site recurrence when compared with open surgery [23]. The rate was 0.5% following laparoscopic surgery and 0.9% following open surgery ($P = .43$), which, along with the findings from the Barcelona Group and a meta-analysis of seven studies with more than 18 months' follow-up by Jackson and colleagues [17], shows that, in the right hands, patients undergoing laparoscopic resections for cancer are not at increased risk for this type of recurrence.

Laparoscopic surgery for rectal cancer

The meta-analysis of 2071 patients by Aziz and colleagues [19] found no significant difference between laparoscopic versus open anterior and abdominoperineal resections in the proportion of patients who had positive radial margins or in the number of lymph nodes harvested, suggesting that laparoscopic and open surgery are comparable in adequacy of resection and oncologic clearance. As expected, operative time was significantly longer with laparoscopic surgery than with open surgery for rectal cancer. Postoperative recovery, in terms of bowel function and shortened hospital stay, was significantly better for patients undergoing laparoscopic resection; in particular, patients undergoing abdominoperineal resections required significantly less parenteral analgesia. There was no significant difference in early and late postoperative complications between laparoscopic and open surgery for rectal cancer, but when only patients undergoing abdominoperineal resections were considered, a significantly lower rate of wound infection was found in the laparoscopic group (0%) than in the open surgery group (13.9%). Only three of the studies included in this meta-analysis were of prospective, randomized design [11,25,26], and only one of these (CLASICC) focused on a group of patients undergoing laparoscopic resection for rectal cancer [11].

Bladder dysfunction (evaluated by the incidence of urinary retention) was not significantly different between the two groups, although concerns have been raised about the potential risk of increased pelvic nerve damage following laparoscopic rectal resection. Quah and colleagues [26] assessed longer-term bladder and sexual dysfunction retrospectively in 40 patients who had undergone laparoscopic surgery and in another 40 patients who had undergone open surgery for rectal cancer. They found a significantly higher rate of sexual dysfunction in men following laparoscopic surgery: 47% of men who had undergone laparoscopic rectal resections reported impotence or impaired ejaculation, compared with 5% of men who had open surgery. There was no difference between the groups in bladder dysfunction or female sexual function. This morbidity may be secondary to iatrogenic disruption of pelvic innervation resulting from laparoscopic surgery. In their study, Jayne and colleagues [27] reported on sexual and bladder dysfunction in a cohort of 147 patients randomly assigned to undergo laparoscopic or open surgery for rectal cancer in the CLASICC trial. The investigators found that, although bladder function was similar in the two groups, overall sexual function was worse in men following laparoscopic surgery (a difference of -11.18; 95% CI, $-22.99-0.63$; $P = .063$). In particular, erectile function tended to be worse in men who had undergone laparoscopic rectal surgery (a difference of -5.84; 95% CI, -10.94 to -0.74; $P = .068$). The authors believed that one possible reason was that total mesorectal excision was performed more commonly in the laparoscopic rectal group than in the open rectal group. No differences in female sexual function were detected in the two groups.

An additional factor to consider in patients undergoing laparoscopic surgery for rectal cancer is the use of neoadjuvant (preoperative) chemoradiotherapy and the impact that this treatment may have on the procedure and its results. A recent study by Rezvani and colleagues [28] retrospectively compared eight patients who received preoperative chemoradiation therapy for rectal cancer with 52 patients who did not. They found a trend toward a higher conversion rate to open surgery and a significantly longer operative duration for laparoscopic resections. There were no changes in mortality or morbidity. Although this is a small and nonrandomized study, further research into the impact of neoadjuvant chemoradiotherapy on the outcomes of laparoscopic surgery for rectal cancer is required. This research is particularly important because neoadjuvant therapy is becoming the mainstay of treatment for this subset of patients who have colorectal cancer.

Cost effectiveness

When compared with open surgery, laparoscopy is clearly associated with an increased cost at the time of the procedure, involving both infrastructure and equipment. Although the infrastructure and set-up costs can be spread over a period of time, the costs of disposable items such as ports, instruments, and staplers used to resect the specimen and create the anastomosis are more fixed. This increased cost has been demonstrated by a number of studies using varying methods and results [29–32]. To compare costs between laparoscopic and open colorectal surgery accurately, the cost implications of preoperative preparation, operative costs, postoperative recovery, follow-up, and the cost of treating complications must be taken into account to determine the health care resources utilized. A study by Braga and colleagues [33] randomly assigned 517 patients undergoing colectomy to either laparoscopic or open resection and compared hospital costs between the two groups. This study took into account the cost of surgical instruments, operation time, routine pre- and postoperative care, postoperative morbidity, and length of hospital stay. They also followed patients for 30 days after hospital discharge to try to determine postoperative morbidity. This study found that although the operative time was 37 minutes longer in the laparoscopic group than in the open group, the overall morbidity rate was significantly lower (18.2% versus 34.7%; $P = .0005$), and the mean length of stay was shorter (9.9 days versus 12.4 days; $P = .0001$). Laparoscopic surgery cost an additional €1171 per patient, but this cost was offset by a saving of €1046 per patient in the laparoscopic group (€401 because of shorter hospital stay and €645 because of the lower cost of treating postoperative complications). The authors found the most expensive complications to treat were infections (wound infection, abscesses, and sepsis), anastomotic leak, and intestinal obstruction. Laparoscopic resections therefore cost an extra €125 per patient when compared with open surgery. In a randomized trial focusing on patients undergoing laparoscopic versus open resections of rectal cancer, the same authors found an additional cost of $351 for patients in the laparoscopic group. The mean follow-up of this study was longer, at 53.6 months [33].

There are limitations in the research investigating the relative costs of laparoscopic versus open surgery for colorectal cancer. Many of the studies looking at cost have compared a mixed group of patients and included both benign and malignant disease. Although at present this evidence is the best available, there is a real need for cost-effectiveness research designed specifically to compare laparoscopic versus open surgery for colorectal cancer. In addition, although much of the cost–benefit analysis has focused on operative and postoperative hospital costs, there are also costs implications of postoperative recovery in the community, the impact of surgery on employment and sick leave, and the socioeconomic impact of impaired performance that must be taken into account. A study by Janson and colleagues [34] in 2004 reported €398 additional cost from lost productivity in patients undergoing open surgery. More research is needed on the impact of laparoscopic surgery on a patient's quality of life and how quality of life, in turn, impacts the cost effectiveness of the procedure.

In the United Kingdom the NICE is an independent organization responsible for providing national guidance for clinical interventions. In the latest review of its guidelines in 2006, the NICE recommended laparoscopic surgery for colorectal cancer in the United Kingdom National Health Service, provided "both laparoscopic and open surgery are suitable for the person and their condition their surgeon has been trained in laparoscopic surgery for colorectal cancer and performs the operation often enough to keep his or her skills up to date" [35]. It did, however, believe that there that was a shortage of surgeons who have completed appropriate training in the technique and who perform this procedure often enough to maintain competence, an issue that currently is under review at the United Kingdom Department of Health.

Learning curve

Although a learning curve of 20 cases has been suggested, the actual learning curve for laparoscopic surgery for colorectal cancer probably is greater than 20 cases [36–39]. It also has been suggested that laparoscopic resection of the rectum is technically more demanding and is associated with a longer learning curve than other laparoscopic colonic resections [37]. What is clear is that studies reporting on laparoscopic versus open surgery for colorectal cancer include surgeons of vastly varying experience. This variation is illustrated by the conversion rate, which was as high as 34% in the recently published multicenter CLASICC trial by Guillou and colleagues [11], the largest comparative randomized trial thus far reporting specifically on a group of patients undergoing laparoscopic surgery for rectal cancer. The inclusion criteria for the large, randomized trials of laparoscopic colorectal surgery such as COST [10] or CLASICC [11] require the operating surgeon to have performed more than 20 laparoscopic resections before submitting patients into the trial. It has been suggested that the learning curve actually may be bimodal, with improvement continuing to more than 100 cases [39].

Summary

This article highlights the individual merits and weaknesses of laparoscopic as compared with open surgery as the primary treatment of colorectal cancer. Although results clearly suggest that laparoscopic surgery for colorectal cancer results in an earlier postoperative recovery, it is more difficult to comment on rarer complications such as deep vein thrombosis, ventral hernia rates, and adhesional small bowel obstruction [40,41]. These areas require further examination within a future trial. To date, results from laparoscopic colorectal resections suggest that the resected specimen is oncologically comparable that obtained with open surgery. Although the 5-year follow-up data of the COST study confirm that patients who have curable colon cancer can safely be offered laparoscopic surgery [23], more long-term data on cancer recurrence and survival at 3 and 5 years postoperatively are eagerly awaited. A final challenge for laparoscopic colorectal surgery will be training a sufficient number of surgeons so that laparoscopic colorectal surgery can be offered reproducibly to large patient populations across health care systems.

References

[1] Nelson H, Petrelli N, Carlin A, et al. Guidelines 2000 for colon and rectal cancer surgery. J Natl Cancer Inst 2001;93(8):583–96.
[2] National Institutes of Health Consensus Development Panel on Gallstones and Laparoscopic Cholecystectomy. Gallstones and laparoscopic cholecystectomy. Surg Endosc 1993; 7(3):271–9.
[3] Heald RJ. Total mesorectal excision is optimal surgery for rectal cancer: a Scandinavian consensus. Br J Surg 1995;82(10):1297–9.
[4] Berends FJ, Kazemier G, Bonjer HJ, et al. Subcutaneous metastases after laparoscopic colectomy. Lancet 1994;344(8914):58.
[5] Nduka CC, Darzi A. Port-site metastasis in patients undergoing laparoscopy for gastrointestinal malignancy. Br J Surg 1997;84(4):583.
[6] Havenga K, Enker WE, McDermott K, et al. Male and female sexual and urinary function after total mesorectal excision with autonomic nerve preservation for carcinoma of the rectum. J Am Coll Surg 1996;182(6):495–502.
[7] Kinn AC, Ohman U. Bladder and sexual function after surgery for rectal cancer. Dis Colon Rectum 1986;29(1):43–8.
[8] Masui H, Ike H, Yamaguchi S, et al. Male sexual function after autonomic nerve-preserving operation for rectal cancer. Dis Colon Rectum 1996;39(10):1140–5.
[9] Kapiteijn E, Marijnen CA, Nagtegaal ID, et al. Preoperative radiotherapy combined with total mesorectal excision for resectable rectal cancer. N Engl J Med 2001;345(9):638–46.
[10] A comparison of laparoscopically assisted and open colectomy for colon cancer. N Engl J Med 2004;350(20):2050–9.
[11] Guillou PJ, Quirke P, Thorpe H, et al. Short-term endpoints of conventional versus laparoscopic-assisted surgery in patients with colorectal cancer (MRC CLASICC trial): multicentre, randomised controlled trial. Lancet 2005;365(9472):1718–26.
[12] Veldkamp R, Kuhry E, Hop WC, et al. Laparoscopic surgery versus open surgery for colon cancer: short-term outcomes of a randomised trial. Lancet Oncol 2005;6(7):477–84.

[13] Lacy AM, Garcia-Valdecasas JC, Delgado S, et al. Laparoscopy-assisted colectomy versus open colectomy for treatment of non-metastatic colon cancer: a randomised trial. Lancet 2002;359(9325):2224–9.

[14] Abraham NS, Young JM, Solomon MJ. Meta-analysis of short-term outcomes after laparoscopic resection for colorectal cancer. Br J Surg 2004;91(9):1111–24.

[15] Schwenk W, Haase O, Neudecker J, et al. Short term benefits for laparoscopic colorectal resection. Cochrane Database Syst Rev 2005;(3):CD003145.

[16] Bonjer HJ, Hop WC, Nelson H, et al. Laparoscopically assisted vs open colectomy for colon cancer: a meta-analysis. Arch Surg 2007;142(3):298–303.

[17] Jackson TD, Kaplan GG, Arena G, et al. Laparoscopic versus open resection for colorectal cancer: a metaanalysis of oncologic outcomes. J Am Coll Surg 2007;204(3):439–46.

[18] Kahnamoui K, Cadeddu M, Farrokhyar F, et al. Laparoscopic surgery for colon cancer: a systematic review. Can J Surg 2007;50(1):48–57.

[19] Aziz O, Constantinides V, Tekkis PP, et al. Laparoscopic versus open surgery for rectal cancer: a meta-analysis. Ann Surg Oncol 2006;13(3):413–24.

[20] Reza MM, Blasco JA, Andradas E, et al. Systematic review of laparoscopic versus open surgery for colorectal cancer. Br J Surg 2006;93(8):921–8.

[21] Thorpe H, Jayne DG, Guillou PJ, et al. Patient factors influencing conversion from laparoscopically assisted to open surgery for colorectal cancer. Br J Surg 2008;95(2):199–205.

[22] Turnbull RB Jr, Kyle K, Watson FR, et al. Cancer of the colon: the influence of the no-touch isolation technique on survival rates. Ann Surg 1967;166(3):420–7.

[23] Fleshman J, Sargent DJ, Green E, et al. Laparoscopic colectomy for cancer is not inferior to open surgery based on 5-year data from the COST Study Group trial. Ann Surg 2007;246(4): 655–62 [discussion: 662–4].

[24] Jayne DG, Guillou PJ, Thorpe H, et al. Randomized trial of laparoscopic-assisted resection of colorectal carcinoma: 3-year results of the UK MRC CLASICC Trial Group. J Clin Oncol 2007;25(21):3061–8.

[25] Araujo SE, da Silva eSousa AH Jr, de Campos FG, et al. Conventional approach × laparoscopic abdominoperineal resection for rectal cancer treatment after neoadjuvant chemoradiation: results of a prospective randomized trial. Rev Hosp Clin Fac Med Sao Paulo 2003;58(3):133–40.

[26] Quah HM, Jayne DG, Eu KW, et al. Bladder and sexual dysfunction following laparoscopically assisted and conventional open mesorectal resection for cancer. Br J Surg 2002;89(12): 1551–6.

[27] Jayne DG, Brown JM, Thorpe H, et al. Bladder and sexual function following resection for rectal cancer in a randomized clinical trial of laparoscopic versus open technique. Br J Surg 2005;92(9):1124–32.

[28] Rezvani M, Franko J, Fassler SA, et al. Outcomes in patients treated by laparoscopic resection of rectal carcinoma after neoadjuvant therapy for rectal cancer. JSLS 2007;11(2):204–7.

[29] Delaney CP, Kiran RP, Senagore AJ, et al. Case-matched comparison of clinical and financial outcome after laparoscopic or open colorectal surgery. Ann Surg 2003;238(1):67–72.

[30] Liberman MA, Phillips EH, Carroll BJ, et al. Laparoscopic colectomy vs traditional colectomy for diverticulitis. Outcome and costs. Surg Endosc 1996;10(1):15–8.

[31] Philipson BM, Bokey EL, Moore JW, et al. Cost of open versus laparoscopically assisted right hemicolectomy for cancer. World J Surg 1997;21(2):214–7.

[32] Senagore AJ, Duepree HJ, Delaney CP, et al. Cost structure of laparoscopic and open sigmoid colectomy for diverticular disease: similarities and differences. Dis Colon Rectum 2002;45(4):485–90.

[33] Braga M, Frasson M, Vignali A, et al. Laparoscopic resection in rectal cancer patients: outcome and cost-benefit analysis. Dis Colon Rectum 2007;50(4):464–71.

[34] Janson M, Bjorholt I, Carlsson P, et al. Randomized clinical trial of the costs of open and laparoscopic surgery for colonic cancer. Br J Surg 2004;91(4):409–17.

[35] National Institute for Health and Clinical Excellence. Available at: http://www.nice.org.uk/ Accessed April 2, 2008.

[36] Bennett CL, Stryker SJ, Ferreira MR, et al. The learning curve for laparoscopic colorectal surgery. Preliminary results from a prospective analysis of 1194 laparoscopic-assisted colectomies. Arch Surg 1997;132(1):41–4 [discussion: 45].

[37] Schlachta CM, Mamazza J, Seshadri PA, et al. Defining a learning curve for laparoscopic colorectal resections. Dis Colon Rectum 2001;44(2):217–22.

[38] Simons AJ, Anthone GJ, Ortega AE, et al. Laparoscopic-assisted colectomy learning curve. Dis Colon Rectum 1995;38(6):600–3.

[39] Tekkis PP, Senagore AJ, Delaney CP, et al. Evaluation of the learning curve in laparoscopic colorectal surgery: comparison of right-sided and left-sided resections. Ann Surg 2005; 242(1):83–91.

[40] Duepree HJ, Senagore AJ, Delaney CP, et al. Does means of access affect the incidence of small bowel obstruction and ventral hernia after bowel resection? Laparoscopy versus laparotomy. J Am Coll Surg 2003;197(2):177–81.

[41] Lumley J, Stitz R, Stevenson A, et al. Laparoscopic colorectal surgery for cancer: intermediate to long-term outcomes. Dis Colon Rectum 2002;45(7):867–72 [discussion: 872–5].

ELSEVIER
SAUNDERS

Surg Oncol Clin N Am
17 (2008) 533–551

SURGICAL
ONCOLOGY CLINICS
OF NORTH AMERICA

Multidisciplinary Treatment of Cancer of the Rectum: A European Approach

R.J. Nicholls, MA, MChir, FRCS[a,b,*],
Paris P. Tekkis, MD, FRCS[a,b]

[a]*Department of Biosurgery and Surgical Technology, St Mary's Hospital,
Imperial College, Praed St, London W2, UK*
[b]*Department of Surgery, St Mark's Hospital, Northwest London Hospitals National Health
Service Trust, Watford Road, Harrow, HA1 3UJ, UK*

Surgery and local recurrence

Local recurrence is the end point of locoregional treatments such as surgery and radiotherapy. In the late 1970s Heald and colleagues [1] developed the technique of total mesorectal excision (TME). They produced evidence that in some cases nests of tumor cells outside lymph nodes could be found in the mesorectum and would have been left behind by a conventional anterior resection. With TME, emphasis subsequently became focused on the circumferential resection margin (CRM) [2]; involvement of the CME is, per se, a predictor of survival [3]. Using TME alone, Heald achieved local recurrence rates of less than 5% [4].

TME is essentially an anatomic dissection of the rectum in the plane between its fascia propria and the surrounding structures. The fascia propria is seen readily on MRI, and the relationship between the fascia propria and the tumor can be gauged preoperatively with an accuracy of more than 90% [5]. Training programs have been established in some European countries [6–8], standardizing the technique of anterior resection to some extent. There is evidence that specialization improves cancer-specific outcome, especially for rectal cancer surgery [9].

The risk factors for local recurrence are pathologic and surgical. The former include T stage and N stage, histologic grade, the level of the tumor, and the presence of vascular or perineural invasion. The latter include the completeness of removal, achieving a clear CRM and an adequate distal

* Corresponding author. Department of Biosurgery and Surgical Technology, St Mary's Hospital, Imperial College, Praed St, London W2, UK.
  E-mail address: j.nicholls@imperial.ac.uk (R.J. Nicholls).

margin of 10 mm or more. There is evidence that achieving a clear CRM is, in part, surgeon related [10]. At present, a 2-mm thickness of normal tissue between the advancing front of the tumor and the CRM of the surgical specimen as determined by histopathologic examination is regarded as clear (R0 resection) [11].

Local recurrence rates are lower after anterior resection than after total anorectal excision [12]. The reasons almost certainly include the greater proximity of the lower rectum to the lateral pelvic wall and the higher incidence of an involved CRM and the greater chance of perforating the rectum during total rectal excision [11]. The surgeon may fail to clear the tumor at the level of the levator ani by employing a dissection as for an anterior resection rather than dividing the levator at its attachment to the pelvic wall and thereby minimizing the chance of an involved margin. The higher incidence of lateral pelvic lymph node involvement with tumors lying below the peritoneal reflection is also likely to be a factor. This incidence ranges from 10% to 25%, depending on the Dukes stage of the primary tumor [13–15]. The sterilization of these lymph nodes by radiotherapy may be one of the explanations for the resulting reduction in local recurrence.

In an epidemiologic study from Malmo, Sweden performed in the 1960s in a region with an autopsy rate of 82% for the whole population, 90% of the patients who had been treated for large bowel cancer were found to have distant metastases. Fifty percent had local recurrence, but only 8% of these had local recurrence without metastases [16]. This finding explains why the failure of locoregional treatments such as surgery and radiotherapy may not influence survival.

Conventional staging systems do not separate the T3 stage into prognostically favorable and unfavorable subgroups in which cancer-specific end points vary according to the degree of penetration into the extrarectal tissues. Thus respective 5-year survival and local recurrence rates are around 40% and 20%, respectively, for an extensive T3 tumor and 80% and 5%, respectively, for a T3 tumor that has penetrated the rectal wall by only a microscopic degree [17,18]. Subdividing the T3 stage into T3a and T3b based on an extrarectal spread of greater or less than 5 mm [19] may improve the quality of trials by more refined staging.

Pretreatment staging

Uniform criteria for entry into clinical trials depend on pretreatment staging. Digital examination is subjective, but it is the clinician's first contact with the tumor. It can gauge its level accurately, immediately indicating whether a restorative resection is possible. It also gives an initial impression whether local excision or adjuvant treatment should be considered, but it cannot give a reliable assessment of T stage. Endoluminal ultrasound is more than 90% accurate in determining whether penetration of the rectal wall has occurred (uT2 versus uT3) and is the imaging modality of choice when considering local excision. Understaging of T1 tumors has been reported in 17% to 31% of cases in large series of ultrasound examinations, however [20,21]. CT is useful for the assessment of disseminated disease but not for locoregional staging.

MRI is the investigation of choice for pretreatment local (T) staging. It correctly anticipates the subsequent histopathologic examination in 85% of T3 and T4 tumors [22,23]. MRI has a sensitivity of 94% and a specificity of 85% in determining the relationship between the advancing border of the tumor and the fascia propria of the rectum [5,24]. Involvement of the fascia propria predicts a positive surgical circumferential margin. MRI also allows the subcategorization of T3 tumors into T3a and T3b [19]. Nodal staging, whether assessed by ultrasound or MRI, is still unreliable, but analysis of the consistency of the node and the regularity of its capsule as demonstrated on MRI may improve its accuracy [25]. More recently, the use of nanoparticle-enhanced MRI (using ultrasmall superparamagnetic iron oxide as a contrast agent) is reported to have sensitivity on the order of 92% and specificity of around 96% for detecting lymph-node metastases [26].

Radiotherapy

Technical advances in radiotherapy with increasingly higher energy irradiation have allowed the delivery of adequate doses to deep structures with minimal release of energy to the superficial tissues. By the 1950s megavoltage photon emission had been achieved, and with the further development of linear accelerators it now is possible to deliver irradiation of up to 20 MeV.

Extensive disease

In the 1960s reports of radiotherapy for unresectable disease demonstrated a temporary improvement of symptoms and a small but significant long-term survival of around 5% [27,28]. Radiotherapy also was shown to render a locally inoperable tumor operable in 30% to 50% of patients, although short-term survival often was disappointing [29–31]. In one report of 100 patients who had locally advanced disease, 79 subsequently underwent resection with a 5-year survival rate of 20% [32].

Primary treatment

In one of the first examples of radiotherapy given as primary treatment, 123 patients without metastatic disease, who were regarded as inoperable mainly because of comorbidity and the surgeon's reluctance to operate, underwent external beam radiotherapy in a dose of 40 Gy. Overall 5-year survival was 21%. Almost all survivors had had a mobile tumor. Of these, 38% survived, compared with only 2% who had a fixed tumor [33]. Using 50-kV contact radiotherapy administered endoluminally, Papillon [34] reported a 5-year survival rate of 78% in a series of 186 carefully selected patients who had a small mobile carcinoma considered clinically to be confined to the rectal wall. The outcome for exophytic tumors was better than for sessile ulcerated tumors (treatment failure, 9.5% versus 26%). In similar lesions the morphology of the tumor subsequently has been shown to influence survival after surgical local excision [35].

Adjuvant and neoadjuvant radiotherapy

In parallel, radiotherapy began to be used as an adjuvant to surgery, usually with survival as the end point. Early randomized trials of preoperative radiotherapy did not include local recurrence as an end point [36–39].

Preoperative radiotherapy and local recurrence: early studies

Local recurrence rates began to be reported in the 1970s. In one early study, preoperative external beam radiotherapy in high dose (50–60 Gy) given to 50 patients was associated with a 50% of tumors confined to the bowel wall (Dukes' stage A), a far higher proportion than would have been expected in a series of patients treated by surgery alone [29]. The same authors also reported lower-than-expected rates of local recurrence, and others had a similar experience [40,41]. Reports of some trials in the 1970s suggested a reduced incidence of lymph node involvement based on examination of the resected operative specimen [32,38,42], but other trials at the time did not support this finding [36,37,43,44].

Postoperative radiotherapy: early studies

Several trials of postoperative adjuvant radiotherapy were reported in the 1980s [45], but there were only a few randomized, controlled trials. A Danish trial randomized patients who had Dukes' stage B and C tumors to surgery only or to surgery with radiotherapy given to 50 Gy over 5 weeks. There was no difference in survival or local recurrence [46]. The Gastrointestinal Tumor Study Group [47] conducted a four-arm study with around 50 patients in each arm. At a median follow-up of 118 weeks, there was no significant difference in local failure in the surgery-only arm (11/57) compared with the surgery and radiotherapy arm (7/47). When chemotherapy was added to surgery and radiotherapy, local recurrence fell to 2 of 39 patients, but toxicity was increased with a small treatment-related mortality [48].

The Medical Research Council reported improved survival after postoperative radiotherapy in a randomized, controlled trial comparing surgery alone in 140 subjects with surgery and radiotherapy (40 Gy in 20 2-Gy fractions over 4 weeks) in 139 subjects. The rates of curative surgery were 40% and 47%, respectively; mortality rates during follow-up were 77% and 69%, respectively [49].

Multidisciplinary treatment in Europe

In 1990 the National Institute of Health published an analysis of adjuvant treatment for rectal cancer [50] and stated that the best current adjuvant therapy was postoperative treatment by both radiotherapy and chemotherapy. This pronouncement was greatly influential, particularly in the United States.

In Europe, by contrast, adjuvant radiotherapy generally has been used as preoperative strategy. Since 1990, randomized, controlled trials have compared preoperative and postoperative radiotherapy and preoperative radiotherapy in low, moderate, and high doses with surgery alone. Variable dose-fractionation regimes have been studied, as has the addition of chemotherapy to radiotherapy for curative rectal cancer (Table 1). Useful reviews of the earlier trials are available [51,52].

Preoperative versus postoperative radiotherapy

Two randomized, controlled trials have compared preoperative versus postoperative radiotherapy. The first included 471 patients accrued between 1980 and 1985 by 13 hospitals in the Uppsala Region in Sweden. Of these patients, 236 were assigned randomly to receive radiotherapy (five cycles of 5 Gy over 2 weeks) followed by surgery within 10 days, and 235 were assigned to surgery followed by 60 Gy over 8 weeks. In the latter group radiotherapy could not be undertaken until 6 weeks after surgery.

There was no difference in postoperative mortality (3% versus 5%), and at a minimum follow-up of 3 years (mean, 6 years), there was no difference in survival. Local recurrence was significantly less, however, in the group receiving preoperative radiotherapy (12% versus 21%; $P < .02$). At 5 years the cumulative probability of local recurrence in the two arms was 14.3% and 26.8% (95% confidence interval [CI], 5%–20%). Distant metastasis subsequently occurred in 36% and 38% of patients, respectively. There was no specific statement on toxicity, but the incidence of delayed healing of the perineal wound in patients undergoing total rectal excision was 33% and 18% in the two groups, respectively. There was no difference in the incidence of anastomotic breakdown. The rate of bowel perforation during surgery was 28% and was not influenced by pre- or postoperative radiotherapy [53,54].

The second trial, the "German trial," included 26 participating centers that enrolled 823 patients under the age of 75 years between 1995 and 2002. Patients who had a T3 or T4 cancer identified by clinical examination, ultrasound, and CT with a tumor lower than 16 cm from the anal verge were assigned randomly to two groups. Both treatment arms included the same regimen of chemoradiotherapy (50.4 Gy over 5 weeks) with fluorouracil (5-FU) (1000 mg/m^2/d) given in the first and fifth weeks. In the preoperative chemoradiotherapy group, surgery was performed 6 weeks later. In the

Table 1
Randomized controlled trials

Trial	Accrual period	Arms	N	Centers	Follow-up (months)	Survival (%)	Local recurrence (%)
Swedish[a] [54]	1980–1985	pRT (5 × 5 Gy) versus postRT (60 Gy)	471	13	72	ND (approx 50)	14.3 versus 26.8
German[a] [55]	1995–2002	pCRT (50.4 Gy + FU) versus postCRT (50.4 Gy + FU)	823	26	45.8	76 versus 74	6 versus 13
Swedish[b] [62]	1987–1990	pRT (5 × 5 Gy) versus S	1147	70	60 minimum	58 versus 48	11 versus 27
Dutch[b] [64]	1996–1999	pRT (5 × 5 Gy) versus S (TME)	1805	108	25 (1–56)	81.8 versus 82[g]	2.4 versus 8.2[g]
Polish[c] [67]	1999–2002	pRT (5 × 5 Gy) versus pCRT (50.4 Gy + FU)	316	19	48 (31–69)	61.2 versus 58	10.6 versus 15.6
British CR07[d] [68]	1998–2005	pRT (5 × 5 Gy) versus S (TME) + selective postRT[f] (45 Gy + FU)	1350	52	36 minimum	80.8 versus 78.7[h]	4.7 versus 11.1[h]
French EORTC 22.921[e] [70]	1993–2003	pRT (45 Gy) pCRT (45 Gy + C) pRT (45 Gy) + postC pCRT (45 Gy + C) + postC	996	40	60	65.8 64.6 67.2 63.2	17.1 8.7 9.6 7.2

Abbreviations: C, French trial: fluorouracil and leucovorin; CRT, chemoradiotherapy; ND, no data; p, preoperative; post, postoperative; RT, radiotherapy; S, surgery.

[a] Preoperative versus postoperative radiotherapy.
[b] Preoperative radiotherapy versus surgery alone.
[c] Preoperative short-course versus preoperative neoadjuvant chemoradiotherapy.
[d] Preoperative radiotherapy versus surgery alone or surgery plus selective postoperative radiotherapy.
[e] Preoperative radiotherapy versus preoperative chemoradiotherapy versus preoperative radiotherapy plus postoperative chemotherapy versus preoperative chemoradiotherapy plus postoperative chemotherapy.
[f] Patients who have positive circumferential resection margins.
[g] Follow-up 25 (1–56) months.
[h] Three-year survival.

postoperative chemoradiotherapy group, a radiation boost of 5.4 Gy was delivered to the postoperative surgical bed. Both groups subsequently received further 5-FU given in four cycles of 5 days each over 4 weeks. This regimen was started 4 weeks after surgery in the preoperative chemoradiotherapy group and 4 weeks after the end of postoperative chemoradiotherapy in the postoperative group. The interval between surgery and the onset of postoperative chemoradiotherapy was not given.

Five-year survival rates were 76% and 74% in the pre- and postoperative groups. Rates of local recurrence were 6% and 13%, respectively ($P < .006$). Acute and long-term toxicity rates were 27% and 40% and 14% and 24%, respectively. There was a significant difference in the stage of disease assessed histopathologically; the incidence of stage III disease was 25% and 40%, respectively. Ninety-two percent of the patients randomly assigned to preoperative chemoradiotherapy received the full treatment according to the protocol, but only 54% in the postoperative group did so. Despite the method of pretreatment staging, only 5% of patients in the postoperative group had a tumor of stage T1 or T2. Nodal status was not significantly different in the two groups (42% versus 39%) [55].

The results from these studies support the conclusion that preoperative radiotherapy reduces the incidence of local recurrence more than postoperative radiotherapy. The German trial also shows that toxicity is greater with postoperative radiotherapy and that compliance with the protocol is less.

Preoperative radiotherapy versus surgery alone

In the United Kingdom, the first Medical Research Council trial randomly assigned 824 patients to surgery only, to surgery with a single preoperative 5-Gy fraction, or to surgery plus radiotherapy to 20 Gy (10 2-Gy fractions) given in 2 weeks before operation. There were no differences in survival or local recurrence among any of the groups [42].

For a 5-year period beginning in 1976, the European Organization for Research and Treatment of Cancer (EORTC) Gastrointestinal Tract Cancer Cooperative Group randomly assigned 466 patients from 13 centers to surgery alone or to preoperative radiotherapy (34.5 Gy in 2.3-Gy fractions over 19 days) followed by surgery at a median of 11 days (range, 1–69 days). Of these patients, 341 had a curative resection. Overall, 5-year survival rates in those having a curative resection were 59.1% and 69.1% ($P < .08$). Local recurrence rates were 30% and 15% ($P < .003$). Significant toxicity occurred only in four patients in the radiotherapy arm [56].

A multicenter trial in western Norway that enrolled 309 patients from 1976 to 1985 used a similar protocol of 31.5 Gy in 18 fractions over 2 to 3 weeks. Five-year survival rates were 57.5% in the surgery-alone arm and 56.7% in the surgery-plus-radiotherapy arm. Local recurrence rates were 21.1% and 13.7%, respectively [57].

The Rectal Cancer Group of the Imperial Cancer Research Fund (ICRF-RCG UK) accrued 468 patients between 1981 and 1985 from 20 contributing centers. Surgery alone was performed in 239 patients; 228 patients received radiotherapy (three 5-Gy fractions over 5 days) followed by surgery within a few days. Follow-up to 5 years or death was achieved in 97% of patients. There was no difference between the arms in 5-year survival of patients having a curative resection (56% versus 52%), but local recurrence was more common after surgery alone (24% versus 17%; $P < .05$). Overall, cardiovascular and thromboembolic complications and treatment mortality were more common in the radiotherapy group, especially among patients treated palliatively (3% versus 13%; $P < .005$) [58].

The Stockholm Colorectal Cancer Study (the Stockholm I trial) enrolled 849 patients from 12 hospitals in the Stockholm-Gotland Health Region between 1980 and 1987. They were assigned randomly to surgery alone or to radiotherapy (five cycles of 5 Gy) given over 5 to 7 days before surgery. There was no difference in survival among the 684 patients treated with curative intent in the two arms, but local recurrence was significantly less in the radiotherapy group. Early mortality, however, was increased in the radiotherapy group (8% versus 2%) [59]. As a result the same group conducted a second trial (Stockholm II), hoping to reduce mortality by changing the method of delivery of radiotherapy from two to four portals and reducing the volume of tissue irradiated. The same protocol was used, and 557 patients (481 of whom were treated with curative resection) were accrued between 1987 and 1993. Two hundred seventy-two patients were assigned to surgery alone, and 285 were assigned to radiotherapy plus surgery. The 10-year survival of patients treated for cure was significantly longer in the radiotherapy group (46% versus 39%; $P < .03$). Local recurrence was significantly greater after surgery alone (12% versus 25%, $P < .001$). In line with the experience in the ICRF-RCG trial [58], subsequent death from cardiovascular causes was higher in the radiotherapy group (13% versus 7%; $P < .07$) [60].

Simultaneously a national Swedish trial, the Swedish Rectal Cancer Trial, was established. This trial accrued patients between 1987 and 1990 from 70 hospitals throughout Sweden, including those admitted into the Stockholm II trial up to 1990. The protocol used in the Stockholm II trial was adopted. The regimen of five 5-Gy cycles was equivalent to 42 Gy when given in 2-Gy fractions five times per week over 4 to 5 weeks [61]. Inclusion criteria were an adenocarcinoma below the promontory in a patient younger than 80 years. Patients who had a tumor that was fixed or suitable for local excision, disseminated disease, a previous malignancy, or who had undergone radiotherapy were excluded.

A total of 1168 patients were enrolled, of whom 1147 were eligible. Of these, 454 in each treatment group underwent a curative resection. Hospital mortality was 3% in the surgery arm and 4% in the radiotherapy plus surgery arm. Mortality was higher (15%) when radiotherapy was given in two beams than when it was given in three or four beams (3%) ($P < .001$). At a minimum follow-up of 5 years, local recurrence rates were 11% (63/553) and 27% (150/557), a reduction of 58% in favor of the radiotherapy arm (95% CI, 46%–69%; $P < .001$). The study also showed a difference in survival, 58% (95% CI, 54%–62%) versus 48% (95% CI, 44%–53%) ($P < .004$) [62].

Late follow-up of this trial at a median of 13 years (range, 3–15 years) showed that these differences were maintained. Overall survival in patients having curative treatment was 38% versus 30%, respectively ($P < .008$), and the rates of local recurrence were 9% versus 26%, respectively ($P < .001$). There was no difference in the incidence of subsequent metastatic disease [63].

A randomized, controlled trial performed by the Dutch Colorectal Cancer Group (the "Dutch trial") accrued patients from 1996 to 1999. By this time TME had been accepted into practice and was used in both arms of the study. Contributing centers included 84 Dutch, 13 Swedish, and 11 other European and Canadian hospitals. Of 1805 eligible patients, 905 were randomly assigned to surgery alone, and 897 were assigned to radiotherapy (five cycles of 5 Gy over 5 days) immediately before surgery. A curative resection was performed in 1653 patients. Twenty-nine of the 897 patients in the radiotherapy arm did not receive this treatment, and 11 of the patients in the surgery-only arm were not operated on. The preoperative staging did not seem to be based on imaging. Patients were followed for a median of 24.9 months (range, 1.1–56 months).

After protocol violations and incomplete treatments were excluded, there were 846 patients in the radiotherapy group. The interval between the end of radiotherapy and surgery exceeded 10 days for 110 of these patients (13%). Survival rates at 2 years were 81.8% after surgery and 82.0% after radiotherapy plus surgery. Distant metastases occurred in 16.8% and 14.8% of patients, respectively. Local recurrence occurred in 8.2% and 2.4% of patients, respectively ($P < .001$). Survival also was related to the following factors: tumor location (>10, 5–10, or < 5 cm from the anal verge; hazard ratio [HR], 1, 2.13, and 2.78, respectively) and stage of disease (I, II, or III; HR, 1, 3.44, and 9.69, respectively). There were no significant differences according to the type of operation [64].

A subsequent follow-up at a median of 6.1 years showed that these early differences were maintained. Although survival was the same in the two arms (63.5% and 64.2%, respectively), local recurrence rates were 10.9% and 5.6%, respectively ($P < .001$). As in the initial report, the location and stage of the tumor were significantly related to survival. In addition, the type of surgery and the presence of a positive CRM became significant factors for survival. The HR was 1.7 for anterior resection versus total rectal excision and 4.03 for negative versus positive margin involvement [65]. Subsequent subgroup analysis has shown that radiotherapy did not result in lower local recurrence in patients who had total rectal excision [66].

Preoperative short-course radiotherapy versus preoperative neoadjuvant chemoradiotherapy

The short-course regimen of five cycles of 5 Gy with surgery within 7 days was compared with preoperative neoadjuvant chemoradiotherapy in a randomized, controlled trial including 316 patients accrued from 19 Polish hospitals between 1999 and 2002, the "Polish trial." Patients who had T3 and T4 tumors, defined by circumferential extent and tethering on digital examination, were enrolled. For mobile tumors, ultrasound, CT, and MRI were used to exclude T1 and T2 lesions. The median follow-up period was 48 months (range, 31–69 months). Of the 316 patients, 155 were randomly assigned to short-course radiotherapy, and 157 were assigned to chemoradiotherapy (50.4 Gy in 28 1.8-Gy fractions plus 5-FU and leucovorin, similar to the regimen in the German trial). Survival rates were 61.2% and 58% in the two arms, local recurrence rates were 10.6% and 15.6%, and circumferential involvement was seen in 12.9% and 4.4% of patients, respectively ($P < .017$). Early toxicity occurred in 3.2% and 18.2% of patients, respectively ($P < .001$), and compliance with the protocol in the two arms was 97.9% and 69.2%, respectively. Late toxic effects occurred in 28.3% and 27.0% of patients, respectively. There were no differences between the two arms in the rates of survival, local recurrence, and late toxicity, but the authors pointed to the low power of the trial. The high incidence (39.5%) in the short-course arm of patients who had T1 or T2 disease raised questions about the accuracy of the pretreatment staging, which was determined largely by clinical examination [67].

Preoperative short-course radiotherapy versus surgery alone or circumferential resection margin–positive surgery and postoperative radiotherapy

The Medical Research Council CR07 trial was designed to compare two different radiotherapy regimens combined with mesorectal excision. A total of 1350 patients from 52 centers were accrued between March 1998 and August 2005. Patients who had resectable adenocarcinoma of the rectum without evidence of metastases were assigned randomly to receive either routine preoperative short-course radiotherapy (25 Gy, 5×5) (PRE) or surgery alone with selective postoperative chemoradiotherapy (POST) given to patients who had involvement of the CRM (45 Gy/5-FU). The median follow-up was 3 years. Eighty-eight percent of the PRE group (595/674) received the allocated treatment. Of the 676 patients in the POST arm, 73 (11%) were CRM-positive, and 51 (70%) of the CRM-positive patients received chemoradiotherapy. Eighty-five percent of the patients who had stage III disease received postoperative chemotherapy. At the time of analysis, 23 patients in the PRE group and 61 patients in the POST group had confirmed local recurrences; 96 and 106, respectively, had distant metastases;

and 115 patients in the PRE group and 146 patients in the POST group had died. The rates of local recurrence at 3 years (the primary end point) were 4.7% for the PRE group and 11.1% for the POST group (HR, 2.47; 95% CI, 1.61–3.79). The rates of disease-free survival were 79.5% and 74.9%, respectively (HR, 1.31; 95% CI, 1.02–1.67), and the rates of overall survival were 80.8% and 78.7%, respectively (HR, 1.25; 95% CI, 0.98–1.59). The advantage of PRE in terms of local recurrence was consistent for tumors located between 0 and 5 cm, 5 to 10 cm, and more than 10 cm from the anal verge (HR, 2.00, 2.14, and 4.97, respectively) [68].

Trial pathologists were trained in histopathologic assessment and in reporting the involvement of the CRM and the plane of surgery; 1232 patients were prospectively assessed for CRM, and 1119 were assessed for the plane of surgery. The CRM was involved (tumor < 1 mm) in 139 of resected specimens (11%); for these patients the 3-year rates of local recurrence, disease-free survival, and overall survival were 18%, 50%, and 57%, respectively. For the 1093 CRM-negative patients, the respective rates were 7%, 81% and 84%. Local recurrence and disease-free survival rates were associated with plane of surgery (log-rank test; $P = .0019$ and $P = .05$, respectively), and in addition there was clear evidence of a reduction in local recurrence rates and improvement in disease-free survival rates in favor of PRE, independent of the quality of surgical assessment. The risk of local recurrence after rectal cancer resection was reduced significantly with an improved surgical dissection plane. The benefit of short-course preoperative radiotherapy also was seen for all planes of dissection. Short-course preoperative radiotherapy and good-quality surgery almost completely eliminated local recurrence [69].

Chemotherapy

There is relatively little information on the effect of adjuvant chemotherapy in rectal cancer, because most of the randomized, controlled trials have focused on radiotherapy. Adjuvant chemotherapy was used in the German trial, but the main aim of this study was related to the effect of radiotherapy, and the chemotherapy regime was similar in each arm [55]. Thus it is not possible to draw conclusions regarding chemotherapy from this study. The EORTC trial 22921 set out to answer the question whether chemotherapy could add any cancer-specific value to radiotherapy combined with surgery. Entry criteria included a T3 or T4 tumor less than 15 cm from the anal verge in patients younger than 80 years. Staging was by clinical examination, ultrasound, and CT. Between 1993 and 2003, 1011 patients from 40 centers (38 within Europe) were assigned randomly to one of four arms. Of the eligible 996 patients, 224 were assigned to radiotherapy plus surgery, 250 were assigned to chemoradiotherapy plus surgery, 251 were assigned to radiotherapy plus surgery plus postoperative adjuvant chemotherapy, and

251 were assigned to chemoradiotherapy plus surgery plus postoperative adjuvant chemotherapy. The radiotherapy regimen (45 Gy in 25 1.8-Gy fractions over 5 weeks) was identical in all groups. Chemotherapy was given in
the same dose in all arms (5-FU, 350 mg/m^2/d, and leucovorin, 20 mg/m^2/d,
given preoperatively over 5 days in weeks 1 and 5 and postoperatively in four
courses every 3 weeks starting 3 to 10 weeks after surgery). Surgery was
performed 3 to 10 weeks after preoperative treatment. The 5-year survival
rates were no different in the four arms (65.8%, 64.6%, 67.2%, and
63.2%, respectively). Local recurrence was higher in the radiotherapy-
plus-surgery arm (17.1%) than in the other three arms, all of which included
chemotherapy given preoperatively, postoperatively, or both preoperatively
and postoperatively (8.7%, 9.6%, and 7.2%, respectively). Adherence to
the chemotherapy protocol was maintained in 82% of patients treated preoperatively but in only 42.9% of those receiving chemotherapy postoperatively.
There was no significant difference in the incidence of late side effects.

The results indicated that chemotherapy given either before or after
surgery reduced local recurrence. There was no evidence that giving chemotherapy both pre- and postoperatively added any advantage to its administration either before or after [70].

Mortality, morbidity, toxicity, and function

Treatment mortality in the ICRF RCG [58] and Stockholm I trials [59]
was greater following radiotherapy plus surgery than after surgery alone
(8% versus 2%, respectively, in the Stockholm I trial, which fell to 1%
and 2%, respectively, in the Stockholm II trial [60], and was 4% versus
3%, respectively, in the Swedish trial [62].) This improvement was associated with a change in the radiotherapy regimen from a two- to four-portal
delivery, which reduced the volume of tissue irradiated. A meta-analysis of
13 randomized, controlled trials of radiotherapy (excluding the Swedish
trial) found no difference in mortality, but subgroup analysis suggested
that mortality was greater when the dose was higher than 30 Gy [51]. In
the Dutch trial there was no difference in mortality between two groups
treated with radiotherapy plus surgery or surgery alone [64]. In the German
trial mortality was 0.7% and 1.2% in both arms receiving radiotherapy
[55].In the Polish trial treatment mortality was not given specifically [67].

Complication rates were higher after radiotherapy plus surgery than after
surgery alone: 57% versus 42%, respectively, in a meta-analysis of 14 trials
[51], 41% versus 28%, respectively, in the Stockholm II trial [60], and 26%
versus 18%, respectively, in the Dutch trial [64]. There were no differences in
complication rates in the two groups in the German trial (34% versus 36%,
respectively) [55] or in any of the arms in the French trial [70].

Among the patients who had actually had the prescribed treatment in the
German trial, the rates for grade 3 and 4 acute toxicity (27% and 40%,

respectively) and for chronic toxicity (14% and 24%, respectively) favored the preoperative radiotherapy regimen [55]. When preoperative short-course radiotherapy and chemoradiotherapy were compared in the Polish trial, early and late toxicity rates were 3.2% and 18.2% and 7.1% and 10.1%, respectively [67].

There is evidence that radiotherapy is associated with worse bowel function. Although there was no difference in urinary function, the Dutch trial reported fecal incontinence rates of 62% and 38%, respectively, and mucous discharge in 27% and 15% of patients, respectively [71]. In the Polish trial, however, there was no difference in bowel function or in the use of antidiarrheal medication between the preoperative short-course radiotherapy group and the chemoradiotherapy group [72].

Tumor response to chemoradiotherapy

Patients in the preoperative arm of the German trial (50.4 Gy plus 5-FU with surgery at 6 weeks) were graded by histopathologic response using a tumor regression grade (TRG) scale of 0 (no regression) to 4 (complete regression) [73]. Of 385 patients, 40 (10%) had complete regression, and 32 (8%) had none. When patients with tumors grade 0 and 1 combined, grades 2 and 3 combined, and grade 4 were analyzed, lymph node metastases were found in 40.7%, 31.9%, and 10% of patients, respectively; disease-free survival rates were 49%, 89%, and 85%, respectively; and local failure rates were 6%, 4%, and 0%, respectively [74,75].

Using the Mandard classification first applied to esophageal carcinoma [76], complete regression occurred in 19% of 144 patients treated with preoperative radiotherapy. When TRG stages 1 and 2 (complete or nearly complete regression) were compared with stages 3 through 5 combined (less complete to no change), 28% versus 42% were lymph node–positive; overall survival rate were 89% versus 68%; disease-free survival rates were 91% versus 58%; and local recurrence rates were 2% versus 17% [77]. A complete histopathologic response occurred in 18 (16%) of 109 patients who received 50.4-Gy radiation plus chemotherapy followed by surgery at 19 to 155 days [78]. This response seemed to be related to the level of the tumor, occurring in 1 of 33 patients who had a tumor located less than 5 cm from the anal verge and in 14 of 70 patients who had a tumor located 6 to 10 cm from the anal verge.

The response is related to the interval between radiotherapy and surgery. No complete regression was seen in 103 patients receiving 41.6 Gy with surgery at 6 days after completion [79]. Tumor response may be increased by an intracavitary boost to external beam radiotherapy. Of the 81 patients in the Lyon trial R96-02 treated by 39 Gy with (43 patients) or without an 85-Gy 50-kV boost (38 patients), 15 (35%) and 26 (68%), respectively, had a complete or nearly complete response. Two-year disease-free survival rates did not differ (86% versus 92%), but seven patients in the boost group were followed without surgery, whereas all the 43 patients in the nonboost group underwent operation [80].

Whether surgery should be performed in patients showing a complete clinical (not necessarily histopathologic) response has been investigated further. In a series of 265 patients who underwent treatment between 1991 and 2002 by preoperative chemoradiotherapy (50.4 Gy plus 5-FU and leucovorin), 71 (26.8%) were deemed to have had a complete clinical response on assessment 8 weeks later. They were followed by monthly examination and at a median follow-up of 57.3 months (range, 12–156 months) two local failures had occurred. (Both were successfully salvaged). The overall 5-year survival rate was 100%, and the disease-free survival rate was 92% [81]. In a subsequent report of 360 patients, 99 (27.5%) had responded completely. In this group the overall recurrence rate was 11%, and there was a disease-specific mortality of only 2% [82]. These results give a glimpse of one aspect of the future treatment of rectal cancer and also relate to the question whether patients who have preoperative radiotherapy are more likely to be treatable by a sphincter-saving procedure.

Early reports had suggested that preoperative radiotherapy could increase the proportion of patients who could be treated by a sphincter-saving procedure [40,41]. This question applies to patients having moderate- to high-dose preoperative radiotherapy with an interval to surgery allowing time for tumor regression. In a review of 4596 patients entered into 10 trials, preoperative radiotherapy was given to 39 Gy or more in eight trials with an interval to surgery of more than 3 weeks in seven trials. Tumor shrinkage occurred in seven trials, but there was no significant increase in the anterior resection rate compared with the controls [83].

A subgroup analysis of patients admitted to the German trial with a low cancer considered by the surgeon before treatment to require a total rectal excision showed that the percentage of patients in the preoperative radiotherapy group who underwent a sphincter-preserving procedure (45/116; 39%) was twice that in the postoperative radiotherapy group (15/78; 19%) [57]. In the R96-02 Lyon trial the addition of an intracavitary boost was associated with sphincter preservation (including no surgery) in 76% patients, compared with 44% of patients who had external beam treatment alone [80]. There is thus some evidence that high-dose preoperative radiotherapy with an interval of some weeks to surgery may influence the type of operation performed.

Summary

The trials show no difference in treatment mortality with surgery alone, with radiotherapy plus surgery, or chemoradiotherapy plus surgery, if a two-portal field is not used. Treatment mortality may be dose related.

Complications and toxicity are greater after preoperative radiotherapy plus surgery than with surgery alone. Both complications and toxicity are more common after postoperative radiotherapy than after preoperative radiotherapy. The rate of local recurrence is lower after preoperative radiotherapy than after surgery alone. Only one trial of preoperative radiotherapy suggested an improvement in survival. Local recurrence is less common after preoperative radiotherapy than after postoperative radiotherapy. There are insufficient data to conclude whether preoperative neoadjuvant chemoradiotherapy is superior to short-course radiotherapy. Chemotherapy in addition to radiotherapy reduces local recurrence. Responders to preoperative chemoradiotherapy have improved cancer-specific outcomes compared with nonresponders. Bowel function is worse after radiotherapy than after surgery alone.

Future studies should consider the following issues:

1. Improving the results of total rectal excision
2. Refining MRI preoperative staging to produce greater uniformity of patients entering clinical trials (Breaking down the T stage into the T3a and T3b stages based on MRI should be part of this refinement)
3. Conducting further trials to compare short-course radiotherapy with neoadjuvant chemoradiotherapy
4. Further testing of chemotherapy as new agents become available
5. Further analyzing the avoidance of surgery after complete response with chemoradiotherapy

References

[1] Heald RJ, Husband EM, Ryall RD. The mesorectum in rectal cancer surgery—the clue to pelvic recurrence? Br J Surg 1982;69(10):613–6.
[2] Quirke P, Durdey P, Dixon MF, et al. Local recurrence of rectal adenocarcinoma due to inadequate surgical resection. Histopathological study of lateral tumour spread and surgical excision. Lancet 1986;2(8514):996–9.
[3] Hall NR, Finan PJ, al-Jaberi T, et al. Circumferential margin involvement after mesorectal excision of rectal cancer with curative intent. Predictor of survival but not local recurrence? Dis Colon Rectum 1998;41(8):979–83.
[4] Heald RJ, Ryall RD. Recurrence and survival after total mesorectal excision for rectal cancer. Lancet 1986;1(8496):1479–82.
[5] Beets-Tan RG, Beets GL, Vliegen RF, et al. Accuracy of magnetic resonance imaging in prediction of tumour-free resection margin in rectal cancer surgery. Lancet 2001;357(9255): 497–504.
[6] Daniels I, Fisher SE, Heald RJ, et al. Accurate staging, selective preoperative therapy and optimal surgery improves outcome in rectal cancer: a review of the recent evidence. Colorectal Dis 2007;9:290–301.
[7] Martling A, Holm T, Rutqvist LE, et al. Effect of training programme on outcome of rectal cancer in the County of Stockholm. Lancet 2000;356:497–504.
[8] Wibe A, Moller B, Norstein J, et al. A national strategic change in treatment policy for rectal cancer—implementation of total mesorectal excision as routine treatment in Norway. A national audit. Dis Colon Rectum 2002;45:857–66.

[9] Iversen L, Harling H, Laurberg S, et al. Influence of caseload and surgical specialty on out-
     come following surgery for colorectal cancer: a review of evidence. Part 2: long-term out-
     come. Colorectal Dis 2007;9:38–46.
[10] Birbeck K, Macklin CP, Tiffin NJ, et al. Rates of circumferential resection margin involve-
     ment vary between surgeons and predict outcomes in rectal cancer surgery. Ann Surg 2002;
     235:449–57.
[11] Nagtegaal ID, van de Velde CJ, Marijnen CA, et al. Low rectal cancer: a call for a change of
     approach in abdominoperineal resection. J Clin Oncol 2005;23:9257–64.
[12] Wibe A, Syse A, Andersen E, et al. Oncological outcome after total mesorectal excision for
     cure for cancer of the lower rectum: anterior vs abdominoperineal resection. Dis Colon Rec-
     tum 2004;47:48–58.
[13] Sauer I, Bacon HE. A new approach for excision of carcinoma of the lower portion of the
     rectum and anal canal. Surg Gynecol Obstet 1952;95:229–42.
[14] Deddish M, Stearns MW. Anterior resection for carcinoma of the rectum and sigmoid area.
     Ann Surg 1961;154:961–6.
[15] Hojo K, Koyama Y, Moriya Y. Lymphatic spread and its prognostic value in patients with
     rectal cancer. Am J Surg 1982;144:350–4.
[16] Berge T, Ekelund G, Mellner C, et al. Carcinoma of the colon and rectum in a defined pop-
     ulation. Acta Chir Scand 1973;(Suppl 4):38–51.
[17] Dukes C, Bussey HJR. The spread of rectal cancer and its effect on prognosis. Br J Cancer
     1958;12:209–20.
[18] Nicholls RJ, Hall C. Treatment of non-disseminated cancer of the lower rectum. Br J Surg
     1996;83(1):15–8.
[19] Merkel S, Mansmann U, Siassi M, et al. The prognostic inhomogeneity of pT3 carcinoma.
     Int J Colorectal Dis 2001;16:298–304.
[20] Mackay SG, Pager CK, Joseph D, et al. Assessment of the accuracy of transrectal ultraso-
     nography in anorectal neoplasia. Br J Surg 2003;90(3):346–50.
[21] Garcia-Aguilar J, Pollack J, Lee SH, et al. Accuracy of endorectal ultrasonography in pre-
     operative staging of rectal tumors. Dis Colon Rectum 2002;45:10–5.
[22] Beets-Tan RG. MRI in rectal cancer: the T stage and circumferential resection margin.
     Colorectal Dis 2003;5:392–5.
[23] Brown G, Radcliffe AG, Newcombe RG, et al. Preoperative assessment of prognostic factors
     in rectal cancer using high-resolution magnetic resonance imaging. Br J Surg 2003;90(3):
     355–64.
[24] Purkayastha S, Tekkis PP, Athanasiou T, et al. Diagnostic precision of magnetic resonance
     imaging for preoperative prediction of the circumferential margin involvement in patients
     with rectal cancer. Colorectal Dis 2007;9:402–11.
[25] Brown G, Richards CJ, Bourne MW, et al. Morphologic predictors of lymph node status in
     rectal cancer with use of high-spatial-resolution MR imaging with histopathologic compar-
     ison. Radiology 2003;227(2):371–7.
[26] Will O, Purkayastha S, Chan C, et al. Diagnostic precision of nanoparticle-enhanced MRI
     for lymph-node metastases: a meta-analysis. Lancet Oncol 2006;7:52–60.
[27] Williams I, Horwitz H. The primary treatment of adenocarcinoma of the rectum by high
     voltage Roentgen rays (1000 kv). Am J Roentgenol 1956;76:919–28.
[28] Wang C, Schulz MD. The role of radiation therapy in the management of carcinoma of the
     sigmoid, rectosigmoid and rectum. Radiology 1962;79:1–5.
[29] Stevens K, Allen CV, Fletcher WS. Preoperative radiotherapy for adenocarcinoma of the
     rectosigmoid. Cancer 1976;37:2866–74.
[30] Economou S, Cole WH. Chemotherapy of cancer of the alimentary tract. Surg Clin North
     Am 1962;42:1147–70.
[31] O'Connell M, Childs DS, Moertel CG, et al. A prospective controlled evaluation of com-
     bined radiotherapy and methanol residue of BCG (MER) for locally resectable or recurrent
     rectal carcinoma. Int J Radiat Oncol Biol Phys 1982;8:115–9.

[32] Boulis Wassif S. Ten years' experience with a multidisciplinary treatment of advanced stages of rectal cancer. Cancer 1983;52:2017–24.

[33] Cummings B, Rider WD, Harwood AR, et al. Radical external beam radiation therapy for adenocarcinoma. Dis Colon Rectum 1983;26:30–6.

[34] Papillon J. Intracavitary irradiation of early rectal cancer for cure. Cancer 1975;36:696–701.

[35] Chambers W, Khan U, Gagliano A, et al. Tumour morphology as a predictor of outcome after local excision of rectal cancer. Br J Surg 2004;91:457–9.

[36] Rider W, Palmer JA, Mahoney LJ, et al. Preoperative irradiation of inoperable cancer of the rectum; report of the Toronto Trial. Can J Surg 1977;20:335–8.

[37] Stearns M, Deddish MR, Quan SHW, et al. Preoperative Roentgen therapy for cancer of the rectum and rectosigmoid. Surg Gynecol Obstet 1974;138:584–92.

[38] Roswit B, Higgins GA, Keehn RJ. Preoperative irradiation for carcinoma of the rectum and rectosigmoid colon. Report of a national VA randomised study. Cancer 1975;35:1597–602.

[39] Higgins G, Donaldson RC, Dannenberg P, et al. Adjuvant therapy for large bowel cancer. Update of VA Surgical Oncology Group Trials. Surg Clin North Am 1981;61:1311–20.

[40] Papillon J. The true role of external-beam irradiation in the initial treatment of cancer of the rectum. Recent Results Cancer Res 1988;110:114–8.

[41] Mohiuddin M, Marks G. High dose preoperative irradiation for cancer of the rectum, 1976–1988. Int J Radiat Oncol Biol Phys 1991;20:37–43.

[42] First report of the MRC working party. Br J Surg 1982;69:513–9.

[43] Hoskins B, Gunderson L, Dosoretz D, et al. Adjuvant postoperative radiotherapy in carcinoma of the rectum and rectosigmoid. Int J Radiat Oncol Biol Phys 1980;6:1379.

[44] Mohiuddin M, Marks G, Kramer S, et al. Adjuvant radiation therapy for rectal cancer. Int J Radiat Oncol Biol Phys 1984;10:977–80.

[45] Withers H, Romsdahl MD, Suxton G. Postoperative radiotherapy for cancer of the rectum and rectosigmoid. American Society for Therapeutic Radiology Proceedings. Int J Radiat Oncol Biol Phys 1980;6:1380.

[46] Balslev I, Pedersen M, Teglbjaerg PS, et al. Postoperative radiotherapy in Dukes B and C carcinoma of the rectum and rectosigmoid. A randomised multicenter study. Cancer 1986; 58:22–8.

[47] Gastrointestinal Tumor Study Group. Prolongation of the disease-free interval in surgically treated rectal carcinoma. N Engl J Med 1985;312:1464–72.

[48] Thomas P, Stablein DM, Lindblad AM, et al. Toxicity associated with adjuvant postoperative therapy for adenocarcinoma of the rectum. Int J Radiat Oncol Biol Phys 1983; 9(Suppl 1):137.

[49] Medical Research Council Working Party. Randomised trial of surgery alone versus radiotherapy followed by surgery for potentially operable locally advanced rectal cancer. Lancet 1996;348:1605–10.

[50] NIH Consensus Conference. Adjuvant therapy for patients with colon and rectal cancer. JAMA 1990;264:1444–50.

[51] Camma C, Giunta M, Fiorica F, et al. Preoperative radiotherapy for resectable rectal cancer. JAMA 2000;284:1008–15.

[52] Colorectal Cancer Collaborative Cancer Group. Adjuvant therapy for rectal cancer: a systematic review of 8,507 patients from 22 randomised trials. Lancet 2001;358:1291–304.

[53] Pahlman L, Glimelius B, Graffman S. Pre- versus postoperative radiotherapy in rectal carcinoma: an interim report from a randomized multicentre trial. Br J Surg 1985;72(12):961–6.

[54] Pahlman L, Glimelius B. Pre- or postoperative radiotherapy in rectal and rectosigmoid carcinoma. Report from a randomized multicenter trial. Ann Surg 1990;211(2):187–95.

[55] Sauer R, Becker H, Hohenberger W, et al. Preoperative versus postoperative chemoradiotherapy for rectal cancer. N Engl J Med 2004;351:1731–40.

[56] Gerard A, Buyse M, Nordlinger B, et al. Preoperative radiotherapy as adjuvant treatment in rectal cancer. Final results of a randomized study of the European Organization for Research and Treatment of Cancer (EORTC). Ann Surg 1988;208(5):606–14.

[57] Dahl O, Horn A, Morild I, et al. Low-dose preoperative radiation postpones recurrences in operable rectal cancer: results of a randomised multicenter trial in western Norway. Cancer 1990;66:2286–94.

[58] Goldberg PA, Nicholls RJ, Porter NH, et al. Long-term results of a randomised trial of short-course low-dose adjuvant pre-operative radiotherapy for rectal cancer: reduction in local treatment failure. Eur J Cancer 1994;30A(11):1602–6.

[59] Cedermark B, Johansson H, Rutqvist LE, et al. The Stockholm I trial of preoperative short term radiotherapy in operable rectal carcinoma. A prospective randomized trial. Stockholm Colorectal Cancer Study Group. Cancer 1995;75(9):2269–75.

[60] Martling A, Holm T, Johansson H, et al. The Stockholm II trial on preoperative radiotherapy in rectal carcinoma: long-term follow-up of a population-based study. Cancer 2001;92: 896–902.

[61] Kirk J, Gray WM, Watson ER. Cumulative radiation effect. Fractionated treatment regimes. Clin Radiol 1971;22:145–55.

[62] Swedish Rectal Cancer Trial Group. Improved survival with preoperative radiotherapy in resectable rectal cancer. N Engl J Med 1997;336:980–7.

[63] Folkesson J, Birgisson H, Pahlman L, et al. Swedish Rectal Cancer Trial: long lasting benefit from radiotherapy on survival and local recurrence rate. J Clin Oncol 2005;23:5644–50.

[64] Kapiteijn E, Marijnen CA, Nagtegaal ID, et al. Preoperative radiotherapy combined with total mesorectal excision for resectable rectal cancer. N Engl J Med 2001;345(9):638–46.

[65] Peeters K, Marijnen CAM, Nagtegaal ID, et al. Increased local control but no survival benefit in irradiated patients with resectable rectal carcinoma. Ann Surg 2007;246:693–701.

[66] Marijnen E, Peeters JCMJ, Putter H, et al. Long term results, toxicity and quality of life in the TME trial. Radiother Oncol 2004;73(Suppl 1):S127.

[67] Bujko K, Nowacki MP, Nasierowska-Guttmejer A, et al. Long-term results of a randomised trial comparing preoperative short-course radiotherapy with preoperative conventionally fractionated chemoradiation for rectal cancer. Br J Surg 2006;93:1215–23.

[68] Sebag-Montefiore D, Steele R, Quirke P, et al. Short course pre-operative radiotherapy results improves outcome when compared with highly selective postoperative chemotherapy. Preliminary results of the MRC CR07 randomised trial. Radiother Oncol 2006;81(S1):S19.

[69] Quirke P, Sebag-Montefiore D, Steele R, et al. The rate of local recurrence after rectal cancer resection is strongly related to the plane of surgical dissection and is further reduced by preoperative short course radiotherapy. Preliminary results of the Medical Research Council (MRC) CR07 Trial. Radiother Oncol 2006;81(S1):S93.

[70] Bosset JF, Collette L, Calais G, et al. Chemotherapy with preoperative radiotherapy for rectal cancer. N Engl J Med 2006;355:1114–23.

[71] Peeters K, van de Velde CJ, Leer JW, et al. Late side effects of short-course preoperative radiotherapy combined with total mesorectal excision for rectal cancer: increased bowel dysfunction in irradiated patients—a Dutch Colorectal Cancer Group study. J Clin Oncol 2005;23:6199–206.

[72] Pietrzak L, Bujko K, Nawacki MP, et al. Quality of life, anorectal and sexual functions after preoperative radiotherapy for rectal cancer: report of a randomised trial. Radiother Oncol 2007;84:217–25.

[73] Dworak O, Keilholz L, Hoffmann A. Pathological features of rectal cancer after preoperative radiotherapy. Int J Colorectal Dis 1997;12:19–23.

[74] Rodel C, Grabenbauer GG, Papadopoulos T, et al. Apoptosis as a cellular predictor for histopathologic response to neoadjuvant radiochemotherapy in patients with rectal cancer. Int J Radiat Oncol Biol Phys 2002;52:294–303.

[75] Rodel K, Martus P, Papadoupolos T, et al. Prognostic significance of tumor regression after preoperative chemoradiotherapy for rectal cancer. J Clin Oncol 2005;23:8688–96.

[76] Mandard A, Dalibard F, Mandard JC, et al. Pathologic assessment of tumor regression after preoperative chemoradiotherapy of esophageal carcinoma: clinicopathological correlations. Cancer 1994;73:2680–6.

[77] Vecchio F, Valentini V, Minsky B, et al. The relationship of pathologic tumor grade (TRG) and outcomes after preoperative therapy in rectal cancer. Int J Radiat Oncol Biol Phys 2005; 62:752–60.

[78] Guillem J, Chessin DB, Shia J, et al. A prospective pathologic analysis using whole-mount sections of rectal cancer following preoperative combined modality therapy: implications for sphincter preservation. Ann Surg 2007;245:88–93.

[79] Bouzourene H, Bosman FT, Seelentag W, et al. Importance of tumor regression assessment in predicting the outcome in patients with locally advanced rectal carcinoma who are treated with preoperative radiotherapy. Cancer 2002;94:1121–30.

[80] Gerard J-P, Chapet O, Nemoz C, et al. Improved sphincter preservation in low rectal cancer with high-dose preoperative radiotherapy: the Lyon R96-02 randomised trial. J Clin Oncol 2004;22:2404–9.

[81] Habr-Gama A, Perez RO, Nadalin W, et al. Operative versus non-operative treatment for stage 0 distal rectal cancer following chemoradiation therapy: long-term results. Ann Surg 2004;240:711–7.

[82] Habr-Gama A. Assessment and management of the cojmplete clinical responce of rectal cancer to chemoradiotherapy. Colorectal Dis 2006;8(Suppl 3):21–4.

[83] Bujko K, Kepka L, Michalki W, et al. Does rectal cancer shrinkage induced by preoperative radiotherapy increase the likelihood of anterior resection? A systematic review of randomised trials. Radiother Oncol 2006;80:4–12.

ELSEVIER
SAUNDERS

Surg Oncol Clin N Am
17 (2008) 553–568

SURGICAL
ONCOLOGY CLINICS
OF NORTH AMERICA

Bilobar Colorectal Liver Metastases: Treatment Options

Daniel Jaeck, MD, PhD, FRCS*, Patrick Pessaux, MD, PhD

*Centre de Chirurgie Viscérale et de Transplantation, Hôpital de Hautepierre,
Hôpitaux Universitaires de Strasbourg, Université Louis Pasteur, Avenue Molière,
67200 Strasbourg, France*

In the United States as well as in Europe, colorectal carcinoma is the second leading cause of cancer-related death [1,2]. More than 50% of patients with colorectal cancer will develop liver metastases during the course of the disease. Hepatic metastases are present in 15% to 25% of patients at the time of diagnosis of colorectal cancer [3], and another 25% to 50% develop liver metastases within 3 years following resection of the primary tumor [4].

Although prospective, randomized clinical trials never have been conducted, ample evidence based on retrospective and comparative studies strongly indicates that hepatic resection is the only available treatment that allows long-term survival. Major reported experience with liver resection is associated with a 25% to 44% 5-year survival [5,6]. Unfortunately, curative resection can only be performed in less than 25% of the patients. Ten years ago, hepatic resection was contraindicated in case of multiple or bilobar nodules. Currently, the trend is to be more aggressive and to increase the indications for surgical resection with the development of new strategies (neoadjuvant chemotherapy including molecular targeted therapy, portal vein embolization [PVE], two-stage resection, or a combination of resection and tumor ablation with radiofrequency or cryotherapy).

The management of bilobar liver metastases demonstrates the advantages of a multidisciplinary approach with step-by-step strategy and regular restaging, to achieve a complete resection (R0) in a large number of patients.

* Corresponding author. Centre de Chirurgie Viscérale et de Transplantation, Hôpital de Hautepierre, Hôpitaux Universitaires de Strasbourg, Université Louis Pasteur, Avenue Molière, 67098 Strasbourg.

E-mail address: daniel.jaeck@chru-strasbourg.fr (D. Jaeck).

1055-3207/08/$ - see front matter © 2008 Elsevier Inc. All rights reserved.
doi:10.1016/j.soc.2008.02.006   *surgonc.theclinics.com*

Is bilobar distribution a prognostic factor?

Initially, multiple or bilobar metastases were considered as a contraindication for hepatic resection. Several studies previously reported established prognostic factors and staging systems that might influence recurrence or survival after hepatic resection for colorectal metastases [7,8]. The prognostic significance of bilobar distribution of multiple metastases is controversial. Some studies report bilobar distribution as a poor prognostic factor [9,10], whereas others suggest that a bilobar distribution of nodules does not affect overall survival [7,8]. After multivariate analysis, the main prognostic factors are patient age, the number and size of largest metastases, carcinoembryonic antigen level, stage of the primary tumor, disease-free interval, and resection margin [7,8]. Ercolani and colleagues [11] reported that the total tumor volume of liver metastases had a stronger influence on survival than did number or location. The long-term outcome was significantly better for patients who had multiple or/and bilobar metastases with a total tumor volume of less than 125 cm^3 than for patients who had single metastasis and total tumor volume more than 380 cm^3.

If complete resection of the metastases can be achieved with tumor-free surgical margins (R0 resection) while maintaining a sufficient volume of residual liver, the number and the bilobar distribution of metastases should not be considered in the selection process, because liver resection still remains the only option for cure.

Preoperative assessment of hepatic involvement

Imaging constitutes a major step in the screening for the presence of disease, its staging, assessment of response to treatment, and detection of tumor recurrence following treatment. Preoperative staging is of great value in patient selection to avoid inappropriate surgery. Evaluation of tumor resectability includes assessment of vascular structures for tumor invasion and vascular abnormalities. The evolution of imaging during the past decades has allowed earlier, more accurate detection and characterization of colorectal liver metastases. The two main difficulties are to distinguish metastases from incidental benign focal liver lesions and to detect small metastases. At the preoperative stage, some bilobar cases may not be recognized if the deposits on one side are too small.

Percutaneous ultrasound is the most widely used imaging technique. The sensitivity exceeds 94% for nodules larger than 2 cm, but it falls to less than 56% for smaller nodules [12]. CT scanning with intravenous contrast (enhanced CT) remains an important step in liver imaging that covers most of the clinical indications. The advent of helical CT has increased the sensitivity of detection of metastases (68% for nodules < 1 cm diameter and 99% for those > 1 cm) [13,14]. Current state-of-the-art multidetector helical CT scanning provides data of the entire chest and abdomen during a single breath-hold, thereby avoiding respiratory misregistration with limited motion artifacts.

With the recent advances in software, hardware, and image acquisition technique, MRI is now the most effective imaging modality for detecting and characterizing liver lesions [15]. MRI is particularly useful in characterizing indeterminate lesions detected by other modalities.

Although helical CT is the modality of choice for staging colorectal liver metastases, up to 25% of the lesions still may be missed [16]. A multimodality strategy is recommended because no single investigation can detect all colorectal liver metastases accurately [17].

In 2005, a meta-analysis, comparing helical CT, MRI, and fluorodeoxyglucose positron emission tomography (FDG-PET) in the detection of colorectal liver metastases showed that the sensitivities on a per-patient basis were 64.7%, 75.8%, and 94.6% respectively [18]. Recent reports, however, have questioned the real sensitivity of FDG-PET [19] and consider MRI and multidetector CT more sensitive than FDG-PET in detecting individual small liver metastases, mostly after neoadjuvant chemotherapy [20,21]. FDG-PET has the advantage of screening the whole body for extrahepatic disease (peritoneal metastases or lymph node involvement), which could be a contraindication for hepatic resection.

Evaluation of hepatic functional reserve

The hepatic functional reserve may be evaluated by measuring the volume of the future remnant liver and assessing the preoperative liver function. Imaging reconstruction techniques in three dimensions are mandatory to evaluate the total volume of the tumors and the volume of nontumoral liver. Three-dimensional reconstruction also shows clearly the relationship between vessels and the tumors. It enables the surgeon to determine an exact operative strategy and to draw it on the computer screen.

Patients who have bilobar metastases often require either extended hepatectomies or multiple resections and therefore are at risk of developing postoperative liver failure. Although the normal liver tolerates removal of up to 60% to 70% of its volume [22], the extent to which the liver parenchyma may be resected in patients who have chemotherapy-associated steatohepatitis [23] has not been defined clearly. Three-dimensional CT has been shown to be the most adequate procedure for measuring liver volumes [24–26]. When the volume of the future remnant liver is less than 40% or when the ratio of remnant liver volume to body weight is less than 0.5% [27], PVE or two-stage hepatectomy has been recommended to improve the safety of the procedure [28,29].

Standard liver biochemistry tests have not been shown to have any predictive value [30]. Other methods have included measurement of uptake of organic anions (such as bromsulphthalein, rose Bengal, and indocyanine green [ICG] [30,31]), the arterial ketone body ratio [32], redox tolerance test [33], the aminopyrine breath test, and the amino acid clearance test [34]. The ICG clearance test seems to be the best discriminating investigation [31,34]. Hepatectomy involving resection of up to 60% of the parenchyma can be justified in patients who have normal liver function with retention of less than 20% of ICG at 15 minutes. Minor hepatectomies can be accomplished even if ICG retention at 15 minutes reaches 23% to 25% [31,34].

When is hepatic resection for bilobar metastases justified?

Surgical resection should be undertaken only if all the liver metastases can be removed (R0 resection) [35]. In case of associated extrahepatic disease, resection is justified in when all the tumoral tissue can be completely removed.

Involvement of lymph nodes in the hepatic pedicle

Several series have reported the prevalence of hepatic lymph node involvement to range from 3% to 33% [36,37]. The management of these patients is controversial. There are two opposite strategies: to consider lymph node involvement as generalized disease contraindicating an hepatic resection or to try to achieve a radical resection including the extrahepatic locations and perform a lymphadenectomy as for hilar cholangiocarcinoma. Hepatic lymph node involvement is recognized as a poor prognostic factor that affects survival [9,38], but in the multi-institutional study by the Association Française de Chirurgie the 5-year survival rate of patients who had lymph node involvement was 12% [7], compared with the expected 0% to 2% without resection [39]. The authors' policy is to perform an hepatic pedicle lymph node dissection limited to the proximal area (near the hilum) during hepatectomy. If involvement is diagnosed by frozen section, an extensive lymphadenectomy is performed from the liver hilum to the origin of the hepatic artery and the celiac axis (distal area) [36]. In patients who have more than three poorly differentiated liver metastases located in segments IV and V, however, a routine extended lymphadenectomy seems indicated [36]. In the authors' experience [36], the 3-year survival rates in patients with and without involvement of the hepatic pedicle lymph nodes were 19% versus 62%, respectively. Moreover, the 3-year survival rate in patients who had hepatoduodenal and retropancreatic lymph node metastases (proximal area) was 38%, compared with 0% survival at 1 year in patients who had lymph node metastases along the common hepatic artery and celiac axis (distal area).

Other extrahepatic involvement

The presence of extrahepatic disease (except pulmonary metastases [40]) traditionally has been considered a contraindication to hepatic resection. Significant advances in surgical techniques and improvement in postoperative support during the past decade have led to extend the indications for hepatectomy. At least two surgical teams have reported encouraging results in patients treated for liver metastases and concomitant peritoneal carcinomatosis [41,42]. Recently, Elias and colleagues [43], in a multivariate analysis, showed that the total number of metastases had a greater prognostic impact than the location of the metastases. These results seem to suggest that the prognosis is determined by the ability to achieve optimal cytoreduction and not by the disease localization. This approach, however, seems justified only for surgical teams experienced in both hepatobiliary surgery and intraperitoneal chemotherapy.

Innovative approaches allowing curative hepatic resection

How to reduce the extent of hepatic resection

Neoadjuvant chemotherapy

The timing and the indications for chemotherapy in patients with colorectal liver metastases are still debated. These patients can be categorized as either presenting with initially resectable disease or presenting with unresectable nodules.

Several studies evaluated the role of neoadjuvant chemotherapy in downstaging liver metastases.

The role of perioperative chemotherapy in patients who had resectable metastases was investigated by the prospective trial 40,983 conducted by the European Organization for the Research and Treatment of Cancer [44]. This study compared surgery alone versus surgery with perioperative chemotherapy (oxaliplatin, leucovorin, and 5-fluorouracil [FOLFOX4]), six cycles before surgery and six cycles after surgery. The six preoperative cycles of FOLFOX4 induced a complete response in 3.8% of patients and a partial response in 40.1% with a decrease in the diameter of the nodules of 29.5%. At 3 years, the disease-free survival was 28.1% in the group treated with surgery alone and 35.4% in the group that received perioperative chemotherapy ($P = .058$). In case of multiple bilobar metastases, the reduction of the size of the nodules could modify and facilitate the liver resection with a minor hepatectomy instead of a major liver resection. Tanaka and colleagues [45] compared the outcome of 48 patients presenting with five or more bilobar metastases treated by a neoadjuvant chemotherapy and surgery with that registered in the 23 patients treated by hepatectomy alone. The 5-year survival rate was 38.9% in the group receiving neoadjuvant chemotherapy compared with 20.7% in the group treated by hepatectomy alone. Moreover, multivariate analysis revealed neoadjuvant chemotherapy to be an independent predictive factor for survival. These results suggest a survival benefit of neoadjuvant chemotherapy in patients with multiple bilobar metastases.

In patients with unresectable liver metastases, data have increasingly shown that neoadjuvant chemotherapy can make some metastases resectable, allowing a hope of prolonged survival [46–49]. In 1996 Bismuth and colleagues [47] reported that an additional 16% of patients who had liver metastases initially considered as unresectable became candidates for hepatic resection with the use of systemic neoadjuvant chemotherapy. There was no mortality in this group of patients, and the morbidity rate was comparable to that observed in patients undergoing liver resection without preoperative chemotherapy. The 3- and 5-year survival rates were 54% and 40%, respectively, comparable to those observed after the resection of initially resectable nodules. These results were confirmed by several other series (Table 1) [48,49]. There is a continuous interest in intra-arterial chemotherapy (in which a catheter is inserted into the hepatic artery) in the treatment of colorectal liver metastases. Intra-arterial chemotherapy has been considered as palliative or adjuvant treatment, but few studies have evaluated this procedure in the neoadjuvant setting [50–52]. These studies reported that curative resection could follow intra-arterial chemotherapy in approximately 5% of cases (see Table 1).

Chemotherapy in combination with new molecular targets (bevacizumab, cetuximab) has been associated with improvement in the response rate and longer median time before progression [53,54]. Whether the inclusion of these target agents could increase the number of patients able to receive a surgical resection is presently unknown and is the subject of ongoing studies.

Local ablation techniques

Local ablation techniques (radiofrequency, cryotherapy, microwave coagulation therapy, interstitial laser photocoagulation, and electrolysis) in combination with surgery increase resectability and curability of patients for whom hepatic resection alone is insufficient. The goal is to resect most of the metastases and to ablate the residual smaller lesions to achieve a R0 status, while preserving adequate liver parenchyma to avoid fatal liver failure.

Table 1
Results after resection of downstaging colorectal liver metastases by chemotherapy

Study	Number of patients	Regimen	% of Resected patients	3-Year survival (%)	5-Year survival (%)
Bismuth et al [47]	300	Systemic	16	54	40
Miyanari et al [48]	64	Systemic	25	56.1	35.1
Adam et al [49]	1104	Systemic	13	52	33
Elias et al [50]	196	Intra-arterial	4.6	NA	NA
Link et al [51]	168	Intra-arterial	5.3	NA	NA
Meric et al [52]	383	Intra-arterial	4.4	NA	NA

Abbreviation: NA, not available.

Cryotherapy involves freezing and thawing of liver tumors by means of a cryoprobe. Hepatic resection combined with cryotherapy for liver metastases not eligible for hepatic resection alone obtained a median survival of 29 months with a 5-year survival rate of 24% [55]. These results are better than those obtained with palliative chemotherapy. Local recurrence at the site of cryotherapy ablation occurs in 5% to 44% of patients [56]. Recurrence has been found to be significantly greater when treating multiple lesions (more than eight), large lesions (>3 cm), and tumors located close to major vessels, because the blood warmth may impair the freezing process [57–59]. The main drawback of this modality is that a laparotomy usually is required; percutaneous or laparoscopic techniques cannot be used.

Radiofrequency ablation involves the percutaneous or intraoperative insertion of an electrode into a nodule under ultrasonic guidance. Radiofrequency energy is emitted through the electrode and generates heat, which leads to coagulative necrosis. Radiofrequency is less expensive than cryotherapy and is associated with fewer complications [60]. Radiofrequency combined with hepatic resection for liver hepatic metastases considered surgically unresectable for cure achieved a median survival of 37.3 months [61]. Abdalla and colleagues [62] reported a retrospective experience using radiofrequency as a component of therapy when patients were considered to have unresectable disease. They concluded that radiofrequency alone or in combination with hepatic resection could not provide survival rates similar to those seen with resection of resectable metastases. The survival of patients treated with radiofrequency alone or in combination with hepatic resection, however, was greater than that of patients receiving only nonsurgical treatment. In fact, there was a selection bias, because the patients who had the worst indications were allocated to radiofrequency, and the patients who had the best indications were allocated to resection. The surgeon who is performing radiofrequency as a curative treatment must be familiar with the performance and the limitations of the equipment to obtain a negative margin for each ablated lesion. It is only under these conditions that radiofrequency may provide good results [63].

Even with a combination of hepatectomy and radiofrequency, some patients are not eligible for curative treatment because one or two liver metastases lie precisely in the surgical plane of the future hepatectomy, and more extensive hepatic resection is unsafe for volumetric reasons. In these patients, a new approach was described using radiofrequency to destroy the liver metastases in the plane of the future hepatectomy resection, followed by hepatic resection through the radiofrequency necrotic zone [64]. In this series, no local recurrence was observed after transmetastasis hepatectomy, suggesting the efficacy of the technique. All patients were alive with a mean follow-up of 19.4 months [65].

Finally, Japanese teams have developed microwave coagulation therapy and reported 5-year survival rates of 20%, 24%, and 24% after microwave therapy alone, microwave therapy in combination with hepatic resection, and hepatic resection alone, respectively [66,67].

Interstitial radiotherapy and ethanol injection currently have been abandoned. Radioactive implants have been used to treat gross residual disease or to sterilize positive margins. The results were poor, with early and late recurrence [68]. The results of percutaneous alcohol injection are far from satisfactory, because early recurrence and partial responses are observed commonly [69]. Contrary to hepatocellular carcinoma, colorectal liver metastases present with dense stroma into which it is difficult to inject alcohol that spreads out into the normal parenchyma. Although the results are somewhat encouraging (Table 2), it should be remembered that local ablation cannot be considered as an alternative to hepatic resection, which still remains the reference standard.

How to increase the volume of the remnant liver parenchyma

Portal vein embolization

One of the prerequisites for hepatectomy, particularly in bilobar metastatic disease, is the need to preserve enough remaining liver parenchyma to avoid life-threatening postoperative liver failure [72]. This concern may occur in the case of a small left lobe when an extended right hepatectomy is mandatory or when major liver resection is necessary in patients who have impaired liver function (eg, caused by previous prolonged chemotherapy). To make hepatectomy feasible and safe in such cases, preoperative PVE can redistribute portal blood flow rich in hepatotrophic substances toward the future remnant liver. At the same time, it induces a shrinkage in the volume of the embolized liver for which resection is planned [73–75]. This atrophy-hypertrophy sequence was observed initially in rabbits following portal branch ligation [76]. In 1990, Makuuchi and colleagues [28] were the first to report PVE in the clinical setting. PVE induces a decrease in hepatocyte growth factor clearance and reroutes hepatotrophic hormones to the unembolized liver. A major hepatectomy then can be performed after the period of liver regeneration. PVE usually is performed

Table 2
Results of local ablation in unresectable liver metastases

Study	Number of patients	Type of procedure	Mean follow-up (months)	Median survival (months)	3-Year survival (%)
Curley et al [61]	123	Radiofrequency	15	NA	NA
Bleicher et al [70]	153	Radiofrequency	11	NA	NA
Elias et al [63]	63	Radiofrequency	27.6	36	47
Finlay et al [71]	75	Cryotherapy	20	33	38
Niu et al [55]	119	Cryotherapy	25	29	43
Tanaka et al [67]	16	Microwave	NA	28	51

Abbreviation: NA, not available.

under a local anesthesia, percutaneously with ultrasound guidance, via a contralateral transhepatic approach to the portal branch to be embolized [73,74]; however, an ipsilateral approach [77] and a direct operative exposure of an ileocolic vein [78] to allow portal vein access have been used also. Cyanoacrylate or others means have been used for PVE. A few liver necrotic complications have been described after PVE, but they have been less severe than after hepatic arterial embolization. Common side effects are minimal and include fever, nausea, mild abdominal pain, and a transient abnormality of liver function tests. Injection is performed under a percutaneous transhepatic approach with isobutyl-2-cyanoacrylate glue (Histoacryl; Braun Medical, Aesculap AG and Co., Tuttlingen, Germany) mixed with iodized oil (lipiodol ultrafide; Guerbet, Aulnay-sous-bois, France). Liver volumetric measurements are obtained with three-dimensional CT scan before and after PVE. Previous studies showed a maximum regeneration in the first week and 70% to 80% of total hypertrophy in 4 to 5 weeks [28,73,75]. In the authors' experience, when the estimated volume of the remnant liver was considered insufficient, a second evaluation 3 to 4 weeks later was performed before excluding the patient from the second-stage hepatectomy [29]. Adequate hypertrophy could be achieved in the majority of patients who had an average increase in functional residual liver volume of approximately 14% of the total liver volume [73–75]. Less than 20% of the patients develop insufficient hypertrophy of the future remnant liver and cannot undergo hepatic resection [73–75]. To minimize the risk of tumor progression during the regeneration phase, it seems safer to maintain chemotherapy. Indeed, continuing chemotherapy while PVE is performed did not impair the hypertrophy of the future remnant liver nor the postoperative outcome after hepatectomy [79]. In the authors' experience, a group of patients presenting unilobar colorectal liver metastases who had undergone right hepatectomy with PVE was compared with a group without PVE [80]. After multivariate analysis, preoperative PVE (relative risk [RR] = 15.09; P = .006), neoadjuvant chemotherapy (RR = 12.52; P = .024), and the number of lesions (RR = 9.96; P = .041) were significantly associated with a decrease rate of intrahepatic recurrences.

In patients with multiple bilobar colorectal liver involvement, metastases in the future remnant liver should be ablated before PVE, because metastatic nodules in the remnant liver can grow more rapidly than nontumoral liver parenchyma [81]. Progression of metastases in the remnant liver may result in nonresectable disease. The concept of a two-stage hepatectomy has been developed for at least two purposes: (1) to try to resect in two stages the whole tumoral tissue that could not be resected in one stage without a risk of postoperative liver failure [82]; (2) to resect before PVE the tumoral nodules of the future nonembolized liver which is expected to hypertrophy, to avoid the growth of these metastatic nodules after PVE [29].

Two-stage hepatectomy

The aim of the two-stage hepatectomy is to achieve sequentially a complete resection of the metastases in patients otherwise deemed suitable only for palliative therapy. In fact, in such patients a complete resection with a single hepatectomy would have left too small a remnant liver after surgery with a high righ of postoperative liver failure. The goal of the first hepatectomy is to clear the future remnant liver of disease, allowing a second liver resection to become feasible and curative provided that restaging has excluded tumor progression. The rationale is to minimize the risk of liver failure by performing a second and complete resection once regeneration has occurred. To optimize the hepatic hypertrophy of the future remnant liver, a PVE is usually necessary between the two hepatectomies. The optimal interval before performing the second liver resection has not been clarified and currently is calculated based on the rate of liver regeneration. Performing the second hepatectomy 6 to 8 weeks after the first resection allows more than 80% of total liver regeneration to occur. The authors' experience in a two-stage hepatectomy procedure combined with PVE [29] showed that surgical outcome and 3-year survival were similar to those registered in patients presenting with initially resectable disease and to those of other reported series (Table 3).

Currently, there is a consensus for the guidelines for two-stage hepatectomies [85]:

1. Avoid leaving residual tumor in the future remnant liver at the first procedure.
2. If resection alone cannot remove all metastases from the future remnant liver, use local nonresectional techniques (eg, radiofrequency ablation) for tumor destruction to avoid tumor progression during hypertrophy of the remnant liver.
3. At the first operation, avoid dissection of the hepatic pedicle and mobilization of the liver lobe that is to be resected at the second stage.

This approach could increase the indications for surgical resection to as many as 27% of patients who have bilobar tumors [82].

Table 3
Results of two-stage hepatectomy for colorectal liver metastases

Study	Number of patients	Successful two-stage procedure (%)	Median survival (months)	3-Year survival (%)
Jaeck et al [29]	33	76	NA	54
Shimada et al [83]	12	100	NA	NA
Togo et al [84]	11	100	18	45
Adam et al [85]	45	69	35	47

Abbreviation: NA, not available.

Surgical strategy

Medical and surgical advances could provide a multidisciplinary approach for patients with bilobar colorectal liver metastases (Fig. 1). Developments in surgery, chemotherapy, and radiology have been brought together into an integrated, combined-modality framework to optimize the management of colorectal liver metastases. In this framework, currently, patients with resectable bilobar metastases may proceed directly to surgery. Indeed, the place of neoadjuvant chemotherapy in such cases is not yet fully

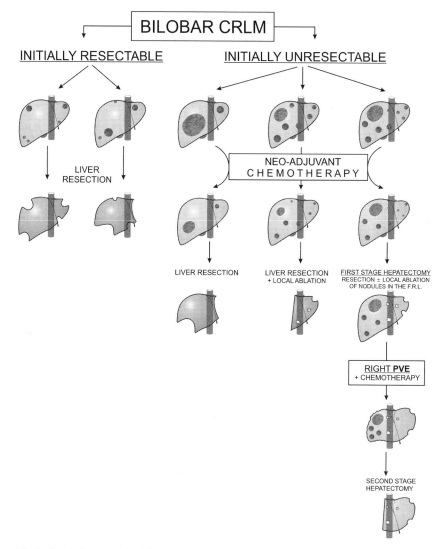

Fig. 1. Surgical strategy for bilobar colorectal liver metastases. CRLM, colorectal liver metastases; FRL, future remnant liver; PVE, portal vein embolization.

evaluated. At the opposite pole, patients with advanced bilobar liver metastases who are not initially candidates for surgical resection require a multidisciplinary approach, including neoadjuvant chemotherapy to allow a curative hepatic resection. Multiple nodules, large nodules, and metastases affecting multiple segments of the liver have usually been considered to be unresectable. Currently, the most important criterion to decide if the patient has resectable disease is the volume of the future remnant liver, independent of the number, the size, and the bilobar status of the liver metastases. This way of thinking allows the surgeons to explore different ways to shift a patient's status from unresectable to resectable. The three most common clinical presentations of initially unresectable liver metastases can be summarized:

1. Patients presenting with a few large bilobar metastases and who develop an objective response to chemotherapy should benefit from liver resection in case of sufficient remnant liver volume.
2. Patients with multiple bilobar liver metastases who had a partial response to chemotherapy should receive a one-stage liver resection combined, if necessary, with local ablation techniques.
3. Patients with multiple bilobar liver metastases and too small a future remnant liver are candidates for a two-stage hepatectomy with PVE.

In conclusion, the multidisciplinary approach makes it possible to expand significantly the population of patients with bilobar colorectal liver metastases who can be treated with curative intent, even if they initially were considered unresectable.

References

[1] Jemal A, Siegel R, Ward E, et al. Cancer statistics, 2007. CA Cancer J Clin 2007;57:43–66.
[2] Remontet L, Estève J, Bouvier AM, et al. Cancer incidence and mortality in France over the period 1978–2000. Rev Epidemiol Sante Publique 2003;51:3–30.
[3] Fong Y, Kemeny N, Paty P, et al. Treatment of colorectal cancer: hepatic metastasis. Semin Surg Oncol 1996;12:219–52.
[4] Steele GJ, Ravikumar TS. Resection of hepatic metastases from colorectal carcinoma: biologic perspectives. Ann Surg 1989;210:127–38.
[5] Simmonds PC, Primrose JN, Colquitt JL, et al. Surgical resection of hepatic metastases from colorectal cancer: a systematic review of published studies. Br J Cancer 2006;94:982–99.
[6] Jaeck D, Bachellier P, Guiguet M, et al. Long-term survival following resection of colorectal hepatic metastases: Association Française de Chirurgie. Br J Surg 1997;84:977–80.
[7] Nordlinger B, Guiguet M, Vaillant JC, et al. Surgical resection of colorectal carcinoma metastases to the liver: a prognostic scoring system to improve case selection based on 1568 patients. Cancer 1996;77:1254–62.
[8] Fong Y, Fortner J, Sun RL, et al. Clinical score for predicting recurrence after hepatic resection for metastatic colorectal cancer: analysis of 1001 consecutive cases. Ann Surg 1999;230: 309–21.
[9] Hughes KS, Simons R, Songhorabodi S, et al. Resection of the liver for colorectal carcinoma metastases: a multi-institutional study of indications for resection. Surgery 1988;103:278–88.

[52] Meric F, Patt YZ, Curley SA, et al. Surgery after downstaging of unresectable hepatic tumors with intra-arterial chemotherapy. Ann Surg Oncol 2000;7:490–5.

[53] Hurwitz H, Fehrenbacher L, Novotny W, et al. Bevacizumab plus irinotecan, fluorouracil, and leucovorin for metastatic colorectal cancer. N Engl J Med 2004;350:2335–42.

[54] Cunningham D, Humblet Y, Siena S, et al. Cetuximab monotherapy and cetuximab plus irinotecan in irinotecan-refractory metastatic colorectal cancer. N Engl J Med 2004;351: 337–45.

[55] Niu R, Yan TD, Zhu JC, et al. Recurrence and survival outcomes after hepatic resection with or without cryotherapy for liver metastases from colorectal carcinoma. Ann Surg Oncol 2007;14:2078–87.

[56] Sotsky TK, Ravikumar TS. Cryotherapy in the treatment of liver metastases from colorectal cancer. Semin Oncol 2002;29:183–91.

[57] Adam R, Akpinar E, Johann M, et al. Place of cryotherapy in the treatment of malignant liver tumors. Ann Surg 1997;225:39–50.

[58] Ruers TJ, Joosten J, Jager GJ, et al. Long-term results of treating hepatic colorectal metastases with cryotherapy. Br J Surg 2001;88:844–9.

[59] Seifert JK, Morris DL. Prognostic factors after cryotherapy for hepatic metastases from colorectal cancer. Ann Surg 1998;228:201–8.

[60] Mulier S, Mulier P, Ni Y, et al. Complications of radiofrequency coagulation of liver tumours. Br J Surg 2002;89:1206–22.

[61] Curley SA, Izzo F, Delrio P, et al. Radiofrequency ablation of unresectable primary and metastatic hepatic malignancies: results in 123 patients. Ann Surg 1999;230:1–8.

[62] Abdalla EK, Vauthey JN, Ellis LM, et al. Recurrence and outcomes following hepatic resection, radiofrequency ablation, and combined resection/ablation for colorectal liver metastases. Ann Surg 2004;239:818–25.

[63] Elias D, Baton O, Sideris L, et al. Hepatectomy plus intraoperative radiofrequency ablation and chemotherapy to treat technically unresectable multiple colorectal liver metastases. J Surg Oncol 2005;90:36–40.

[64] Ouellet JF, Pessaux P, Pocard M, et al. Transmetastasis curative liver resection immediately following radiofrequency destruction. J Surg Oncol 2002;81:108–10.

[65] Elias D, Manganas D, Benizri E, et al. The trans-metastasis hepatectomy (through metastases previously ablated with radiofrequency): results of a 13-case study of colorectal cancer. J Surg Oncol 2006;93:8–12.

[66] Shibata T, Niinobu T, Ogata N, et al. Microwave coagulation therapy for multiple hepatic metastases from colorectal carcinoma. Cancer 2000;89:276–84.

[67] Tanaka K, Shimada H, Nagano Y, et al. Outcome after hepatic resection versus combined resection and microwave ablation for multiple bilobar colorectal metastases to the liver. Surgery 2006;139:263–73.

[68] Armstrong JG, Anderson LL, Harrison LB, et al. Treatment of liver metastases from colorectal cancer with radioactive implants. Cancer 1994;73:1800–4.

[69] Amin Z, Brown SG, Lees WR. Local treatment of colorectal liver metastases. A comparison of interstitial laser photocoagulation (ILP) and percutaneous alcohol injection (PAI). Clin Radiol 1993;48:166–71.

[70] Bleicher RJ, Allegra DP, Nora DT, et al. Radiofrequency ablation in 447 complex unresectable liver tumors: lessons learned. Ann Surg Oncol 2003;10:52–8.

[71] Finlay IG, Seifert JK, Stewart GJ, et al. Resection with cryotherapy of colorectal hepatic metastases has the same survival as hepatic resection alone. Eur J Surg Oncol 2000;26:199–202.

[72] Bismuth H, Houssin D, Castaing D. Major and minor segmentectomies "réglées" in liver surgery. World J Surg 1982;6:10–24.

[73] De Baere T, Roche A, Elias D, et al. Preoperative portal vein embolization for extension of hepatectomy indications. Hepatology 1996;24:1386–91.

[74] Azoulay D, Castaing D, Smail A, et al. Resection of nonresectable liver metastases from colorectal cancer after percutaneous portal vein embolization. Ann Surg 2000;231:480–6.

[75] Abdalla EK, Hicks ME, Vauthey DN. Portal vein embolization: rationale, technique and future prospects. Br J Surg 2001;88:165–75.

[76] Rous P, Larimore L. Relation of the portal blood to liver maintenance. A demonstration of liver atrophy conditional on compensation. J Exp Med 1920;31:609–32.

[77] Nagino M, Nimura Y, Kondo S, et al. Selective percutaneous transhepatic embolization of the portal vein in preparation for extensive liver resection: the ipsilateral approach. Radiology 1996;200:559–63.

[78] Tsuge H, Mimura H, Kawata N, et al. Right portal embolization before extended right hepatectomy using laparoscopic catheterization of the ileocolic vein: a prospective study. Surg Laparosc Endosc 1994;4:258–63.

[79] Goere D, Farges O, Leporrier J, et al. Chemotherapy does not impair hypertrophy of the left liver after right portal vein obstruction. J Gastrointest Surg 2006;10:365–70.

[80] Oussoultzoglou E, Bachellier P, Rosso E, et al. Right portal vein embolization before right hepatectomy for unilobar colorectal liver metastases reduces the intrahepatic recurrence rate. Ann Surg 2006;244:71–9.

[81] Elias D, De Baere T, Roche A, et al. During liver regeneration following right portal embolization the growth rate of liver metastases is more rapid than that of the liver parenchyma. Br J Surg 1999;86:784–8.

[82] Adam R, Laurent A, Azoulay D, et al. Two-stage hepatectomy: a planed strategy to treat irresectable liver tumors. Ann Surg 2000;232:777–85.

[83] Shimada H, Tanaka K, Masui H, et al. Results of surgical treatment for multiple (≥ 5 nodules) bilobar hepatic metastases from colorectal cancer. Langenbecks Arch Surg 2004;389: 114–21.

[84] Togo S, Nagano Y, Masui H, et al. Two-stage hepatectomy for multiple bilobar liver metastases from colorectal cancer. Hepatogastroenterology 2005;52:913–9.

[85] Adam R, Miller R, Pitombo M, et al. Two-stage hepatectomy approach for initially unresectable colorectal hepatic metastases. Surg Oncol Clin N Am 2007;16:525–36.

ELSEVIER
SAUNDERS

Surg Oncol Clin N Am
17 (2008) 569–586

SURGICAL
ONCOLOGY CLINICS
OF NORTH AMERICA

Treatment of Pancreatic Adenocarcinoma: A European Perspective

Dirk J. Gouma, MD*, Olivier R.C. Busch, MD, Thomas M. van Gulik, MD

Department of Surgery, Academic Medical Center of the University of Amsterdam, Meibergdreef 9, 1105 AZ Amsterdam, the Netherlands

Pancreatic tumors are the fifth most common cause of cancer-related death in the Western world [1,2]. The incidence in Europe as well as the United States is around 10 to 12 cases per 100,000 population per year [1,2]. The majority of pancreatic tumors are adenocarcinoma. The etiology is still unknown. A model of genetic progression and the accumulation of multiple genetic changes resulting in PanIN-1A (*K-ras* mutations), PanIN-2 (loss *p16* expression) and PanIN-3 lesions (loss of *SMAD4* expression) and subsequently invasive carcinoma now is generally accepted, and the critical pathways are being investigated [3–5]. Predisposing factors are chronic pancreatitis, hereditary pancreatitis, familial pancreatic carcinoma (5%–10%), and genetic syndromes as Peutz-Jeghers syndrome, familial atypical multiple melanoma syndrome, and familial adenomatous polyposis. Intraductal papillary mucinous neoplasms (IPMN) also is considered a premalignant state [5,6]. Despite investigations of critical pathways, surgical resection still offers the only chance for cure. After surgical treatment, however, the overall 5-year survival rate is around 4% to 15% and has hardly improved during the last decades [7,8]. One of the pioneers in pancreas surgery in Europe, M. Trede, covering 25 years of experience, concluded that, with the modalities currently available, timely diagnosis and definitive cure are rare [9].

The diagnostic strategy/staging, surgical management, and adjuvant treatment of pancreatic cancer have changed worldwide during the past decades. These changes are discussed in this article, with specific attention given to European studies and contributions.

* Corresponding author.
E-mail address: d.j.gouma@amc.uva.nl (D.J. Gouma).

doi:10.1016/j.soc.2008.02.005

Diagnostic strategy and staging

The aim of the current diagnostic strategies is to select patients for potential curative resections. Others, more pessimistically, have suggested that the main goal of staging should be a selection to achieve optimal palliation and that staging might help avoid unnecessary operations and identify patients for nonsurgical palliation [7].

Many modalities, such as ultrasound plus Doppler, CT scans, magnetic resonance cholangiopancreaticography (MRCP), endoscopic ultrasound (EUS), endoscopic retrograde cholangiopancreaticography (ERCP) or percutaneous transhepatic cholangiography (PTC) with intraductal ultrasound, positron emission tomography, brush and fine-needle biopsy, and diagnostic laparoscopy, are available in most referral centers. The question remains, however, which of these tests are necessary, first to establish the diagnosis and second to obtain accurate staging in terms of local tumor extent and metastasis. Because the clinical presentation often is obstructive jaundice, ultrasound generally is used as the first test to exclude benign disease, in particular common bile duct stones (gallbladder stones), and nearly always shows dilated bile ducts and sometimes a pancreatic mass and/or liver metastasis. In the past ERCP frequently was used in Europe as the next diagnostic test. A study from the Netherlands showed that 30% of patients underwent ERCP before a CT scan was performed [10]. Because of the improved quality of spiral CT and MRCP, there is general agreement that ERCP is no longer justified in the diagnostic work-up. Data about the accuracy of CT scanning, EUS, and MRI/MRCP in detecting a pancreatic mass and showing the presence of liver metastases and local resectability are widely variable because of variations in technical performance and patient selection [11]. A meta-analysis comparing CT scanning, MRI, and ultrasound showed comparable results for these tests in demonstrating a pancreatic mass, with overall sensitivities of 76%, 91%, and 84%, respectively, and specificities of 75%, 85%, and 82%, respectively [12]. Differentiating focal pancreatitis from pancreatic carcinoma by these cross-sectional imaging modalities remains a problem in about 5% to 8% of patients [13].

A recent meta-analysis of EUS in patients who had biliary obstruction showed excellent results for bile duct stones but less impressive results for malignancy [14]. EUS combined with fine-needle aspiration can confirm the diagnosis, but, unfortunately, a negative biopsy does not exclude malignancy [15]. Therefore a pancreatic mass shown on one of the previously mentioned imaging techniques, especially in a patient who does not have a history of chronic pancreatitis, should be considered an indication for surgery even if the fine-needle aspiration is negative.

Staging generally is performed noninvasively using the same imaging modalities. The specificities of MRI and CT for detecting liver metastases are 92% and 82%, respectively. The introduction of multidetector CT angiography will further improve the ability to predict resectability [16]. EUS also is highly accurate in detecting vascular infiltration; in a meta-analysis, the pooled sensitivity was 73% (95% confidence interval [CI], 68.8–76.9), and the pooled specificity was 90.2% (95% CI, 87.9–92.2), but the success rate is highly dependent on the experience of the endoscopist [17]. Positron emission tomography might be helpful in detecting metastases. It will show the primary pancreatic lesion, but false-positive findings caused by chronic pancreatitis have been reported [18]. Because of its availability in general practice and its cost effectiveness CT scanning presently is the most important diagnostic tool for staging in Europe. The use of EUS depends on local expertise but should be used routinely if the tumor cannot be visualized.

Small, superficial liver metastases as well as peritoneal deposits can be missed easily by these techniques, and diagnostic laparoscopy has been used widely to improve staging [19,20]. Diagnostic laparoscopy can be combined with laparoscopic ultrasound, which has been reported to be sensitive for the detection of intrahepatic metastases and for the evaluation of enlarged lymph nodes and also tumor ingrowth in vascular structures surrounding peripancreatic tumors [21]. In the early period, the additional value of diagnostic laparoscopy in patients who had carcinoma of the pancreatic head was reported to be between 18% and 82% [19–21]. The improved accuracy of CT scanning has limited the added value of laparoscopic staging, and recent studies showed a relatively low percentage ($< 15\%$) of liver metastasis found on laparoscopic staging after a high-quality helical CT scan [20].

The authors investigated the added value of diagnostic laparoscopy as well as the consequences for treatment in terms of outcome. Patients who had pathologically proven metastasis during laparoscopy were assigned randomly to palliative treatment by endoscopic stenting or a surgical bypass procedure. The hospital-free survival was shorter in the endoscopically treated patients than in patients treated with surgical bypass [22]. This study again showed a limited benefit of diagnostic laparoscopy (added value: 13%) in preventing laparotomy; more importantly, it showed no improved hospital-free survival after subsequent nonsurgical palliation, and diagnostic laparoscopy was abandoned [23,24]. Of course, there might be an indication for performing laparoscopy in a well-defined group of selected patients who have a high risk of advanced disease (eg, who have ascites or extremely elevated CA 19-9 levels).

Preoperative biliary drainage

The increased risk of surgery in jaundiced patients was recognized by Whipple and colleagues [25], who proposed a two-stage approach for surgery in jaundiced patients (surgical drainage followed by resection 4 weeks later). After the introduction of percutaneous and endoscopic drainage, ERCP/PTC and subsequent biliary drainage were included in the routine diagnostic work-up. Internal biliary drainage has been shown to improve liver function and nutritional status, to reduce systemic endotoxemia and cytokine release, and subsequently to improve immune response in multiple experimental models [26–30]. Clinical studies and randomized, controlled trials could not confirm the positive effect of preoperative biliary drainage [30–34]. Some studies even reported a deleterious effect, resulting in part from complications associated with the drainage procedure such as infections caused by contamination of the biliary system [35,36].

A meta-analysis to examine the effectiveness of preoperative biliary drainage in jaundiced patients who had tumors showed no difference in overall mortality between patients who had preoperative biliary drainage and those who had immediate surgery. The overall complication rate was higher with preoperative biliary drainage than with immediate surgery (57% versus 42%, respectively) [37]. From this meta-analysis the authors concluded that preoperative biliary drainage should not be performed routinely, but around 90% of patients in The Netherlands still undergo preoperative drainage. Therefore, a prospective, randomized trial addressing the effects of preoperative biliary drainage on patients who have obstructive jaundice caused by distal obstruction is being performed currently as a multicenter study [38]. At present there is no indication for routine preoperative drainage, but this procedure can be performed in selected patients, depending on severity of jaundice (serum bilirubin > 300 μmol/L), for logistical reasons (eg, prolonged preoperative staging or referral, waiting list status, or the use of preoperative chemoradiotherapy).

Surgical treatment

Indications for surgical treatment/resection

The selection of patients for resection is heavily dependent on local treatment philosophy and criteria for accepting patients for resection. Indications currently are changing in Europe.

In some countries, tumor ingrowth in the portal/mesenteric vein seen on CT scan is not a contraindication for performing a resection, and a nonradical (R1) resection might be justified as optimal palliative treatment [39]. In a collective report on portal-mesenteric vein resections (in 1646 patients), resection did not increase mortality, but the median survival was 13 months. The investigators concluded that by time tumor has involved the vein, cure is unlikely, but palliative treatment is adequate [40]. The present authors believe that resection should not be performed if a macroscopic radical resection cannot be obtained, because it provides only limited survival benefits, if any, and increases morbidity [41,42]. Ingrowth seen at CT scan of more than 180° is considered incurable, with limited survival time, and therefore resection is not performed [42,43].

Until recently there was consensus that patients who had metastases should not undergo resection. A recent study, however, showed acceptable survival after pancreatic resection combined with liver resection for limited metastatic disease [44]. Currently there is no corroborating evidence, and this policy is not generally accepted. Surgery for recurrent pancreatic carcinoma has also been adopted in Europe, and in a very selected subgroup of patients this procedure was performed safely; patients might benefit [45].

Surgical procedure

The standard procedure for pancreatic carcinoma is a partial pancreaticoduodenectomy. This procedure can be performed by a Kausch-Whipple resection or the pylorus-preserving Whipple procedure. The different types of resection, standard versus extended, have been defined and described after a consensus meeting [46]. Two randomized, controlled trials from Germany and The Netherlands showed the no relevant differences in outcome, in terms of morbidity, mortality, recurrence, and survival, between pylorus-preserving pancreaticoduodenectomy and the classic Whipple procedure [47,48]. This finding was confirmed recently by a meta-analysis from six randomized, controlled trials showing no difference in overall mortality (odds ratio, 0.49%; 95% CI, 0.17–1.40; $P = .18$) and morbidity (odds ratio, 0.89; 95% CI, 0.48–1.62; $P = .69$) and survival (hazard ratio, 0.74; 95% CI, 0.52–1.07) [49]. The classic Whipple procedure is preferred only for tumors that might infiltrate the area of the pylorus and gastric antrum.

There also is discussion about the extent of the lymphadenectomy, standard versus extended resection. Four randomized, controlled trials have shown no benefit in survival and increased morbidity (eg, an increased rate of delayed gastric emptying and diarrhea) after extended lymph node dissection [50–54]. This finding was confirmed in a recent meta-analysis of overall survival (hazard ratio, 0.93, 95% CI, 0.77–1.13) and in another review [55,56]. The regional resection, including standard portal vein and mesenteric artery resection, did not lead to prolonged survival and therefore should be abandoned. Today the indication for total pancreatectomy is limited to patients who have extensive IPMN.

A pancreatic corpus-and-tail resection should be performed for lesions in the corpus and tail. Currently there is a trend to perform an extended tail resection, the radical antegrade pancreatosplenectomy [57,58]. Results of a European study on laparoscopic pancreatic resection showed that its role remains controversial and probably is limited to benign lesions [59].

Reconstruction after resection

The most life-threatening complication after resection is leakage of the pancreaticoenteric anastomosis, and this complication might be related to the type of reconstruction, which generally is performed by a pancreaticojejunostomy or pancreaticogastrostomy. The pancreaticogastrostomy became popular in France, and retrospective studies have suggested that the leakage rate is lower after pancreaticogastrostomy than after pancreaticojejunostomy [60]. Randomized, controlled trials from the same center and from Italy comparing pancreaticojejunostomy and pancreaticogastrostomy showed no difference in mortality and leakage rate, however [61,62]. In a systematic analysis of 13 nonrandomized observational studies, the rate of pancreatic fistula was significantly lower for pancreaticogastrostomy than for pancreaticojejunostomy (3.7% versus 16.5%, respectively), but the meta-analysis of three randomized, controlled trials showed no difference in the fistula rate (13.8% versus 15.8%, respectively), clearly showing that patient selection and local experience might play a role [63].

Another meta-analysis combining all these randomized, controlled trials and large cohort studies found that pancreaticogastrostomy was safer [64]. The methodologic flaws of this meta-analysis have been discussed extensively, and it has been suggested that attention should be paid to the randomized, controlled trials showing no difference and that pancreatic surgeons should use the technique with which they are familiar [65].

A recent randomized, controlled trial from China comparing the standard pancreaticojejunostomy with a new binding pancreaticojejunostomy showed no leakage in the 106 patients randomly assigned to the binding technique [66]. These excellent results have to be confirmed in other studies.

Perioperative somatostatin and analogues or probiotics

The role of somatostatin and its analogues in reducing postoperative complications after pancreatic surgery has been discussed for more than a decade. Trials have been performed in many European countries, and outcomes have ranged from a reduction in overall complications and a reduction in mortality to no difference in outcome [67–70]. It has been suggested that these differences might result in part from patient selection (eg, risk factors for leakage; the inclusion of pancreatic versus ampullary tumors) and from the experience level of the participating centers. In a meta-analysis summarizing 10 trials, somatostatin did not reduce overall mortality (odds ratio, 1.17; 95% CI, 0.70–1.94) but did reduce pancreatic-specific complications (odds ratio, 0.56; 95% CI, 0.39–0.81; $P = .002$) [71]. Currently the authors use somatostatin only in patients at high risk for leakage (eg, patients who have a soft pancreas and patients without pancreatic duct dilatation). A recent study did show that selective administration of octreotide had clinical and cost benefits in high-risk glands [72].

A small randomized, controlled trial evaluated the early administration of enteral nutrition with a combination of different lactobacilli and showed a reduction of bacterial infections from 40% (in controls) to 12.5% [73]. Prophylactic treatment with probiotics might have a role in preventing surgical infection, but more evidence is needed before routine use is advocated [74].

Management of complications

Classification

Pancreatic surgery has advanced considerably during the past decades, but morbidity is still substantial, and complications are reported in 30% to 60% of patients, depending on the definition used. In 1988, Trede and Schwall [75] published a landmark paper on the management of the most important complications (ie, postoperative hemorrhage and anastomotic leakage). Although the clinical symptoms have not changed during the past decades, the management of these complications has moved from extended surgical procedures to less invasive radiologic intervention. Comparison of reported series on management of complications is difficult because of the differences in definitions used. Therefore an International Study Group on Pancreatic Surgery, including a number of European centers, introduced a system of well-defined definitions for pancreatic fistula and leakage, postoperative hemorrhage, and delayed gastric emptying [76–78].

Because the definition also includes limited, nonspecific, and often clinically irrelevant complications, a grading system (A, B, and C) has been introduced to indicate the clinical relevance and management. The comment, "It is a consensus we cannot ignore," is hopeful, but these systems still must be validated in daily practice [79,80]. Others have proposed a system for grading the severity of complications according to the clinical management, and this system was validated recently in a cohort of patients from Johns Hopkins [81,82].

Pancreatic leakage

The pancreatoenteric anastomosis is the Achilles' heel of the operation. The rate of leakage/fistula is reported to range from 2% to more than 20% and is related to the type of tumor (ampullary and duodenal tumors versus pancreatic cancer), the duct size, the pancreas consistency, the use of routine drainage after surgery, and, probably most important, the experience of the surgeon. Especially when sepsis is limited, leakage generally is treated successfully by percutaneous drainage of the collection or through the drain placed near the anastomosis during surgery. If a clinical deterioration occurs, however, relaparotomy must be performed, and one must choose surgical drainage, disconnection of the anastomosis combined with drainage of the pancreatic duct, or completion pancreatectomy [83]. The authors reported a series showing that completion pancreatectomy in an early phase after resection was associated with low mortality (zero), but the procedure, of course, results in insulin-dependent diabetes mellitus [84]. A new alternative, preservation of a small remnant (3–4 cm tail) to prevent brittle diabetes, was associated with higher morbidity and mortality [84].

At the same time others reported a series with a low leakage rate and suggested that completion pancreatectomy was no longer useful. Recently, however, the same group concluded that completion pancreatectomy is indicated for patients who have severe leakage/sepsis, clinical deterioration, or hemorrhage [85,86].

Hemorrhage

The incidence of postoperative hemorrhage varies widely, from 1% to 6%. For patients who have a delayed (massive) hemorrhage, a "sentinel bleed" often is found, particularly in patients who have a septic complication. A sentinel bleed absolutely requires urgent investigation and treatment. For hemodynamically stable patients, a contrast CT scan should be performed to confirm the pseudoaneurysm. The next step is angiography to perform embolization (in the splenic artery) or stenting (in a branch of the hepatic artery) [87–89]. Despite general acceptance of embolization, most patients still need urgent surgical intervention. Even after successful embolization, adequate management of intra-abdominal collections is crucial to prevent recurrent bleeding. The overall mortality for delayed hemorrhage is reported to be as high as 40%.

Delayed gastric emptying

Although not fatal, delayed gastric emptying has a major clinical impact because it has been reported in 14% to 60% of patients and increases hospital stay extensively. Fortunately in more recent studies the rate of delayed gastric emptying was reduced to less than 20%. It has been shown to be related to intra-abdominal infections but not to the type of resection (pylorus-preserving versus standard Whipple procedure) [47,48]. A number of studies supported the routine use of prokinetic drugs such as erythromycin [90]. Recently a study from Germany and a randomized, controlled trial from Japan showed that the type of reconstruction is important: there was a lower incidence of delayed gastric emptying after an antecolic reconstruction than after a retrocolic reconstruction [91,92].

Hospital volume and mortality

Numerous studies have shown that the postoperative mortality rate of pancreatic surgery is lower in high-volume centers than in low-volume centers [93,94]. This volume–outcome effect has underlined the importance of centralization. Although not generally accepted in the rest of the world, most states in the United States do centralize successfully. In European countries centralization has been discussed more recently. The first studies that plead for centralization were received with reluctance [95–97]. During the past years many European countries analyzed this volume–mortality relationship using national databases, and all showed this positive correlation [95–100]. The scientific validity of these publications is questioned, however, because they should reflect selection bias, being based on data from large academic centers, single states, or selected patients.

Two systematic reviews of the data from independent national routine health registries on hospital volume and mortality showed convincing evidence of an inverse relationship between hospital volume and mortality [101,102]. A study reporting on a 10-year ongoing plea for centralization among the surgical community in The Netherlands did not show a reduction of the mortality rate after pancreatic resection or a change in the referral pattern [101]. Currently other methods, such as reimbursement strategies by the government or health insurance companies and the introduction of performance indicators, are being introduced to achieve this centralization.

Neoadjuvant and adjuvant treatment

The prognosis of patients who have pancreatic cancer is poor, even in the selected group of patients who undergo resection [7,8]. Adjuvant therapy by chemoradiotherapy therefore has been investigated in a number of clinical trials, with conflicting results. In a study by the Gastrointestinal Tumor Study Group, chemoradiotherapy after resection was compared with resection alone. This trial was closed early because of better survival observed in the arm with adjuvant chemoradiotherapy [103]. Adjuvant chemoradiotherapy was considered for many years as the standard of care after resection of pancreatic carcinoma in the United States. In the European Organization for Research and Treatment of Cancer study, a nonsignificant advantage of postoperative chemoradiotherapy was suggested after short-term follow-up and subgroup analysis for pancreatic cancer [104]. The long-term results, however, did not show any benefit for chemoradiation [105]. The results of the European Study Group for Pancreatic Cancer-1 trial showed a survival benefit for patients treated with adjuvant chemotherapy (5-fluorouracil [5-FU]/leucovorin) versus no chemotherapy (20.1 months versus 15.5 months, respectively) [106]. Chemoradiotherapy did not have any benefit on survival in this study. Another randomized, controlled trial comparing gemcitabine versus observation showed a median disease-free survival of 13.4 months versus 6.9 months, respectively. Improvement was seen in all subgroups, including patients who had microscopic nonradical resections (R1) and R0 resections. There was no significant difference in overall survival between the gemcitabine and the control group [107]. Because of the relatively favorable results of adjuvant chemotherapy in both European studies, this treatment option should be considered after resection in all patients who have pancreatic carcinoma, as suggested in a recent review and meta-analysis of adjuvant strategies for pancreatic cancer [108,109].

Palliative treatment

Unfortunately, most patients who have pancreatic cancer (approximately 80%) will have palliative treatment. Therefore palliation of symptoms still is the major focus in improving outcome of patients. The decision to aim for palliative treatment/surgery can be made at two different time points during the disease. The first decision generally is made after the staging procedures; the choice must be made to undertake potentially curative surgery, palliative surgery, or nonsurgical (endoscopic) palliation. A second step in the selection of treatment is made during surgery and can involve attempt at a resection with curative intent (R0 resection), a resection for optimal palliation (R1 resection), or other surgical procedures for palliative treatment.

The three most important symptoms that should be treated to improve quality of life in advanced pancreatic cancer are obstructive jaundice, duodenal obstruction, and pain [110]. Obstructive jaundice is found in 70% to 90% of patients, and relief of the obstructive jaundice dramatically improves the patient's quality of life. Biliary drainage can be achieved nonsurgically by endoscopic or percutaneous placement of a biliary stent or surgically by performing a biliary bypass [110,111]. Four prospective, randomized, controlled trials have been performed, three of which compared surgical biliary drainage and endoscopic drainage [112–115]. The success rate for short-term relief of biliary obstruction is comparable for surgical and nonsurgical drainage procedures and ranges between 80% and 100%.

Surgical treatment is associated with higher initial morbidity, longer hospital stay, and probably higher initial mortality, but long-term results are better. Endoscopic treatment is associated with a lower initial mortality and morbidity but more frequently leads to late biliary complications and reinterventions caused by clotting of the stent, infection, and gastric outlet obstruction. Therefore surgical palliation should be preferred in relatively fit patients who are expected to survive for more than 6 months [116]. A surgical bypass can be performed by a hepaticojejunostomy alone or a by double bypass, including a gastroenterostomy.

From two randomized, controlled trials it might be concluded that a prophylactic gastrojejunostomy is preferable to a biliary bypass alone, because of the significantly reduced risk of late gastric outlet obstruction and the low morbidity and mortality rates [117,118]. In the authors' study, none of the patients who received a gastrojejunostomy developed late gastric outlet obstruction during follow-up, compared with 19% of patients who did not undergo a gastrojejunostomy in the initial procedure [118]. Endoscopic duodenal stenting now has been accepted as an alternative nonsurgical palliative treatment [119]. Combined endoscopic biliary and duodenal stenting is successful in more than 80% of patients in allowing toleration of soft solids or a full diet [120,121]. Therefore the debate whether prophylactic gastrojejunostomy should be performed remains of interest.

At the time of diagnosis, approximately 40% to 80% of patients already report pain.

Pain management should be pharmacologic and consists of analgesics such as nonsteroidal anti-inflammatory drugs and oral or transdermal narcotic analgesics. The next step is a celiac plexus nerve block. Currently the celiac plexus block can be performed percutaneously, by endoscopic ultraso-nography, or during laparotomy [122–124]. Only a few randomized, con-trolled trials have compared percutaneous neurolytic celiac plexus blockade versus placebo, and the best evidence regarding prevention of pain comes from the recent study by Wong and colleagues [122]. The three different procedures never have been compared in a randomized, controlled trial. Although effective, bilateral splanchnicectomy is not used frequently in most centers.

Palliative resection

Several reports have discussed the indications for performing a pancreato-duodenectomy as a palliative treatment option. This controversial question results from the observation in recent literature that morbidity and mortal-ity rates after pancreatoduodenectomy are decreasing. Retrospectively, three studies investigated the role of a pancreatoduodenectomy for pallia-tion by comparing the outcomes of patients who had nonradical resections with the outcomes of patients who underwent a single or double bypass for a locally invasive tumor without metastases [125–127]. Survival is signifi-cantly longer after a palliative resection than after bypass. This difference probably reflects patient selection and the limited comparability of the two groups. The available data confirm that, when radical resectability is questionable, a resection can offer relatively good palliation, so in many cen-ters a more aggressive approach currently is advocated for patients who have a doubtful resectable tumor. Because of the relative safety of pancre-atic resection, an even more aggressive approach was adopted in Germany, and a highly selected group of patients who had metastases (liver, perito-neal, or M1 lymph nodes) underwent resection; the report suggested pallia-tion was adequate [44].

Palliative chemotherapy and radiotherapy

Several phase II studies have investigated the role of radiotherapy in non-metastatic, locally advanced pancreatic cancer. With modern conformal radiotherapy, high doses, up to 72 Gy, can be delivered without unaccept-able toxicity [128]. Although pain relief often is achieved, overall results usu-ally are disappointing. Median survival times are reported between 5.5 and 11 months. Combined chemoradiotherapy also has been investigated, and infusion of 5-FU in addition to radiotherapy is the most commonly used multimodality treatment. Recently the efficacy of gemcitabine, known to be a potent enhancer of tumor radioresponse in vitro, has been investigated. A real improvement in the results has not been observed with this combina-tion [129].

For metastatic pancreatic cancer, gemcitabine is considered the standard chemotherapy. Gemcitabine was superior to 5-FU in a randomized trial. It showed a modest gain in median overall survival: 5.7 versus 4.2 months

[130]. Moreover, the probability of 1-year survival was 18% with gemcitabine versus 2% with 5-FU, and a clinical benefit response of 24% was
reported for gemcitabine versus 5% for 5-FU. After this trial, several studies
were performed to improve the efficacy of gemcitabine by combining it with
other molecular alterations (eg, growth factor receptors, angiogenic factors,
and other signaling molecules). In a recent meta-analysis of 20 phase III trials involving 6296 patients, no significant difference was found in overall
survival (relative risk [RR], 0.93; 95% CI, 0.84–1.03). A slight improvement
was found in progression-free survival (RR, 0.91; 95% CI, 0.84–0.98) and
overall response rate (RR, 1.57; 95% CI, 1.17–1.94) [131]. Therefore gemcitabine remains the standard treatment.

The overall higher response rate, however, supports the hypothesis that
this new class of cancer drugs can earn a place in systemic pancreatic cancer
treatment in the future.

References

[1] Parkin DM, Bray F, Ferlay J, et al. Global cancer statistics 2002. CA Cancer J Clin 2005;55:
    74–108.
[2] Lowenfels AB, Maisonneuve P. Epidemiology and risk factors for pancreatic cancer. Best
    Pract Res Clin Gastroenterol 2006;20:197–209.
[3] Klein WM, Hruban RH, Klein-Szanto AJ, et al. Direct correlation between proliferative
    activity and dysplasia in pancreatic intraepithelial neoplasia (PanIN): additional evidence
    for a recently proposed model of progression. Mod Pathol 2002;15:441–7.
[4] Lochan R, Daly AK, Reeves HL, et al. Genetic susceptibility in pancreatic ductal
    adenocarcinoma. Br J Surg 2008;95:22–32.
[5] Ducreux M, Boige V, Goéré D, et al. Pancreatic cancer: from pathogenesis to cure. Best
    Pract Res Clin Gastroenterol 2007;21:997–1014.
[6] Vitone LJ, Greenhalf W, McFaul CD, et al. The inherited genetics of pancreatic cancer and
    prospects for secondary screening. Best Pract Res Clin Gastroenterol 2006;20:253–83.
[7] Gudjonsson B. Carcinoma of the pancreas: critical analysis of costs, results of resections,
    and the need for standardized reporting. J Am Coll Surg 1995;181:483–503.
[8] Kuhlmann KF, De Castro SM, Wessling JC, et al. Surgical treatment of pancreatic
    adenocarcinoma; actual survival and prognostic factors in 343 patients. Eur J Cancer
    2004;40:549–58.
[9] Trede M, Richter A, Wendl K. Personal observations, opinions, and approaches to cancer
    of the pancreas and the periampullary area. Surg Clin North Am 2001;81:595–610.
[10] Tilleman EH, Benraadt J, Bossuyt PM, et al. [Diagnosis and treatment of pancreatic
    carcinoma in the region of Amsterdam Comprehensive Cancer Care Center in 1997].
    Ned Tijdschr Geneeskd 2001;145:1358–62 [in Dutch].
[11] Michl P, Pauls S, Gress T. Evidence-based diagnosis and staging of pancreatic cancer. Best
    Pract Res Clin Gastroenterol 2006;20:227–51.
[12] Bipat S, Phoa SS, Van Delden OM, et al. Ultrasonography, computed tomography and
    magnetic resonance imaging for diagnosis and determining resectability of pancreatic
    adenocarcinoma: a meta-analysis. J Comput Assist Tomogr 2005;29:438–45.
[13] Van Gulik TM, Reeders JW, Bosma A, et al. Incidence and clinical findings of benign,
    inflammatory disease in patients resected for presumed pancreatic head cancer. Gastroint-
    est Endosc 1997;46:417–23.

[14] Garrow D, Miller S, Sinha D, et al. Endoscopic ultrasound: a meta-analysis of test performance in suspected biliary obstruction. Clin Gastroenterol Hepatol 2007;5: 616–23.

[15] Hunt GC, Faigel DO. Assessment of EUS for diagnosing, staging, and determining resectability of pancreatic cancer: a review. Gastrointest Endosc 2002;55:232–7.

[16] Zamboni GA, Kruskal JB, Vollmer CM, et al. Pancreatic adenocarcinoma: value of multidetector CT angiography in preoperative evaluation. Radiology 2007;245:770–8.

[17] Puli SR, Singh S, Hagedorn CH, et al. Diagnostic accuracy of EUS for vascular invasion in pancreatic and periampullary cancers: a meta-analysis and systematic review. Gastrointest Endosc 2007;65:788–97.

[18] Pakzad F, Groves AM, Ell PJ. The role of positron emission tomography in the management of pancreatic cancer. Semin Nucl Med 2006;36:248–56.

[19] Bemelman WA, De Wit LD, Van Delden OM, et al. Diagnostic laparoscopy combined with laparoscopic ultrasonography in staging of cancer of the pancreatic head region. Br J Surg 1995;82:820–4.

[20] Pisters PW, Lee JE, Vauthey JN, et al. Laparoscopy in the staging of pancreatic cancer. Br J Surg 2001;88:325–37.

[21] Nieveen van Dijkum EJ, de Wit LT, van Delden OM, et al. Staging laparoscopy and laparoscopic ultrasonography in more than 400 patients with upper gastrointestinal carcinoma. J Am Coll Surg 1999;189:459–65.

[22] Nieveen van Dijkum EJ, Romijn MG, Terwee CB, et al. Laparoscopic staging and subsequent palliation in patients with peripancreatic carcinoma. Ann Surg 2003;237:66–73.

[23] Tilleman EH, Kuiken BW, Phoa SS, et al. Limitation of diagnostic laparoscopy for patients with a periampullary carcinoma. Eur J Surg 2004;30:658–62.

[24] Tilleman EH, Busch OR, Bemelman WA, et al. Diagnostic laparoscopy in staging pancreatic carcinoma: developments during the past decade. J Hepatobiliary Pancreat Surg 2004; 11:11–6.

[25] Whipple AO, Parsons WB, Mullins CR. Treatment of carcinoma of the ampulla of Vater. Ann Surg 1935;102:763–79.

[26] Gouma DJ, Coelho JC, Fisher JD, et al. Endotoxemia after relief of biliary obstruction by internal and external drainage in rats. Am J Surg 1986;151:476–9.

[27] Gouma DJ, Coelho JC, Schlegel JF, et al. The effect of preoperative internal and external biliary drainage on mortality of jaundiced rats. Arch Surg 1987;122:731–4.

[28] Bemelmans MH, Gouma DJ, Greve JW, et al. Effect of antitumour necrosis factor treatment on circulating tumour necrosis factor levels and mortality after surgery in jaundiced mice. Br J Surg 1993;80:1055–8.

[29] Kimmings AN, van Deventer SJ, Obertop H, et al. Endotoxin, cytokines, and endotoxin binding proteins in obstructive jaundice and after preoperative biliary drainage. Gut 2000;46:725–31.

[30] Kimmings N, Sewnath ME, Mairuhu WM, et al. The abnormal lipid spectrum in malignant obstructive jaundice in relation to endotoxin sensitivity and the result of preoperative biliary drainage. Surgery 2001;129:282–91.

[31] McPherson GA, Benjamin IS, Hodgson HJ, et al. Pre-operative percutaneous transhepatic biliary drainage: the results of a controlled trial. Br J Surg 1984;71:371–5.

[32] Pitt HA, Gomes AS, Lois JF, et al. Does preoperative percutaneous biliary drainage reduce operative risk or increase hospital cost? Ann Surg 1985;201:545–53.

[33] Hatfield AR, Tobias R, Terblanche J, et al. Preoperative external biliary drainage in obstructive jaundice. A prospective controlled clinical trial. Lancet 1982;2:896–9.

[34] Sewnath ME, Birjmohun RS, Rauws EA, et al. The effect of preoperative biliary drainage on postoperative complications after pancreaticoduodenectomy. J Am Coll Surg 2001;192: 726–34.

[35] Sohn TA, Yeo CJ, Cameron JL, et al. Do preoperative stents increase postpancreaticoduodenectomy complications? J Gastrointest Surg 2000;4:258–67.

[36] Povoski SP, Karpeh MS Jr, Conlon KC, et al. Association of preoperative biliary drainage with postoperative outcome following pancreaticoduodenectomy. Ann Surg 1999;230: 131–42.

[37] Sewnath ME, Karsten TM, Prins MH, et al. A meta-analysis on the efficacy of preoperative biliary drainage for tumours causing obstructive jaundice. Ann Surg 2002;236: 17–27.

[38] Van der Gaag NA, de Castro SM, Rauws EA, et al. Preoperative biliary drainage for periampullary tumors causing obstructive jaundice; DRainage vs. (direct) OPeration (DROP-trial). BMC Surg 2007;7:3.

[39] Michalski CW, Kleeff J, Bachmann J, et al. Second-look operation for unresectable pancreatic ductal adenocarcinoma at a high-volume center. Ann Surg Oncol 2008;15: 186–92.

[40] Siriwardana HP, Siriwardena AK. Systematic review of outcome of synchronous portal-superior mesenteric vein resection during pancreatectomy for cancer. Br J Surg 2006;93: 662–73 [review].

[41] Van Geenen RC, Ten Kate FJ, De Wit LT, et al. Segmental resection and wedge excision of the portal or superior mesenteric vein during pancreatoduodenectomy. Surgery 2001;129: 158–63.

[42] Phoa SS, Tilleman EH, Van Delden OM, et al. Value of CT criteria in predicting survival in patients with potentially resectable pancreatic head carcinoma. J Surg Oncol 2005;91: 33–40.

[43] Phoa SS, Reeders JW, Stoker J, et al. CT criteria for venous invasion in patients with pancreatic head carcinoma. Br J Radiol 2000;73:1159–64.

[44] Shrikhande SV, Kleeff J, Reiser C, et al. Pancreatic resection for M1 pancreatic ductal adenocarcinoma. Ann Surg Oncol 2007;14:118–27.

[45] Kleeff J, Reiser C, Hinz U, et al. Surgery for recurrent pancreatic ductal adenocarcinoma. Ann Surg 2007;245:566–72.

[46] Pedrazzoli S, Beger H, Obertop H, et al. A surgical and pathological based classification of resection of pancreatic cancer: summary of an international workshop on surgical procedures in pancreatic cancer. Dig Surg 1999;16:337–45.

[47] Tran KT, Smeenk HG, Van Eijck CH, et al. Pylorus preserving pancreaticoduodenectomy versus standard Whipple procedure: a prospective, randomized, multicenter analysis of 170 patients with pancreatic and periampullary tumors. Ann Surg 2004;240:738–45.

[48] Seiler CA, Wagner M, Bachmann T, et al. Randomized clinical trial of pylorus-preserving duodenopancreatectomy versus classical Whipple resection-long term results. Br J Surg 2005;92:547–56.

[49] Diener MK, Knaebel HP, Heukaufer C, et al. A systematic review and meta-analysis of pylorus-preserving versus classical pancreaticoduodenectomy for surgical treatment of periampullary and pancreatic carcinoma. Ann Surg 2007;245:187–200.

[50] Pedrazzoli S, DiCarlo V, Dionigi R, et al. Standard versus extended lymphadenectomy associated with pancreatoduodenectomy in the surgical treatment of adenocarcinoma of the head of the pancreas: a multicenter, prospective, randomized study. Lymphadenectomy Study Group. Ann Surg 1998;228:508–17.

[51] Farnell MB, Pearson RK, Sarr MG, et al. A prospective randomized trial comparing standard pancreatoduodenectomy with pancreatoduodenectomy with extended lymphadenectomy in resectable pancreatic head adenocarcinoma. Surgery 2005;138:618–28 [discussion: 628–30].

[52] Yeo CJ, Cameron JL, Sohn TA, et al. Pancreaticoduodenectomy with or without extended retroperitoneal lymphadenectomy for periampullary adenocarcinoma: comparison of morbidity and mortality and short-term outcome. Ann Surg 1999;229:613–22 [discussion: 622–4].

[53] Yeo CJ, Cameron JL, Lillemoe KD, et al. Pancreaticoduodenectomy with or without distal gastrectomy and extended retroperitoneal lymphadenectomy for periampullary

adenocarcinoma, part 2: randomized controlled trial evaluating survival, morbidity, and mortality. Ann Surg 2002;236:355–66 [discussion: 366–8].

[54] Nimura Y, Nagino M, Kato H, et al. Regional versus extended lymph node dissection in radical pancreaticoduodenectomy for pancreatic cancer: a multicenter, randomized controlled trial. HPB 2004;6:2.

[55] Michalski CW, Kleeff J, Wente MN, et al. Systematic review and meta-analysis of standard and extended lymphadenectomy in pancreaticoduodenectomy for pancreatic cancer. Br J Surg 2007;94:265–73.

[56] Farnell MB, Aranha GV, Nimura Y, et al. The role of extended lymphadenectomy for adenocarcinoma of the head of the pancreas: strength of the evidence. J Gastrointest Surg 2008;134:706–15.

[57] Strasberg SM, Drebin JA, Linehan D. Radical antegrade modular pancreatosplenectomy. Surgery 2003;133:521–7.

[58] Shimada K, Sakamoto Y, Sano T, et al. Prognostic factors after distal pancreatectomy with extended lymphadenectomy for invasive pancreatic adenocarcinoma of the body and tail. Surgery 2006;139:288–95.

[59] Mabrut JY, Fernandez-Cruz L, Azagra JS, et al. Hepatobiliary and Pancreatic Section (HBPS) of the Royal Belgian Society of Surgery; Belgian Group for Endoscopic Surgery (BGES); Club Coelio. Laparoscopic pancreatic resection: results of a multicenter European study of 127 patients. Surgery 2005;137:597–605.

[60] Oussoultzoglou E, Bachellier P, Bigourdan JM, et al. Pancreaticogastrostomy decreased relaparotomy caused by pancreatic fistula after pancreaticoduodenectomy compared with pancreaticojejunostomy. Arch Surg 2004;139:327–35.

[61] Duffas JP, Suc B, Msika S, et al. French Associations for Research in Surgery. A controlled randomized multicenter trial of pancreatogastrostomy or pancreatojejunostomy after pancreatoduodenectomy. Am J Surg 2005;189:720–9.

[62] Bassi C, Falconi M, Molinari E, et al. Reconstruction by pancreaticojejunostomy versus pancreaticogastrostomy following pancreatectomy: results of a comparative study. Ann Surg 2005;242:767–71 [discussion: 771–3].

[63] Wente MN, Shrikhande SV, Müller MW, et al. Pancreaticojejunostomy versus pancreaticogastrostomy: systematic review and meta-analysis. Am J Surg 2007;193:171–83 [review].

[64] McKay A, Mackenzie S, Sutherland FR, et al. Meta-analysis of pancreaticojejunostomy versus pancreaticogastrostomy reconstruction after pancreaticoduodenectomy. Br J Surg 2006;93:929–36 [review].

[65] Dixon E, Fingerhut A, Bassi C, et al. Meta-analysis of pancreaticojejunostomy versus pancreaticogastrostomy reconstruction after pancreaticoduodenectomy. Br J Surg 2006; 93:1435 [authors' comment Br J Surg 2006; 93:929–36].

[66] Peng SY, Wang JW, Lau WY, et al. Conventional versus binding pancreaticojejunostomy after pancreaticoduodenectomy: a prospective randomized trial. Ann Surg 2007;245: 692–8.

[67] Büchler M, Friess H, Klempa I, et al. Role of octreotide in the prevention of postoperative complications following pancreatic resection. Am J Surg 1992;163:125–30 [discussion: 130–1].

[68] Pederzoli P, Bassi C, Falconi M. et al, and the Italian Study Group. Efficacy of octreotide in the prevention of complications of elective pancreatic surgery. Br J Surg 1994;81:265–9.

[69] Gouillat C, Chipponi J, Baulieux J, et al. Randomized controlled multicentre trial of somatostatin infusion after pancreaticoduodenectomy. Br J Surg 2001;88:1456–62.

[70] Suc B, Msika S, Piccinini M, et al. Octreotide in the prevention of intra-abdominal complications following elective pancreatic resection: a prospective multicenter randomized controlled trial. Arch Surg 2004;139:288–94.

[71] Connor S, Alexakis N, Garden OJ, et al. Meta-analysis of the value of somatostatin and its analogues in reducing complications associated with pancreatic surgery. Br J Surg 2005;92: 1059–67.

[72] Vanounou T, Pratt WB, Callery MP, et al. Selective administration of prophylactic octreotide during pancreaticoduodenectomy: a clinical and cost-benefit analysis in low- and high-risk glands. J Am Coll Surg 2007;205:546–57.

[73] Rayes N, Seehofer D, Theruvath T, et al. Effect of enteral nutrition and synbiotics on bacterial infection rates after pylorus-preserving pancreatoduodenectomy: a randomized, double-blind trial. Ann Surg 2007;246:36–41.

[74] Van Santvoort HC, Besselink MG, Timmerman HM, et al. Probiotics in surgery. Surgery 2008;143:1–7 [review].

[75] Trede M, Schwall G. The complications of pancreatectomy. Ann Surg 1988;207:39–47.

[76] Bassi C, Dervenis C, Butterini G, et al. Postoperative pancreatic fistula: an International Study Group on Pancreatic Fistula definition. Surgery 2005;138:8–13.

[77] Wente MN, Veit JA, Bassi C, et al. Postpancreatectomy hemorrhage (PPH): an International Study Group of Pancreatic Surgery (ISGPS) definition. Surgery 2007;142:20–5.

[78] Wente MN, Bassi C, Dervenis C, et al. Delayed gastric emptying (DGE) after pancreatic surgery: a suggested definition by the International Study Group of Pancreatic Surgery (ISGPS). Surgery 2007;142:761–8.

[79] Fernández-del Castillo C. Consensus defining postpancreatectomy complications: an opportunity we cannot ignore. Surgery 2007;142:771–2.

[80] Pratt WB, Callery MP, Vollmer CM Jr. Risk prediction for development of pancreatic fistula using the ISGPF classification scheme. World J Surg 2008;32:419–28.

[81] Strasberg SM, Linehan DC, Clavien PA, et al. Proposal for definition and severity grading of pancreatic anastomosis failure and pancreatic occlusion failure. Surgery 2007;141:420–6.

[82] DeOliveira ML, Winter JM, Schafer M, et al. Assessment of complications after pancreatic surgery: A novel grading system applied to 633 patients undergoing pancreaticoduodenectomy. Ann Surg 2006;244:931–7 [discussion: 937–9].

[83] Van Berge Henegouwen MI, De Wit LT, Van Gulik TM, et al. Incidence, risk factors, and treatment of pancreatic leakage after pancreaticoduodenectomy: drainage versus resection of the pancreatic remnant. J Am Coll Surg 1997;185:18–24.

[84] De Castro SM, Busch OR, Van Gulik TM, et al. Incidence and management of pancreatic leakage after pancreatoduodenectomy. Br J Surg 2005;92:1117–23.

[85] Büchler MW, Wagner M, Schmied BM, et al. Changes in morbidity after pancreatic resection: toward the end of completion pancreatectomy. Arch Surg 2003;138:1310–4 [discussion: 1315].

[86] Muller MW, Friess H, Kleeff J, et al. Is there still a role for total pancreatectomy. Ann Surg 2007;246:966–74 [discussion: 974–6].

[87] De Castro SM, Kuhlmann KF, Busch OR, et al. Delayed massive hemorrhage after pancreatic and biliary surgery: embolization or surgery? Ann Surg 2005;241:85–91 [Comment in: Ann Surg 2006;243:138–9; author reply 139].

[88] Heiss P, Bachthaler M, Hamer OW, et al. Delayed visceral arterial hemorrhage following Whipple's procedure: minimally invasive treatment with covered stents. Ann Surg Oncol 2008;15:824–32.

[89] Yekebas EF, Wolfram L, Cataldegirmen G, et al. Postpancreatectomy hemorrhage: diagnosis and treatment: an analysis in 1669 consecutive pancreatic resections. Ann Surg 2007;246:269–80.

[90] Lytras D, Paraskevas KI, Avgerinos C, et al. Therapeutic strategies for the management of delayed gastric emptying after pancreatic resection. Langenbecks Arch Surg 2007;392:1–12 [Epub Oct 5, 2006. Review].

[91] Hartel M, Wente MN, Hinz U, et al. Effect of antecolic reconstruction on delayed gastric emptying after the pylorus-preserving Whipple procedure. Arch Surg 2005;140:1094–9.

[92] Tani M, Terasawa H, Kawai M, et al. Improvement of delayed gastric emptying in pylorus-preserving pancreaticoduodenectomy: results of a prospective, randomized, controlled trial. Ann Surg 2006;243:316–20.

[93] Lieberman MD, Kilburn H, Lindsey M, et al. Relation of perioperative deaths to hospital volume among patients undergoing pancreatic resection for malignancy. Ann Surg 1995; 222:638–45.

[94] Birkmeyer JD, Siewers AE, Finlayson EV, et al. Hospital volume and surgical mortality in the United States. N Engl J Med 2002;346:1128–37.

[95] Gouma DJ, De Wit LT, Van Berge Henegouwen MI, et al. (Hospital experience and hospital mortality following partial pancreaticoduodenectomy in The Netherlands). Ned Tijdschr Geneeskd 1997;141:1738–41 [in Dutch].

[96] Gouma DJ, Van Geenen RC, Van Gulik TM, et al. Rates of complications and death after pancreaticoduodenectomy: risk factors and the impact of hospital volume. Ann Surg 2000; 232:786–95.

[97] Nordback L, Parviainen M, Räty S, et al. Resection of the head of the pancreas in Finland: effects of hospital and surgeon on short-term and long-term results. Scand J Gastroenterol 2002;37:1454–60.

[98] Roeder N, Wenke A, Heumann M, et al. (Volume outcome relationship: consequences of reallocation of minimum volume based on current German surgical regulations). Chirurg 2007;78:1018–27 [in German].

[99] Topal B, Van de Sande S, Fieuws S, et al. Effect of centralization of pancreaticoduodenectomy on nationwide hospital mortality and length of stay. Br J Surg 2007;94:1377–81.

[100] Balzano G, Zerbi A, Capretti G, et al. Effect of hospital volume on outcome of pancreaticoduodenectomy in Italy. Br J Surg 2008;95:357–62.

[101] Van Heek NT, Kuhlmann KF, Scholten RJ, et al. Hospital volume and mortality after pancreatic resection: a systematic review and an evaluation of intervention in The Netherlands. Ann Surg 2005;242:781–8 [discussion: 788–90].

[102] Chowdhury MM, Dagash H, Pierro A. A systematic review of the impact of volume of surgery and specialization on patient outcome. Br J Surg 2007;94:145–61 [review].

[103] Gastrointestinal Tumor Study Group. Further evidence of effective adjuvant combined radiation and chemotherapy following curative resection of pancreatic cancer. Cancer 1987;59:2006–10.

[104] Klinkenbijl JH, Jeekel J, Sahmoud T, et al. Adjuvant radiotherapy and 5-fluorouracil after curative resection of cancer of the pancreas and periampullary region. Phase III trial of the EORTC GITCCG. Ann Surg 1999;230:776–84.

[105] Smeenk HG, van Eijck CH, Hop WC, et al. Long-term survival and metastatic pattern of pancreatic and periampullary cancer after adjuvant chemoradiation or observation: long-term results of EORTC trial 40891. Ann Surg 2007;246:734–40.

[106] Neoptolemos JP, Stocken DD, Friess H, et al. A randomized trial of chemoradiotherapy and chemotherapy after resection of pancreatic cancer. N Engl J Med 2004;350:1200–10.

[107] Oettle H, Post S, Neuhaus P, et al. Adjuvant chemotherapy with gemcitabine vs observation in patients undergoing curative-intent resection of pancreatic cancer: a randomized controlled trial. JAMA 2007;297:267–77.

[108] Ghaneh P, Smith R, Tudor-Smith C, et al. Neoadjuvant and adjuvant strategies for pancreatic cancer. Eur J Surg Oncol 2008;34:297–305.

[109] Boeck S, Ankerst DP, Heinemann V. The role of adjuvant chemotherapy for patients with resected pancreatic cancer: systematic review of randomized controlled trials and meta-analysis. Oncology 2008;72:314–21.

[110] Nieveen van Dijkum EJ, Kuhlmann KF, Terwee CB, et al. Quality of life after curative or palliative surgical treatment of pancreatic and periampullary carcinoma. Br J Surg 2005;92: 471–7.

[111] Davids PH, Groen AK, Rauws EA, et al. Randomised trial of self expanding metal stents versus polyethylene stents for distal malignant biliary obstruction. Lancet 1992;340:1488–92.

[112] Bornmann PC, Harries-Jones EP, Tobias R, et al. Prospective controlled trial of transhepatic biliary endoprosthesis versus bypass surgery for incurable carcinoma of head of pancreas. Lancet 1986;1:69–71.

[113] Shepherd HA, Royle G, Ross AP, et al. Endoscopic biliary endoprosthesis in the palliation of malignant obstruction of the distal common bile duct: a randomized trial. Br J Surg 1988; 75:1166–8.

[114] Andersen JR, Sorensen SM, Kruse A, et al. Randomised trial of endoscopic endoprosthesis versus operative bypass in malignant obstructive jaundice. Gut 1989;30:1132–5.

[115] Smith AC, Dowsett JF, Russell RC, et al. Randomised trial of endoscopic stenting versus surgical bypass in malignant low bile duct obstruction. Lancet 1994;344:1655–60.

[116] Müller MW, Friess H, Köninger J, et al. Factors influencing survival after bypass procedures in patients with advanced pancreatic adenocarcinomas. Am J Surg 2008;195:221–8.

[117] Lillemoe KD, Cameron JL, Hardacre JM, et al. Is prophylactic gastrojejunostomy indicated for unresectable periampullary cancer? A prospective randomized trial. Ann Surg 1999;230:322–8.

[118] vanHeek NT, de Castro SM, van Eijck CH, et al. The need for a prophylactic gastrojejunostomy for unresectable periampullary cancer: a prospective randomized multicenter trial with special focus on assessment of quality of life. Ann Surg 2003;238:894–902.

[119] Telford Jj, carrlock DL, Baron TH, et al. Palliation of patients with malignant gastric outlet obstruction with the enteral Wallstent: outcomes of a multicenter study. Gastrointest Endosc 2004;60:916–20.

[120] Multignami N, Tringali A, Shah SG, et al. Combined endoscopic stent insertion in malignant biliary and duodenal obstruction. Endoscopy 2007;39:440–7.

[121] Graber I, Dumas R, Filoche B, et al. The efficacy and safety of duodenal stenting: a prospective multicenter study. Endoscopy 2007;39:784–8.

[122] Wong GY, Schroeder DR, Corns PE, et al. Effect of neurolytic celiac plexus block on pain relief, quality of life, and survival in patients with unresectable pancreatic cancer: a randomized controlled trial. JAMA 2004;291:1092–9.

[123] Lillemoe KD, Cameron JL, Kaufman HS, et al. Chemical splanchnicectomy in patients with unresectable pancreatic cancer. A prospective randomized trial. Ann Surg 1993;217:447–55.

[124] Michaels A, Dragnov PV. Endoscopic ultrasonography guided celiac plexus neurolysis. World J Gastroenterol 2007;13:3575–80 [review].

[125] Reinders ME, Allema JH, van Gulik TM, et al. Outcome of microscopically nonradical, subtotal pancreaticoduodenectomy (Whipple's resection) for treatment of pancreatic head tumors. World J Surg 1995;19:410–4 [discussion: 414–5].

[126] Lillemoe KD, Cameron JL, Yeo CJ, et al. Pancreaticoduodenectomy. Does it have a role in the palliation of pancreatic cancer? Ann Surg 1996;223:718–25.

[127] Kuhlmann K, de Castro S, van Heek T, et al. Microscopically incomplete resection offers acceptable palliation in pancreatic cancer. Surgery 2006;139:188–96.

[128] Ceha HM, Van Tienhoven G, Gouma DJ, et al. Feasibility and efficacy of high dose conformal radiotherapy for locally advanced pancreatic cancer. Cancer 2000;89:2222–9.

[129] De Lange SM, Van Groeningen CJ, Meijer OW, et al. Gemcitabine-radiotherapy in patients with locally advanced pancreatic cancer. Eur J Cancer 2002;38:1212–7.

[130] Burris HA III, Moore MJ, Andersen J, et al. Improvements in survival and clinical benefit with gemcitabine as first-line therapy for patients with advanced pancreas cancer: a randomized trial. J Clin Oncol 1997;15:2403–13.

[131] Bria E, Milella M, Gelibter A, et al. Gemcitabine-based combinations for inoperable pancreatic cancer: have we made real progress? A meta-analysis of 20 phase 3 trials. Cancer 2007;110:525–33.

ELSEVIER
SAUNDERS

Surg Oncol Clin N Am
17 (2008) 587–606

SURGICAL
ONCOLOGY CLINICS
OF NORTH AMERICA

Intraductal Papillary Mucinous Neoplasms of the Pancreas: Indication, Extent, and Results of Surgery

Alain Sauvanet, MD

Service de Chirurgie Digestive, Hôpital Beaujon, Université Paris VII, AP-HP,
100 Bd du Général Leclerc, 92118 Clichy-Cedex, France

Although recognized before the 1980s [1], intraductal and papillary mucinous neoplasm (IPMN) of the pancreas was first described as a distinct entity in 1982 [2] and since then has become an important surgical topic. Today it is fully accepted that IPMN is a precursor of pancreatic adenocarcinoma and involves successive stages of dysplasia, as described in the World Health Organization (WHO) classification of pancreatic neoplasms [3,4]. To date, pancreatic resection before occurrence of invasive carcinoma is the only treatment avoiding the disastrous prognosis of the latter condition. Conversely, long-term prognosis after pancreatic resections for noninvasive IPMN is good, so the indications for pancreatic surgery have increased to prevent adenocarcinoma [5,6]. Even if pancreatic resections are associated with a very low mortality today, they still carry an important morbidity of up to 50% [7–10]. Furthermore, IPMN is observed mainly in the seventh decade, so indications for "preventive" surgery can be difficult to determine, especially in patients carrying a significant surgical risk [5]. IPMN also has emerged as an indication for uncommon techniques of pancreatic resection, including total pancreatectomy and limited resection (enucleation, resection of the ventral pancreas, or medial pancreatectomy) [9,11,12], thus giving the pancreatic surgeon a wider armamentarium than possible for other indications.

The aims of surgery differ according to the presence of malignancy. For malignant IPMN and especially for invasive malignancy, radical resection is essential but entails a substantial operative risk and long-term pancreatic insufficiency. For benign IPMN, in theory, the operative risk and the loss of pancreatic function should be minimal. Thus, surgery for malignant and

E-mail address: alain.sauvanet@bjn.ap-hop-paris.fr

benign IPMN differs in patient selection, surgical technique, and accepted risk of long-term functional disorders. These differences underline the need for (1) a good knowledge of both the pathology and the natural history of the disease; (2) an accurate diagnosis of the disease and its severity, particularly differentiating invasive from noninvasive IPMN (this point is more important in asymptomatic patients in whom IPMN is an incidental finding); and (3) an accurate appreciation of extent of the disease in the pancreatic gland. This article details the indications, surgical techniques, and results of surgery in IPMN.

Pathology and natural history of intraductal and papillary mucinous neoplasms of the pancreas

The WHO classification of pancreatic neoplasms published in 1996 [3] and modified in 2000 [4] reported four successive stages of IPMN: mild dysplasia (IPMN adenoma), moderate dysplasia (border-line IPMN), severe dysplasia (IPMN carcinoma in situ), and invasive carcinoma. Only the last stage of the disease is associated with the adverse prognostic factors identified in ductal adenocarcinoma (poor differentiation, lymph node metastases, lymphatic/vascular embolism, perineural invasion, and peritoneal or hepatic metastases).

Median age at diagnosis ranges from 61 to 68 years [5,6,11,13–24]. In three series [10,16,21] and in one multi-institutional report [25], the median age of patients who had mild or moderate dysplasia was 2 to 6 years younger than that of patients who had carcinoma, but most other series reported no differences in age [6,19,20,23,26,27]. There are no substantial data in the literature to determine how many years are required for benign IPMN to evolve before becoming symptomatic. Because IPMN rarely is diagnosed before the age of 40 years [5,13,14,22,27,28], it probably appears in most patients during the fourth or fifth decade of life.

The risk of malignant transformation depends on the pathologic subtype. In surgical series, the prevalence of malignant transformation (both carcinoma in situ and invasive carcinoma) ranges from 10% to 59% when IPMN is confined to the branch ducts (branch-duct type IPMN) (Fig. 1) and from 56% to 92% when IPMN involves the main duct exclusively (main-duct type IPMN) (Fig. 2) or both the main duct and the branch ducts (mixed-type IPMN) (Fig. 3) (Table 1). One prospective study evaluated the 5-year incidence of carcinoma (both invasive and noninvasive) as 63% for main-duct type and mixed-type IPMN versus 15% for branch-duct type IPMN [13].

It has been suggested recently that IPMN could be a particular subtype of familial pancreatic cancer [37]. Although there are no available data suggesting that relatives of patients who have IPMN should be screened, the relationship between IPMN and familial pancreatic cancer should be clarified in

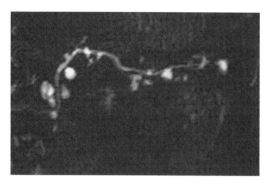

Fig. 1. MR cholangiopancreatography: diffuse branch-duct type IPMN. This patient was not operated because lack of symptoms, absence of morphologic signs suggestive of malignancy, and involvement of the whole pancreatic gland.

the future to determine if the poor prognosis of pancreatic cancer could be prevented in a larger proportion of patients.

Most frequent symptoms are epigastric pain (in 50%–70% of patients), weight loss (in 30%–50% of patients), acute pancreatitis (in 20%–40% of patients), diabetes (in 10%–30% of patients), jaundice (in 10%–25% of patients), and steatorrhea (in 5%–20% of patients) [7,13,15,19,20,27]. Asymptomatic patients, however, represent 5% to 40% of patients in surgical series [6,7,13,17,19,27]. This rate is more important, ranging from 57% to 98%, in patients included in observational studies, but a lack of symptoms generally is a condition for enrollment in these studies [36,38–40].

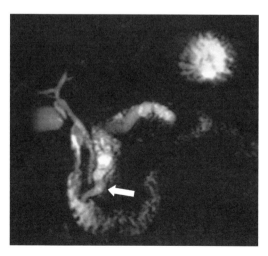

Fig. 2. MR cholangiopancreatography: diffuse main-duct type IPMN. Presence of a diffuse main duct dilatation. A gap (*arrow*) is visible in the cephalic part of the main duct, corresponding to carcinoma in situ on pathologic examination of the specimen of pancreaticoduodenectomy.

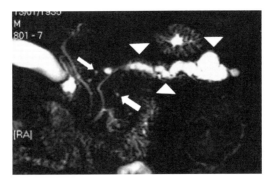

Fig. 3. MR cholangiopancreatography: mixed-type IPMN predominating in the distal pancreas. The main duct of the distal pancreas (*arrowheads*) is dilated. This patient underwent distal pancreatectomy with transection margin involved by mild dysplasia on the only branch ducts. Some small, dilated branch ducts (*arrows*) were deliberately left in place in the head.

Preoperative assessment

Diagnosis of intraductal and papillary mucinous neoplasm and malignancy complicating intraductal and papillary mucinous neoplasms

The symptoms and ductal abnormalities of IPMN are not specific. The only specific morphologic finding of IPMN is mucus oozing through major or minor papilla [20]. The symptoms and ductal abnormalities seen in IPMN also can be observed in ductal adenocarcinoma, ampullary tumors, chronic pancreatitis, and in some rare benign cystic conditions [41]. The former two diagnoses usually indicate surgery for IPMN. Conversely, the latter two usually do not justify a pancreatic resection. Misdiagnosis can be particularly detrimental in patients who have incidental IPMN. In the author's group, other pancreatic and periampullary lesions represented 7% of the pancreatectomies performed for suspicion of IPMN, but this percentage declined to only 4% in their most recent experience, probably because of better knowledge of the disease and recent advances in imaging [41]. False-positive diagnoses of IPMN occurred mainly in patients who had chronic pancreatitis [41].

Many authors have studied the clinical, biologic, and morphologic signs predictive of malignancy. The most strongly identified signs are reported in Table 2. There is not consensus about some of the other signs, which have been identified in only a few studies or even in a single study. Jaundice is the strongest sign suggestive of malignancy [6,8,16,17,19,20,32], including branch-duct IPMN [8]. Weight loss and diabetes also were identified as predictive of malignancy in several studies [7,10,11,16,19,35,42], whereas steatorrhea seems to be less strongly associated with malignancy [19]. Available data concerning pain are contradictory: some studies identified pain as significantly more frequent in benign disease [7,8,17], but in another study it was associated with malignancy [11]. Acute pancreatitis might be more

Table 1

Distribution of malignancy (noninvasive and invasive) in intraductal and papillary mucinous neoplasms of the pancreas according to subtype of intraductal and papillary mucinous neoplasms in surgical series

Authors and year [reference]	No. of patients	Main-duct type or mixed type		Branch-duct type	
		In situ (%)	Invasive (%)	In situ (%)	Invasive (%)
Kobari et al 1999 [15]	30	69	23	25	6
Terris et al 2000 [29]	43	20	36	15	0
Doi et al 2002 [30]	38	84		46	
Bernard et al 2002 [31]	53	25	51	17	8
Sugiyama et al 2003 [32]	62	13	57	50	9
Kitagawa et al 2003 [20]	63	11	54	4	31
Sohn et al 2004 [16]	129	NA	45	NA	30
Salvia et al 2004 [7]	147	18	42	NA	NA
Couvelard et al 2005 [33]	154	25	32	13	10
Ban et al 2006 [34]	80	57	23	8	2
Fujino et al 2006 [35]	57	88		33	
Schmidt et al 2007 [19]	156	28	28	6	14
Yang et al 2007 [17]	43	26	39	20	0
Nagai et al 2007 [11]	72	30	52	15	37
Murakami et al 2007 [26]	62	25	36	12	6
Imaizumi et al 2007 [18]	244	39	33	30	10
Rodriguez et al 2007 [8]	145[a]	NA	NA	11	11
Peraez-Luna et al 2007 [36]	77[a]	NA	NA	5	6

Abbreviation: NA, not available.

[a] Series including only operated patients with branch-duct type IPMN. These two groups also reported patients with branch-duct IPMN who deliberately did not undergo operation because of the absence of findings suggestive of malignant transformation.

Table 2
Predictive factors of malignancy in intraductal and papillary mucinous neoplasms of the pancreas

Factor	Presentation	Authors and year [reference]
Clinical	Jaundice	Kitagawa et al 2003 [20]
		Sugiyama et al 2003 [32]
		Sohn et al 2004 [16]
		Wada et al 2005 [6]
		Yang et al 2007 [17]
		Rodriguez et al 2007 [8]
		Schmidt et al 2007 [19]
	Weight loss	Paye et al 2000 [10]
		Sohn et al 2004 [16]
		Nagai et al 2007 [11]
		Schmidt et al 2007 [19]
	Diabetes mellitus	Taouli et al 2000 [42]
		Salvia et al 2004 [7]
		Fujino et al 2006 [35]
	Steatorrhea	Schmidt et al 2007 [19]
Biologic	Abnormal liver tests	Kitagawa et al 2003 [20]
		Yang et al 2007 [17]
Imaging	Location in the head	Murakami et al 2007 [26]
		Yokoyama et al 2007 [22]
	Main duct diameter	
	≥ 6 mm	Fujino et al 2006 [35]
		Murakami et al 2007 [26]
		Nagai et al 2007 [11]
	≥ 7 mm	Sugiyama et al 2003 [32]
	≥ 8 mm	Murakami et al 2007 [26]
	≥ 10 mm	Taouli et al 2000 [42]
	Length of main duct dilatation	O'Toole et al 2007 [43]
	Presence of a pancreatic mass	O'Toole et al 2007 [43]
		Vullierme et al 2007 [44]
	Branch duct diameter	
	≥ 26 mm	Murakami et al 2007 [26]
	≥ 30 mm	Imaizumi et al 2007 [18]
		Nagai et al 2007 [11]
	Presence of mural nodules	Sugiyama et al 2003 [32]
		Schmidt et al 2007 [19]
	Height of mural nodules ≥ 3 mm	Imaizumi et al 2007 [18]
	Atypical cytopathology	Schmidt et al 2007 [19]
		Murakami et al 2007 [26]
		Pelaez-Luna et al 2007 [36]

frequent in benign IPMN [13]. The serum CA 19-9 level was not predictive of malignancy [11,17,35] except in one study [20].

Morphologically, the signs most strongly suggestive of malignancy are ductal abnormalities, including the diameter of the main pancreatic duct (with a threshold ranging from 6–10 mm), the presence of mural thickening or mural nodules, and, for branch-duct IPMN, a cyst diameter exceeding 25 or 30 mm. These criteria cannot differentiate benign from malignant IPMN with absolute accuracy. Mural nodules within cysts (Fig. 4) must be differ-entiated from mucus plugs (Fig. 5). The authors' group found that only the identification of an infiltrating mass by CT or endoscopic ultrasound was suggestive of invasive carcinoma [43,44]. Cyst size must be considered with caution, because one Japanese series reported several cases of invasive malignant branch-duct type IPMN in cysts smaller than 30 mm [11]. The presence of mucus at duodenal endoscopy also is associated with contradic-tory results [20,25]. A positron emission tomography scan could be useful to differentiate benign from malignant IPMN with an 80% sensitivity for de-tecting noninvasive carcinoma and a 95% sensitivity for detecting invasive carcinoma [45]; however, these scores have been evaluated in a only few pa-tients and have not yet been confirmed by another group. Atypical cytopa-thology of the pancreatic fluid harvested endoscopically was reported recently to be useful in diagnosing malignant IPMN [19,26,36].

The studies that evaluated these predictive factors had several limitations. (1) Some studies relied only on clinicopathologic factors, without precise as-sessment of preoperative radiologic findings [6,17,20,22,27], so they did not analyzed all the morphologic factors on an intent-to-diagnose basis. (2) For the other studies, the preoperative assessment was not uniform; in particu-lar, endoscopic ultrasound was not used routinely, and MRI was used only in most recent series. (3) Patients who had invasive malignancy sometimes were pooled with patients who had carcinoma in-situ [14]. Carcinoma-in-situ is not correlated with extent of surgery and the long-term prognosis, because no lymphadenectomy is required for carcinoma in situ, and the survival observed after resection for carcinoma in situ is equivalent to that for earlier stages of noninvasive disease [18]. (4) Some studies identified these factors using only univariate analysis, whereas others also used multi-variate analysis. (5) A preoperative distinction between passive main duct dilatation (in the setting of branch-duct type IPMN) and main-duct type

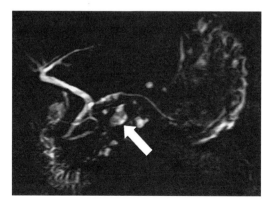

Fig. 4. MR cholangiopancreatography: branch-duct type IPMN with mural nodules. An irreg-ular gap is present in the largest branch duct (*arrow*). The gap is in continuity with the cyst wall, proving that it developed from the cystic wall.

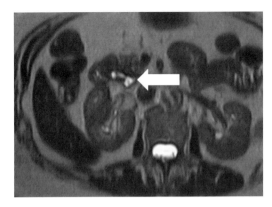

Fig. 5. MR cholangiopancreatography: branch-duct type IPMN of the uncinate process with mucus plug. A gap in the dilated branch duct (*arrow*) is surrounded by fluid signal, proving that it did not develop from the cyst wall.

(or mixed-type) IPMN, which could be useful for defining accurate indications for surgery, was not assessed by the majority of studies. Neither clinical factors (except for diabetes, which seems to be more frequent in main-duct type IMPN [15]) nor MRI [46] allow these two entities to be differentiated accurately. Also, endoscopic ultrasound tends to overestimate the diagnosis of main-duct type IPMN in up to 20% of branch-duct type IPMN [43].

Evaluation of topography

Accurate preoperative evaluation of topography is needed to plan the most suitable type of pancreatectomy, resecting all or almost all the neoplastic epithelium while preserving the healthy pancreas or segments involved only by obstructive pancreatitis. IPMN is located most frequently in the pancreatic head, so pancreaticoduodenectomy is the most common procedure, performed in approximately 60% of cases (Table 3). Distal pancreatectomy is performed in 20% of cases. Conversely, the rate of total pancreatectomy varies greatly, between 6% and 28%, whereas other types of resection (mainly limited resections) are performed in 0% to 40% of cases. This variation between series may be related to (1) reluctance to perform total pancreatectomy in some groups and (2) difficulties in determining precisely the extent of the disease within the pancreatic gland. Indeed, total pancreatectomy can be excessive in some patients if the extent of surgery is guided only by the preoperative imaging [10,35]. The rate of total pancreatectomy probably can be limited to 10% or less if a partial pancreatectomy performed on the side of the most important and typical abnormalities (usually located in the pancreatic head) is extended to the opposite side step by step as indicated by results of frozen sectioning [5,33]. The only theoretical disadvantage of this approach is the risk of tumor spillage if tumor is

Table 3
Distribution of type of pancreatic resections in surgical series

Authors and year [reference]	No. of patients	Pancreaticoduodenectomy (%)	Distal pancreatectomy (%)	Total pancreatectomy (%)	Others (%)
Falconi et al 2001 [47]	55	65	18	9	5
Bernard et al 2002 [31]	53	64	21	8	4
Chari et al 2002 [23]	123	50	28	23	–
Sohn et al 2004 [16]	134	71	12	15	2
D'Angelica et al 2004 [27]	63	66	23	10	2
Couvelard et al 2005 [33]	154	62	17	9	12
Fujino et al 2006 [35]	57	53	23	28	2
Wada et al 2007 [6]	100	61	26	13	–
Yokoyama et al 2007 [22]	100	57	25	6	12
Schmidt et al 2007 [19]	156	56	29	10	5
Murakami et al 2007 [26]	62	50	5	5	40

transected; however, only exceptional cases of postoperative peritoneal carcinomatosis or mucinous ascites have been reported, suggesting that this
risk is small [5,48]. For tumor apparently located in the distal pancreas,
the usual predominance of IPMN in the pancreatic head and the higher
rate of intrapancreatic recurrence after distal pancreatectomy [22] than after
pancreaticoduodenectomy suggest that frozen sectioning of the transection
margin should be performed early during the operation to determine if
the pancreatectomy should be extended to the pancreatic head and, if so,
to discuss an alternative procedure to avoid total pancreatectomy.

To limit the extent of pancreatic resection and the risk of postoperative
pancreatic insufficiency, dilatation caused by chronic obstruction by mucus,
which does not involve IPMN, should be identified. Chronic obstruction by
mucus can be located upstream or downstream from the segment of pancreas involved by IPMN. Downstream dilatation is a specific and common
finding in IPMN. In two studies, the author's group found that imaging
overestimated the extent of the disease in 7% to 21% of patients [10,43].

Aims, drawbacks, and indications of surgery

Surgery for IPMN has several goals: (1) resection of the neoplastic disease to treat malignant transformation or to prevent it; (2) limiting operative
risk; (3) limiting the occurrence and severity of postoperative pancreatic insufficiency; and (4) treating symptoms. In theory, resection of neoplastic disease should include pancreatectomy according to carcinologic principles in
case of invasive components and complete resection of noninvasive IPMN
[18]. The need for complete resection of noninvasive IPMN is still debated,
however, particularly in surgery for benign IPMN [5,16,23,28,35,49].

The operative risk is limited by adequate selection of patients. The mortality rate of both distal and medial pancreatectomy is less than 1%, even
when the significant morbidity of a pancreatic fistula is involved [12,50–53].
The series of limited pancreatic resections (including enucleation, resection
of the ventral pancreas, and head resection with segmental duodenectomy)
is small, but mortality in these procedures also seems to be very low
[9,11,12,18,54] In surgery for IPMN, postoperative mortality has been
observed after total pancreatectomy [35,55] and pancreaticoduodenectomy
[10,16,27]. In pancreatic adenocarcinoma, several studies have identified
age [56–58], renal failure [58–60], diabetes [58,61], and chronic liver disease
[58,62] as predictive factors of mortality after pancreaticoduodenectomy,
but these factors have not been demonstrated to be predictive of mortality
in patients who have IPMN, especially benign disease.

Postoperative pancreatic insufficiency is observed after hemi- or total
pancreatectomy. New-onset diabetes occurs in 5% to 10% of cases after
pancreaticoduodenectomy [63–66] and in 10% to 25% of cases after distal
pancreatectomy [12,51,67]. Enzyme supplementation is needed to treat

exocrine insufficiency after 50% to 60% of pancreaticoduodenectomies [63–66] and after fewer than 5% to 15% of distal pancreatectomies [12,67]. These rates reflect the experience in patients undergoing operation for a variety of tumors. The highest reported rates are probably realistic in patients who have IPMN, because the disease by itself can lead to pancreatic insufficiency [12]. In patients who have IPMN, the postoperative occurrence or worsening of pancreatic dysfunction could be prevented by preserving pancreatic segments with normal ductal system or with ductal dilatation without involvement by IPMN. Indeed, functional results are much better in patients who have limited resections. For example, the rate of postoperative diabetes is less than 10% after medial pancreatectomy and seems nonsignificant after enucleation [9,12,68].

Total pancreatectomy results in definitive pancreatic insufficiency. Apancreatic diabetes is characterized by instability, low insulin requirements, and frequent onset of hypoglycemia (caused by the lack of endogenous glucagon) [55,69]. Some series reported distant rehospitalization or even death caused by hypoglycemia [35,55]. Exocrine function usually is corrected by enzyme replacement associated with a proton-pump inhibitor to prevent early enzyme inactivation by gastric acid [69]. Continuous administration of proton-pump inhibitors also is needed to prevent the risk of marginal ulcer on the gastrojejunostomy [53,69].

The very high risk of malignancy associated with main duct involvement has led all authors to agree about the need for routine pancreatic resection in this setting, provided the operative risk is acceptable [70]. The management of branch-duct type IPMN is more controversial. Some authors reported a high risk (50%) of malignancy in this setting and therefore recommended routine resection [11]. Conversely, a relatively low risk of malignancy (approximately 15%) usually is observed with branch-duct type IPMN, and the whole pancreatic gland is involved by the disease in 15% to 20% of patients [19,39]. These findings and the morbidity of pancreatic surgery has led some authors to prefer close follow-up with imaging in asymptomatic patients who have branch-duct IPMN, provided there are no findings suggestive of malignancy at initial assessment (cyst diameter < 20–30 mm according to series, absence of thick wall, and absence of mural nodules) [14,36,38–40]. Recently, some authors also proposed obtaining a negative cytologic study on pancreatic fluid harvested endoscopically before undertaking this observational approach [19], but others have reported preoperative cytology to be unreliable and disappointing [71]. A conservative approach is supported by longitudinal follow-up studies that estimated the incidence of morphologic changes (increase in cyst size, emergence of mural nodules, or main duct dilatation) leading to surgery to range from 6% to 18% with a 34- to 61-month median follow-up [38–40,46,72]; furthermore, in these studies, the actuarial incidence of malignancy in branch-duct type IPMN ranged from 0% to 15% with a median follow-up ranging from 32 to 61 months [36,38–40]. This discrepancy between the incidences of morphologic changes and malignancy suggests that criteria allowing differentiation between malignant and benign branch-duct IPMN have a high sensitivity for detecting malignancy but need better specificity to limit the indications of surgery for ultimately benign lesions [36,43].

Recurrent epigastric pain and attacks of acute pancreatitis usually lead to surgery. There are very few data in the literature about the influence of surgery on these symptoms. In one series of 22 patients who mainly underwent hemipancreatectomies with a mean follow-up of 2.5 years, the rate of symptomatic recurrence was 13%, including only one patient (5%) who experienced a single documented attack of acute pancreatitis [73]. In another series including 28 limited pancreatic resections (enucleation or medial pancreatectomies), no patient developed recurrent pain with a median 25-month follow-up [9]. In inoperable patients, endoscopic pancreatic sphincterotomy can be considered, but its value was not evaluated [49]. Several authors consider diabetes, steatorrhea, and jaundice suggestive of malignancy and therefore these symptoms usually lead to pancreatectomy. Jaundice is treated by surgery. Diabetes and steatorrhea can persist or even be worsened by surgery, but they have lower priority than treatment of malignancy.

Techniques and results of surgery for intraductal and papillary mucinous neoplasms of the pancreas

Malignant intraductal and papillary mucinous neoplasms

Surgical exploration must be performed even if CT reveals findings of arterial invasion because obliteration of the periarterial fat plane can be caused by inflammation instead of by tumor extension [44]. Surgery for malignant and especially invasive IPMN should include regional lymphadenectomy and vascular resection if needed [18]. For cephalic invasive IPMN, pancreaticoduodenectomy with and without pylorus preservation gives equivalent results [74]. To limit the risk of gastric ischemia, preservation of the pylorus and continuity of the right gastric vessels is preferred if a total or a completion pancreatectomy is needed at the same time or during reoperation.

The actuarial 5-year survival after resection of invasive IPMN ranges between 35% and 60% [6,7,11,16,18,22,23,26,27]. Most deaths are related to cancer recurrence, and most recurrences are metastatic, indicating a role for adjuvant therapy [23,27,28]. More rarely, only intrapancreatic recurrences occur, even several years later, which can lead to reoperation for completion pancreatectomy [22]. Last, some patients develop extrapancreatic cancer [22,75,76].

It has been suggested that long-term survival is better after total pancreatectomy than after partial pancreatectomy when performed for malignant IPMN [77,78]. In these studies, however, the number of patients was limited, and frozen sectioning of the transection margin was not done routinely, so some patients developed early recurrence after partial pancreatectomy caused by invasive/in situ carcinoma on the transection margin. To date, most authors routinely have used frozen sectioning of the pancreatic margin and extended or even complete pancreatectomy when frozen sectioning reveals invasive or noninvasive carcinoma [22,33]. There is, however, no consensus about the role of total pancreatectomy for invasive IPMN when the transection margin is involved by dysplasia: some authors advocate extending pancreatectomy until a disease-free margin on the main pancreatic duct is obtained [22,33], but most others, considering that long-term prognosis is affected mainly by the invasive component, do not recommend extending the pancreatectomy in this setting provided there is no invasive disease on the margin [6,16,23,28].

The prognosis after resection for invasive IPMN is similar to that observed after pancreatectomy for common ductal adenocarcinoma after stratification according to tumor stage [6,24,35]. The main adverse prognostic factors are an increased CA-19.9 concentration two times normal or higher [24], a nonradical (R1) resection [16,23], lymph node involvement [24,27], advanced tumor stage [6], presence of vascular invasion [27], and tubular (versus colloid) type of invasion [27]. The apparently better prognosis observed after pancreatectomy for invasive IPMN than after pancreatectomy for ductal adenocarcinoma probably reflects the inclusion of less advanced disease. For example, the rate of lymph node involvement in invasive IPMN ranges from 12% to 54% [7,14,16,18,24,27,79], versus 60% to 70% in common ductal adenocarcinoma [6,24].

Benign intraductal and papillary mucinous neoplasms

Noninvasive IPMN can be treated by a pancreatic resection tailored to the extent of the disease into the pancreatic gland [18,68]. Although pancreaticoduodenectomy and distal pancreatectomy usually are necessary to treat benign IPMN, more limited resections, including pancreatic head resection with segmental duodenectomy [54], enucleation [9,68], medial pancreatectomy [9,12,68], and resection of ventral pancreas for a lesion located in the uncinate process (Fig. 6) [80], can be proposed in some cases, particularly in localized branch-duct type IPMN. All types of limited pancreatic resection must be preceded by extensive morphologic and biologic assessment to ensure that there is no sign suggesting malignancy, because limited resections do not allow any lymph node clearance [9,54].

Frozen sectioning of the pancreatic margin is necessary to determine the extent of resection of any type of pancreatectomy. With experienced pathologists, frozen sectioning of the pancreatic margin is very reliable, with accuracy as high as 94% [33]. Frozen sectioning of the resected specimen also can be used during limited resection to exclude invasive malignancy [9]. Today there is no consensus about the threshold of IPMN lesions needing

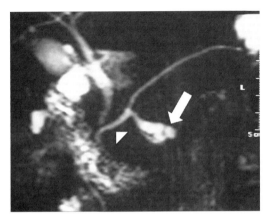

Fig. 6. MR cholangiopancreatography: IPMN limited to a branch duct of the uncinate process
(*arrow*). The main duct (*arrowhead*) is slightly dilated downstream. This patient underwent successful local resection with negative margins on the communicating duct.

extend resection. In the author's group, any degree of main-duct IPMN and/
or borderline branch-duct IPMN is an indication for extended resection [33].
In another group, all degrees and subtypes of IPMN lesions were considered
positive [5]. Some patients present with eroded epithelium in the main duct
[33,47]; this finding is suggestive of multifocal lesions and probably should
lead to extending the resection for a few centimeters and obtaining another
frozen sectioning.

Patients who have benign IPMN have a very good long-term prognosis
with a 5-year actuarial survival exceeding 95% [6,18,22,27]. Follow-up relies
mainly on abdominal CT scan and MRI [22,73]. MRI is useful to evaluate
residual or recurrent disease, but interpretation of ductal changes can be difficult after pancreaticoduodenectomy because stenosis of the pancreatico-
digestive anastomosis is common [73]. Follow-up can be marked by
intrapancreatic recurrence and extrapancreatic neoplasms.

After partial pancreatectomy for noninvasive IPMN, the prevalence of
intrapancreatic recurrence ranges from 2% to 8% [5,6,22,23]. Intrapancreatic recurrence occurs 1 to 11 years after initial resection, so follow-up
should be prolonged [5,6,16,22]. Some of these recurrences occur in patients
who had a tumor-free margin, thus proving that some IPMN are multifocal
and discontinuous [5,22,24,81]. Diagnosis of discontinuous lesions is difficult; it can be done either preoperatively by peroral pancreatoscopy and intraductal endosonography [82] or intraoperatively by pancreatoscopy with
staged biopsies [35] and intraductal cytology analyzed during the procedure
[81]. These techniques are not in widespread use, and normal findings do not
eliminate the risk of long-term recurrence in the pancreatic remnant [22].
Today, intraoperative frozen sectioning of the pancreatic margin is the
most widely available tool for determining the extent of resection [5,33]. Because the risk of intrapancreatic recurrence seems higher with a positive

margin, obtaining a negative margin should be a reasonable goal [5,49]. The indications for total pancreatectomy for benign IPMN also are controversial. Despite the good life expectancy observed after pancreatectomy for noninvasive IPMN and the risk of intrapancreatic recurrence, some authors are reluctant to perform total pancreatectomy, which involves a decreased quality of life and a risk of severe or even lethal hypoglycemia [35,55,69]. Young age [23], main-duct involvement at frozen sectioning of the pancreatic margin [33], and a socioeconomic condition predicting that postoperative diabetes will be managed satisfactorily [55,69] are factors favoring total pancreatectomy provided appropriate preoperative information has been given and that consent has been obtained.

In some recent series from Asia, 25% to 36% of patients who had IPMN developed synchronously or metachronously extrapancreatic cancers; most of these tumors were gastric and colonic [22,75,76]. Further series are necessary to confirm these findings, particularly in the Western world, and to determine if a specific follow-up of patients operated for noninvasive IPMN is needed.

Summary

The aims of surgery for IPMN are to prevent or to treat malignant transformation (resection of "suspicious" epithelium) while limiting the operative risk and the functional drawbacks of surgery.

Adenocarcinoma (both in situ and invasive) complicating IPMN is seen in 60% to 70% of patients who have main-duct involvement and in 10% to 20% of those who have only branch-duct involvement. Several factors predictive of carcinoma have been identified: these factors are clinical (jaundice, recent onset or worsening of diabetes) or morphologic (main duct > 7 mm or branch-ducts > 30 mm in diameter, presence and height of mural nodules, presence of a pancreatic mass).

When factors predictive of malignancy are present, pancreatic resection should be performed according to oncologic principles including en bloc hemipancreatectomy and lymphadenectomy. Frozen section of the pancreatic margin should be performed routinely. In this setting, whether the presence of noninvasive IPMN on the pancreatic margin should lead to extended (or even to complete) pancreatectomy or can be considered as acceptable (because of the bad prognosis of the invasive component) remains unanswered.

For benign IPMN, the extent of resection should be tailored to the extent of the disease, general condition of the patient, result of routine frozen section of pancreatic margin, and presence or absence of main-duct involvement. The rate of intrapancreatic recurrence seems higher when the transection margin is involved, so obtaining a negative margin should be a reasonable goal. For benign and localized IPMN, a limited resection (enucleation, resection of the uncinate process, or medial pancreatectomy) can treat symptoms efficiently while preserving pancreatic function. Except after total pancreatectomy for noninvasive IPMN, follow-up is needed for detection of recurrence. To date, the reported risk of intrapancreatic recurrence is less than 8%. Otherwise, patients undergoing operation for IPMN are at higher risk of developing extrapancreatic neoplasms, mainly gastric and colonic tumors.

Acknowledgments

The author thanks Pr. Philippe Lévy and Dr. Marie-Pierre Vullierme for their help in the preparation of the manuscript.

References

[1] Tollefson MK, Libsch KD, Sarr MG, et al. Intraductal papillary mucinous neoplasm: did it exist prior to 1980? Pancreas 2003;26:55–8.

[2] Ohhashi K, Murakami Y, Murayama M, et al. For cases of mucous secreting pancreatic cancer. Progress of Digestive Endoscopy 1982;20:348–51.

[3] Kloppel G, Solcia E, Longnecker DS, et al. Histological typing of tumors of the exocrine pancreas. In: WHO international histological classification of tumours. Berlin: Springer; 1996.

[4] Longnecker DS, Adler G, Hruban RH, et al. Intraductal papillary mucinous neoplasms of the pancreas. In: Hamilton SR, Aaltonen LA, editors. World Health Organization classification of tumors. Pathology and genetics of tumors of the digestive system. Lyon (France): IARC Press; 2000. p. 237–40.

[5] White R, D'Angelica M, Katabi N, et al. Fate of the remnant pancreas after resection of noninvasive intraductal papillary mucinous neoplasm. J Am Coll Surg 2007;204:987–95.

[6] Wada K, Kozarek RA, Traverso LW. Outcomes following resection of invasive and noninvasive intraductal papillary mucinous neoplasms of the pancreas. Am J Surg 2005;189:632–6.

[7] Salvia R, Fernandez-del Castillo C, Bassi C, et al. Main intraductal papillary mucinous neoplasm of the pancreas. Clinical predictors of malignancy and long term survival following resection. Ann Surg 2004;239:678–87.

[8] Rodriguez JR, Salvia R, Crippa S, et al. Branch-duct intraductal papillary mucinous neoplasms: observation in 145 patients who underwent resection. Gastroenterology 2007;133: 72–9.

[9] Sauvanet A, Blanc B, Couvelard A, et al. Limited pancreatic resections for non-invasive intraductal papillary and mucinous neoplasms (IPMN) of the pancreas [abstract]. HPB Surgery 2007;9(Suppl 2):29.

[10] Paye F, Sauvanet A, Terris B, et al. Intraductal papillary mucinous tumors of the pancreas: pancreatic resections guided by preoperative morphological assessment and intraoperative frozen section examination. Surgery 2000;127:536–44.

[11] Nagai K, Doi R, Kida A, et al. Intraductal papillary mucinous neoplasms of the pancreas: clinicopathologic characteristics and long-term follow-up after resection. World J Surg 2008; 32:271–8.

[12] Crippa S, Bassi C, Warshaw AL, et al. Middle pancreatectomy: indications, short- and long-term operative outcomes. Ann Surg 2007;246:69–76.

[13] Lévy P, Jouannaud V, O'Toole D, et al. Natural history of intraductal papillary mucinous tumors of the pancreas: actuarial risk of malignancy. Clin Gastroenterol Hepatol 2006;4: 460–8.

[14] Jang JY, Kim SW, Lee SE, et al. Treatment guidelines for branch duct type intraductal papillary mucinous neoplasms of the pancreas: when can we operate or observe? Ann Surg Oncol 2008;15:199–205.

[15] Kobari M, Egawa S, Shibuya K, et al. Intraductal papillary mucinous tumors of the pancreas comprise 2 clinical subtypes: differences in clinical characteristics and surgical management. Arch Surg 1999;134:1131–6.

[16] Sohn TA, Yeo CJ, Cameron JL, et al. Intraductal papillary mucinous neoplasms of the pancreas: an updated experience. Ann Surg 2004;239:788–97.

[17] Yang AD, Melstrom LG, Bentrem DJ, et al. Outcomes after pancreatectomy for intraductal papillary mucinous neoplasms of the pancreas: an institutional experience. Surgery 2007; 142(4):529–37.

[18] Imaizumi T, Hatori T, Harada N, et al. Intraductal papillary mucinous neoplasm of the pancreas; resection and cancer prevention. Am J Surg 2007;194:595–9.

[19] Schmidt CM, White PB, Waters JA, et al. Intraductal papillary mucinous neoplasms: predictors of malignant and invasive pathology. Ann Surg 2007;246:644–54.

[20] Kitagawa Y, Unger TA, Taylor S, et al. Mucus is a predictor of better prognosis and survival in patients with intraductal papillary mucinous tumor of the pancreas. J Gastrointest Surg 2003;7:12–9.

[21] Z'graggen K, Rivera JA, Compton CC, et al. Prevalence of activating K-ras mutations in the evolutionary stages of neoplasia in intraductal papillary mucinous tumors of the pancreas. Ann Surg 1997;226:491–500.

[22] Yokoyama Y, Nagino M, Oda K, et al. Clinicopathologic features of re-resected cases of intraductal papillary mucinous neoplasms (IPMNs). Surgery 2007;142:136–42.

[23] Chari ST, Yadav D, Smyrck TC, et al. Study of recurrence after surgical resection of intraductal papillary mucinous neoplasm of the pancreas. Gastroenterology 2002;123:1500–7.

[24] Maire F, Hammel P, Terris B, et al. Prognosis of malignant intraductal papillary mucinous tumours of the pancreas after surgical resection. Comparison with pancreatic ductal adenocarcinoma. Gut 2002;51:717–22.

[25] Suzuki Y, Atomi Y, Sugiyama M, et al. Cystic neoplasm of the pancreas: a Japanese multi-institutional study of intraductal papillary mucinous tumor and mucinous cystic tumor. Pancreas 2004;28:241–6.

[26] Murakami Y, Uemura K, Hayashidani Y, et al. Predictive factors of malignant or invasive intraductal papillary-mucinous neoplasms of the pancreas. J Gastrointest Surg 2007;11: 338–44.

[27] D'Angelica M, Brennan MF, Suriawinata AA, et al. Intraductal papillary mucinous neoplasms of the pancreas: an analysis of clinicopathologic features and outcome. Ann Surg 2004;239:400–8.

[28] Raut CP, Cleary KR, Staerkel GA, et al. Intraductal papillary mucinous neoplasms of the pancreas: effect of invasion and pancreatic margin status on recurrence and survival. Ann Surg Oncol 2006;13:582–94.

[29] Terris B, Ponsot P, Paye F, et al. Intraductal papillary mucinous tumors of the pancreas confined to secondary ducts show less aggressive pathologic features as compared with those involving the main pancreatic duct. Am J Surg Pathol 2000;24:1372–7.

[30] Doi R, Fujimoto K, Wada M, et al. Surgical management of intraductal papillary mucinous tumor of the pancreas. Surgery 2002;132:80–5.

[31] Bernard P, Scoazec JY, Joubert M, et al. Intraductal papillary-mucinous tumors of the pancreas: predictive criteria of malignancy according to pathological examination of 53 cases. Arch Surg 2002;137:1274–8.

[32] Sugiyama M, Izumisato Y, Abe N, et al. Predictive factors for malignancy in intraductal papillary-mucinous tumours of the pancreas. Br J Surg 2003;90:1244–9.

[33] Couvelard A, Sauvanet A, Kianmanesh R, et al. Frozen sectioning of the pancreatic cut surface during resection of intraductal papillary mucinous neoplasms of the pancreas is useful and reliable: a prospective evaluation. Ann Surg 2005;242:774–8.

[34] Ban S, Naitoh Y, Mino-Kenudson M, et al. Intraductal papillary mucinous neoplasm (IPMN) of the pancreas: its histopathologic difference between 2 major types. Am J Surg Pathol 2006;30:1561–9.

[35] Fujino Y, Suzuki Y, Yoshikawa T, et al. Outcomes of surgery for intraductal papillary mucinous neoplasms of the pancreas. World J Surg 2006;30:1909–14.

[36] Pelaez-Luna M, Suresh T, Chari T, et al. Do consensus indications for resection in branch duct intraductal papillary mucinous neoplasm predict malignancy? A study of 147 patients. Am J Gastroenterol 2007;102:1759–64.

[37] Canto MI, Goggins M, Ralph H, et al. Screening for early pancreatic neoplasia in high-risk individuals. A prospective controlled study. Clin Gastroenferol Hepatol 2006;4: 766–81.

[38] Tanno S, Nakano Y, Nishikawa T, et al. Natural history of branch duct intraductal papillary-mucinous neoplasms of the pancreas without mural nodules: long-term follow-up results. Gut 2008;57:339–43.

[39] Salvia R, Crippa S, Falconi M, et al. Branch-duct intraductal papillary mucinous neoplasms of the pancreas: to operate or not to operate? Results of a prospective protocol on the management of 109 consecutive patients. Gut 2007;56:1086–90.

[40] Rautou PE, Levy P, Vullierme MP, et al. Morphological changes in branch duct intraductal papillary mucinous neoplasms of the pancreas: a mid-term follow-up study. J Clinical Gastroenterol Hepatol 2008;[epub ahead of print].

[41] Hammel P, Bouattour M, Rebours V, et al. Misdiagnosis in patients undergoing surgery for intraductal papillary mucinous neoplasias (IPMN) [abstract]. Gastroenterology 2007;132: A531.

[42] Taouli B, Vilgrain V, Vullierme MP, et al. Intraductal papillary mucinous tumors of the pancreas: helical CT with histopathologic correlation. Radiology 2000;217:757–64.

[43] O'Toole D, Couvelard A, Palazzo L, et al. Accuracy of EUS in the topographical diagnosis and in predicting malignancy in patients with intraductal papillary mucinous tumours (IPMN): comparative blind study with histology in 103 operated patients [abstract]. Gastroenterology 2007;132:A84.

[44] Vullierme MP, Giraud-Cohen M, Hammel P, et al. Malignant intraductal papillary mucinous neoplasm of the pancreas: in situ versus invasive carcinoma surgical resectability. Radiology 2007;245:483–90.

[45] Sperti C, Bissoli S, Pasquali C, et al. 18-Fluorodeoxyglucose positron emission tomography enhances computed tomography diagnosis of malignant intraductal papillary mucinous neoplasms of the pancreas. Ann Surg 2007;246:932–9.

[46] Irie H, Yoshimitsu K, Aibe H, et al. Natural history of pancreatic intraductal papillary mucinous tumor of branch duct type: follow-up study by magnetic resonance cholangiopancreatography. J Comput Assist Tomogr 2004;28:117–22.

[47] Falconi M, Salvia R, Bassi C, et al. Clinicopathological features and treatment of intraductal papillary mucinous tumour of the pancreas. Br J Surg 2001;88:376–81.

[48] Takahashi H, Nakamori S, Nakahira S, et al. Surgical outcomes of noninvasive and minimally invasive intraductal papillary-mucinous neoplasms of the pancreas. Ann Surg Oncol 2006;13:955–60.

[49] Azar C, Van de Stadt J, Rickaert F, et al. Intraductal papillary mucinous tumours of the pancreas. Clinical and therapeutic issues in 32 patients. Gut 1996;39:457–64.

[50] Pannegeon V, Pessaux P, Sauvanet A, et al. Pancreatic fistula after distal pancreatectomy: predictive risk factors and value of conservative treatment. Arch Surg 2006;141:1071–6.

[51] Lillemoe KD, Kaushal S, Cameron JL, et al. Distal pancreatectomy: indications and outcomes in 235 patients. Ann Surg 1999;229:693–700.

[52] Bilimoria MM, Cormier JN, Mun Y, et al. Pancreatic leak after left pancreatectomy is reduced following main pancreatic duct ligation. Br J Surg 2003;90:190–6.

[53] Sauvanet A, Partensky C, Sastre B, et al. Medial pancreatectomy: a multi-institutional retrospective study of 53 patients by the French Pancreas Club. Surgery 2002;132:836–43.

[54] Nakao A, Fernandez-Cruz L. Pancreatic head resection with segmental duodenectomy: safety and long-term results. Ann Surg 2007;246:923–31.
[55] Billings BJ, Christein JD, Harmsen WS, et al. Quality-of-life after total pancreatectomy: is it really that bad on long-term follow-up. J Gastrointest Surg 2005;9:1059–67.
[56] Muscari F, Suc B, Kirzin S, et al. Risk factors for mortality and intra-abdominal complications after pancreatoduodenectomy: multivariate analysis in 300 patients. Surgery 2005;139: 591–8.
[57] Lightner AM, Glasgow RE, Jordan TH, et al. Pancreatic resection in the elderly. J Am Coll Surg 2004;198:697–706.
[58] Ho V, Heslin MJ. Effect of hospital volume and experience on in-hospital mortality for pancreaticoduodenectomy. Ann Surg 2003;237:509–14.
[59] Adam U, Makowiec F, Riediger H, et al. Risk factors for complications after pancreatic heard resection. Am J Surg 2004;187:201–8.
[60] Gouma DJ, Van Geenen RCI, Van Gulik TH. Rates of complications and death after pancreaticoduodenectomy: risk factors and the impact of hospital volume. Ann Surg 2000;232: 786–95.
[61] Birkmeyer J, Samuel RG, Finlayson G, et al. Effect of hospital volume in in-hospital mortality with pancreaticoduodenectomy. Surgery 1999;125:250–6.
[62] Billingsley KG, Hur K, Henderson WG, et al. Outcome after pancreaticoduodenectomy for periampullary cancer: an analysis from the Veterans Affairs National Surgical Quality Improvement Program. J Gastrointest Surg 2003;7:484–91.
[63] Lemaire E, O'Toole D, Sauvanet A, et al. Functional and morphological changes in the pancreatic remnant following pancreaticoduodenectomy with pancreaticogastric anastomosis. Br J Surg 2000;87:434–8.
[64] Yamaguchi K, Tanak M, Chijiiwa K, et al. Early and late complications of pylorus-preserving pancreatoduodenectomy in Japan 1998. J Hepatobiliary Pancreat Surg 1999;6:303–11.
[65] Rault A, SaCunha A, Klopfenstein D, et al. Pancreaticojejunal anastomosis is preferable to pancreaticogastrostomy after pancreaticoduodenectomy for longterm outcomes of pancreatic exocrine function. J Am Coll Surg 2005;201:239–44.
[66] Ishikawa O, Ohigashi H, Eguchi H, et al. Long-term follow-up of glucose tolerance function after pancreaticoduodenectomy: comparison between pancreaticogastrostomy and pancreaticojejunostomy. Surgery 2004;136:617–23.
[67] Balzano G, Zerbi A, Veronesi P, et al. Surgical treatment of benign and borderline neoplasms of the pancreatic body. Dig Surg 2003;20:506–10.
[68] Kanazumi N, Nakao A, Kaneko T, et al. Surgical treatment of intraductal papillary-mucinous tumors of the pancreas. Hepatogastroenterology 2001;48:967–71.
[69] Heidt DG, Burant C, Simeone DM. Total pancreatectomy: indications, operative technique, and postoperative sequelae. J Gastrointest Surg 2007;11:209–16.
[70] Tanaka M, Chari S, Adsay V, et al. International consensus guidelines for management of intraductal papillary mucinous neoplasms and mucinous cystic neoplasms of the pancreas. Pancreatology 2005;6:17–32.
[71] Maire F, Couvelard A, Hammel P, et al. Intraductal papillary mucinous tumors of the pancreas: the preoperative value of cytologic and histopathologic diagnosis. Gastrointest Endosc 2003;58:701–6.
[72] Sai JK, Suyama M, Kubokawa Y, et al. Management of branch duct-type intraductal papillary mucinous tumor of the pancreas based on magnetic resonance imaging. Abdom Imaging 2003;28:694–9.
[73] Sugiyama M, Abe N, Tokuhara M, et al. Magnetic resonance cholangiopancreatography for postoperative follow-up of intra ductal papillary-mucinous tumors of the pancreas. Am J Surg 2003;13:251–5.
[74] Diener MK, Knaebel HP, Heukaufer C, et al. A systematic review and meta-analysis of pylorus-preserving versus classical pancreaticoduodenectomy for surgical treatment of periampullary and pancreatic carcinoma. Ann Surg 2007;245:187–200.

[75] Choi MG, Kim SW, Han SS, et al. High incidence of extra pancreatic neoplasms in patients with Intraductal papillary mucinous neoplasms. Arch Surg 2006;141:51–6.

[76] Eguchi H, Ishikawa O, Ohigashi H, et al. Patients with pancreatic intraductal papillary mucinous neoplasms are at high risk of colorectal cancer development. Surgery 2006;139: 749–54.

[77] Cuillerier E, Cellier C, Palazzo L, et al. Outcome after surgical resection of intraductal papillary and mucinous tumors of the pancreas. Am J Gastroenterol 2000;95:441–5.

[78] Zamora C, Sahel J, Cantu DG, et al. Intraductal papillary or mucinous tumors (IPMN) of the pancreas: report of a case series and review of the literature. Am J Gastroenterol 2001;96: 1441–7.

[79] Yamao K, Ohashi K, Nakamura T, et al. The prognosis of intraductal papillary mucinous tumors of the pancreas. Hepatogastroenterology 2000;47:1129–34.

[80] Nakagohri T, Kenmochi T, Kainuma O, et al. Inferior head resection of the pancreas for intraductal papillary mucinous tumors. Am J Surg 2000;179:482–4.

[81] Eguchi H, Ishikawa O, Ohigashi H, et al. Role of intraoperative cytology combined with histology in detecting continuous and skip type intraductal cancer existence for intraductal papillary mucinous carcinoma of the pancreas. Cancer 2006;107:2567–75.

[82] Hara T, Yamaguchi T, Ishihara T, et al. Diagnosis and patient management of intraductal papillary-mucinous tumor of the pancreas by using peroral pancreatoscopy and intraductal ultrasonography. Gastroenterology 2002;122:34–43.

Surg Oncol Clin N Am
17 (2008) 607–633

SURGICAL
ONCOLOGY CLINICS
OF NORTH AMERICA

Liver Resection for Hepatocellular Carcinoma

Richard Bryant, MD[a], Alexis Laurent, MD, PhD[a],
Claude Tayar, MD[a], Jeanne Tran van Nhieu, MD[b],
Alain Luciani, MD, PhD[c], Daniel Cherqui, MD[a],*

[a]*Department of Gastrointestinal and Hepatobiliary Surgery, Hopital Henri Mondor*
(APHP) – University of Paris, 94000 Creteil, France
[b]*Department of Pathology, Hopital Henri Mondor (APHP) – University of Paris,*
94000 Creteil, France
[c]*Department of Radiology, Hopital Henri Mondor (APHP) – University of Paris,*
94000 Creteil, France

Hepatocellular carcinoma (HCC) is the fifth most common cancer world-wide. In 90% of cases it is associated with chronic liver disease (CLD), most often at the stage of cirrhosis. Surgical treatment for HCC includes both resection and liver transplantation, but such options can be offered only to approximately 30% of patients [1].

In the rarer situation of HCC without CLD, transplantation has a limited role, and resection is the treatment of choice, most often consisting of a major hepatectomy [2,3]. In the presence of cirrhosis, liver transplantation is considered the treatment of choice because it both removes the tumor and eliminates the associated liver disease [1,4]. It can be proposed only for patients who have small tumors without vascular invasion (a single tumor < 5 cm or two or three tumors < 3 cm). Progress in screening for HCC has allowed the identification of an increasing number of patients meeting these criteria [5–7]. The shortage of liver donors restricts the availability of transplantation, however [8].

Hepatic resection in the setting of cirrhosis has long been limited by increased mortality and morbidity and by an elevated risk of recurrence through the appearance of new lesions associated with the underlying CLD [9]. Recent progress in techniques of liver resection and a better understanding of the risk factors involved have allowed an improvement in the

---

* Corresponding author.
E-mail address: daniel.cherqui@hmn.aphp.fr (D. Cherqui).

1055-3207/08/$ - see front matter © 2008 Elsevier Inc. All rights reserved.
doi:10.1016/j.soc.2008.02.002 *surgonc.theclinics.com*

results of partial liver resection for HCC both in terms of operative risk and long-term results [8–15]. This improvement has led to a renewed interest in liver resection for HCC, which remains the reference treatment for HCC in the normal liver and for which the indications for HCC in the cirrhotic liver are increasing.

The indications and the results for liver resection for HCC depend on the stage of the tumor at diagnosis, the functional reserve of the liver, and the use of suitably adapted surgical techniques. This article briefly discusses liver resection for HCC without CLD; then the majority of this article discusses liver resection for HCC with CLD.

Liver resection for hepatocellular carcinoma without chronic liver disease

About 10% of hepatocellular carcinomas are found in livers that are perfectly healthy or are affected by minimal fibrosis [1,2]. They present in younger patients without a male predominance. In most cases there is no identifiable cause, but a certain number of patients may have serologic markers of hepatitis B infection or hemochromatosis despite having a histologically normal liver. Fibrolamellar HCC is a particular histologic type of HCC that occurs in young females with a normal alpha-fetoprotein level and is more commonly associated with nodal metastases than the other forms of HCC [16–18].

In patients without known risk factors there is, of course, no screening and therefore at diagnosis the tumor is typically large and symptomatic. The most common symptoms are abdominal pain, the presence of a mass or heaviness in the right upper quadrant, or deterioration in the general condition. Rarely, the presentation is with jaundice or ascites, usually associated with an unresectable tumor.

Diagnosis is based on imaging and possibly confirmed with a biopsy of the tumor. Some authors biopsy hepatic tumors routinely; others do so only if the results will alter the management. If a biopsy is performed, it always should be done across normal liver to limit the risk of bleeding or tumor dissemination [19], and a biopsy of nontumoral liver should be associated to assess the underlying liver.

Morphologic evaluation is based on imaging including abdominal ultrasound, three-phase CT, and MRI of the liver. The choice between CT and MRI depends on local expertise and availability. The two methods, often associated, are equivalent in their evaluation of large lesions and in the identification of small lesions, particularly in identifying additional lesions contralateral to the primary tumor. New-generation, multidetector CT machines allow very high-quality vascular reconstructions and have obviated the need for preoperative diagnostic angiography. HCC without CLD typically presents as a single, large tumor that is hypervascular and heterogenous because of the presence of zones of necrosis. Imaging should specify the size of the tumor, its precise segmental location, and its relations to vascular structures, should identify endoluminal venous invasion (portal or hepatic venous tumor thrombus, which is characteristic of HCC) or the presence of satellite nodules or more distant additional lesions, and should include a volumetric study. Exclusion of dissemination, whether extrahepatic, pulmonary, nodal (rare except in fibrolamellar HCC), or adrenal, is essential. The role of fluorodeoxyglucose positron emission tomography in HCC has not been well evaluated.

Formal contraindications to the resection of HCC without CLD are the presence of extrahepatic metastases and the presence of multiple bilobar lesions. Invasion of the biliary confluence or tumor thrombus in the portal trunk or inferior vena cava are relative contradictions, as discussed later.

Resection is the treatment of choice for HCC without CLD. The role of transplantation remains very limited because of the advanced stage at diagnosis with its associated elevated risk of recurrence and the better tolerance of partial hepatic resection with a healthy liver [1,2,17]. Therefore, in the absence of alternative therapeutic options, the indications for resection should be broad.

Because of the usually advanced stage at presentation, a major hepatectomy, often extended, usually is required for the resection of HCC without CLD (Fig. 1). Such a hepatectomy may be performed with low morbidity and mortality because of the regenerative capacities of the normal liver. Preoperative volumetric studies should ensure that the functional residual volume after resection is at least 30% of the initial volume of the total liver. If this is not the case, portal vein embolization should be performed, as discussed later [12,20]. The resection should be anatomic and aim to obtain a margin greater than 1 cm. The techniques of resection are detailed later in the discussion of resection with CLD. A large incision is necessary. Rarely, a thoracoabdominal approach may be useful for a very large posterior tumor [21]. Operative exploration confirms the health of the

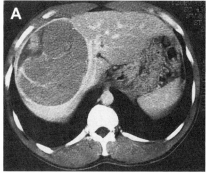 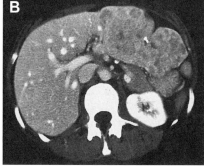

Fig. 1. HCC in normal liver. (*A*) Right-sided tumor: right hepatectomy extended to segment 4. (*B*) Left-sided fibrolamellar carcinoma with calcification: left hepatectomy.

nontumoral liver and evaluates the tumor characteristics. Intraoperative ultrasound evaluates the relations of the tumor to vascular structures and searches for additional lesions or unrecognized vascular invasion.

In cases of invasion of the inferior vena cava or the principal hepatic veins, total vascular exclusion of the liver may be necessary. With very large tumors, a hepatectomy without initial mobilization (anterior approach) is recommended (see later discussion) [22].

Five-year survival after resection of HCC without CLD is in the order of 50% to 60% [2,3,17,23]. The prognosis for fibrolamellar HCC normally is not different from that of other HCCs except when nodal metastases are present; in that case, the outlook is significantly worse [18]. Recurrences after resection of HCC without CLD often are widespread from the outset, and the treatment is palliative [17]. Screening for recurrences with regular imaging is justified, nevertheless, because certain isolated intrahepatic recurrences may be suitable for percutaneous ablation or iterative resection. In rare cases a limited recurrence occurring several months or years after the initial resection may be an indication for salvage liver transplantation.

Resection for hepatocellular carcinoma with chronic liver disease

About 90% of HCCs are associated with CLD. Any chronic hepatopathy can be complicated by HCC, but the most frequent causes are viral hepatitis B and C, alcoholism, and hemochromatosis [1]. Recently, nonalcoholic steatohepatitis has been recognized as a risk factor for HCC [24].

The complications of resection with CLD are related to the decreased regenerative abilities related to the fibrosis and, to a lesser degree, to the activity of the hepatitis. The patient is exposed to the risk of postoperative hepatic insufficiency that may result in death or chronic decompensation of the cirrhosis. Resection of HCC in the cirrhotic liver requires rigorous patient selection including evaluation of the tumor stage and of the functional hepatic reserve. Resection may be considered if a resection with curative intent can be performed with acceptable morbidity and mortality.

During the past decade important progress has been made in the quality of imaging techniques, better patient selection and preparation, the use of better-adapted surgical techniques, and optimized postoperative care. Better patient selection and reduced operative bleeding have reduced the operative mortality from more than 10% in the 1980s to less than 5% in most specialized centers today [8–15]. Certain teams have even reported zero mortality rates [11]. Certain studies also suggest that a lower recurrence rate and improved long-term survival can be achieved with an anatomic resection rather than a simple tumorectomy [25,26]. Long-term results also can be improved with treatment of the underlying liver disease, particularly with antiviral treatment. Also, screening for recurrence with regular postoperative imaging is justified by the availability of treatment methods [1,27,28].

Patient selection

Tumor staging

The morphologic evaluation is based on imaging, including screening abdominal ultrasound and hepatic cross-sectional imaging with triple-phase CT and/or MRI. Imaging should detail the size of the tumor, its precise segmental location, its vascular relations, and the presence of endoluminal venous invasion (portal or hepatic venous tumor thrombus characteristic of HCC) or satellite or distant nodules and should include volumetric studies. Metastatic disease should be excluded, in particular with CT of the thorax.

The indications for resection depend on the size of the lesions, their number, their location, and the estimated residual liver volume. The best candidates for resection are patients who have a single peripheral lesion allowing conservation of a residual liver volume of more than 50% [12,20]. HCC screening programs allow the identification of tumors matching these criteria at an early stage (<5 cm). In these cases, resection, transplantation, and percutaneous treatments are competing alternatives. The location of the tumor therefore is an important consideration in the choice of treatment. With a peripheral lesion, a resection may be performed with curative intent and in an anatomic fashion without sacrificing a large volume of parenchyma. Conversely, a central lesion smaller than 5 cm may require the sacrifice of a more significant volume of parenchyma with the risk of postoperative hepatic insufficiency, so that a percutaneous treatment or transplantation would be favored.

A large number of patients, however, still present at a more advanced stage with a tumor larger than 5 cm, above the limit for transplantation or percutaneous treatment. In these cases a major hepatic resection is the only possibility, and functional analysis and volumetric studies of the liver therefore are essential [29–31]. Arterial chemoembolization has been proposed by some as adjuvant treatment before resection of HCC in cirrhosis. This strategy may reduce the size of the lesion ("downstaging") [32] but has not been shown to prolong survival and is not used routinely [33]. Chemoembolization also may be used to potentiate the effect of portal embolization, if it is performed several weeks before the portal embolization (Figs. 2–5) [34].

The presence of satellite nodules often is evidence of locoregional metastatic spread caused by microscopic vascular invasion. This finding worsens the prognosis but is not a contraindication to surgery. The presence of bilobar lesions normally indicates multicentric carcinogenesis, suggesting that a resection is unlikely to be curative. Nevertheless, a limited resection (or destruction by radiofrequency) of a single lesion contralateral to the major hepatectomy may be performed if it is discovered intraoperatively [35].

As is the case for HCC without CLD, contraindications to resection of HCC with CLD include extrahepatic metastases, multiple bilobar lesions,

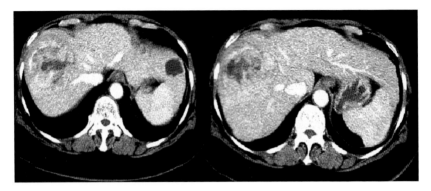

Fig. 2. HCC in cirrhosis. Large right-sided HCC (6 cm) in hepatitis B virus–associated cirrhosis. Patient is Child-Pugh's class A and has no signs of portal hypertension.

invasion of the biliary confluence, and extensive tumor thrombus of the portal venous trunk or the inferior vena cava.

Three particular cases merit special mention: HCC with vascular extension, biliary extension, or tumor rupture.

The presence of tumor thrombus in a major portal branch (sectorial or lobar), or less commonly in the hepatic veins, is seen often in advanced HCC. Such vascular invasion carries a poor prognosis, because it is associated with tumor dissemination, intrahepatic in the case of portal vein invasion and systemic in the case of hepatic vein invasion [36–38]. Nevertheless, in selected patients who are in good general condition and who have preserved hepatic function, resection may be considered because it may offer good palliation and, occasionally, prolonged survival. More rarely, extension to the portal bifurcation or the inferior vena cava may lead to a rescue procedure. Unblocking the portal venous trunk or the inferior vena cava therefore is necessary. In the latter case a thoracoabdominal approach is necessary with exposure and clamping of the intrapericardial inferior vena cava [37].

An HCC also can fistulate into the biliary tree. In this case, the presentation is of a liver tumor with obstructive jaundice. Treatment consists of liver resection with exploration and unblocking of the bile duct containing the tumor material [39].

Some HCCs present with an acute hemoperitoneum caused by tumor rupture. The reference treatment is urgent arterial embolization for hemostasis [40]. If the clinical course is favorable, a subsequent resection may be considered [41].

Estimation of functional hepatic reserve

Aside from evaluation of the tumor, an estimation of hepatic function is essential in selecting candidates for hepatic resection with CLD (Box 1;

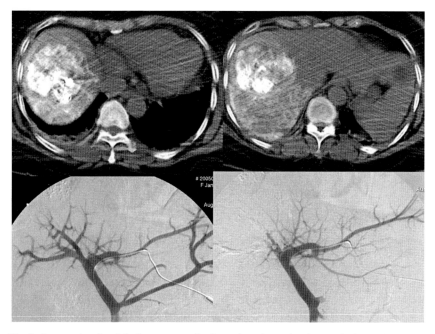

Fig. 3. Preparation for right hepatectomy in the patient shown in Fig. 2, who has a large HCC and cirrhosis. The top panel shows transarterial chemoembolization. CT at 3 weeks shows lipiodol accumulation in the tumor. The lower panel shows right portal vein embolization. Percutaneous puncture of a left portal vein branch allows access to the right portal vein, which is embolized with cyanoacrylate glue or coils.

Table 1). Hepatectomy with CLD is associated with significantly higher mortality and morbidity. The major risk is postoperative hepatic insufficiency, followed by chronic decompensation of the cirrhosis. Predictive criteria for the development of postoperative hepatic insufficiency are related essentially to preoperative hepatic function and the histologic grade of the underlying CLD. The evaluation of preoperative hepatic function is based on the Child-Pugh score [1,9,14], which is stratified into three groups: A (normal hepatic function), B (mild-to-moderate hepatocellular insufficiency), and C (severe hepatocellular insufficiency) (see Table 1). Most authors agree that in cirrhotic patients only those in Child-Pugh class A are suitable for a hepatic resection. Some authors, particularly in Asia, use global tests of hepatic function, in particular the indocyanine green retention test. This test involves injecting the dye and measuring its residual concentration after 15 minutes. For Makuuchi [11], the indocyanine green retention at 15 minutes defines the acceptable extent of resection: major hepatectomy is possible with up to 15% retention, and limited resection is mandated with retention above 20%.

Other criteria also need to be considered (see Box 1). In patients who have Child-Pugh class A cirrhosis, portal hypertension is correlated with

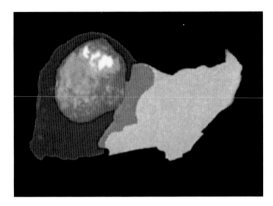

Fig. 4. Volumetric study after right portal vein embolization in the patient shown in Figs. 2 and 3. The left lobe increased by 20% with a functional remnant liver volume of 56%, allowing right hepatectomy (functional remnant volume = total volume − [right liver volume − tumor volume]).

postoperative decompensation of the cirrhosis, particularly in the form of ascites [42]. The portosystemic pressure gradient (wedged minus unwedged hepatic venous pressure) can be measured directly. A gradient greater than 10 mm Hg defines portal hypertension. Such direct measurement by hepatic venous catheterization is the reference method, but it is invasive and rarely used. The degree of portal hypertension is evaluated more commonly by searching for esophageal varices at upper endoscopy and by the presence of splenomegaly or collateral circulations on CT scanning. Thrombocytopenia is associated with splenomegaly and also is an indication of portal hypertension. A major hepatic resection is contraindicated in the presence of portal hypertension. A limited resection may be considered when the portal

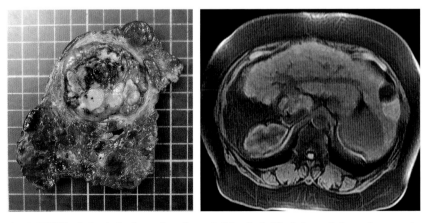

Fig. 5. HCC in cirrhosis (in the patient shown in Figs. 2–4). The left panel shows the operative specimen, an encapsulated 6-cm tumor on macronodular cirrhosis. The right panel shows the follow-up CT 6 months after right hepatectomy.

Box 1. Selection criteria for liver resection for hepatocellular carcinoma in chronic liver disease (F3 or F4 fibrosis on liver biopsy)

For a major resection (≥ three segments)
Child-Pugh class A
Indocyanine green retention at 15 minutes < 15% (mainly used in Asia)
No esophageal varices
Platelets > 100,000/mm^3
Transaminases ≤ two times normal
Hypertrophy of the contralateral liver after portal vein embolization
Functional residual liver volume > 50% (functional residual volume = total liver volume − [resected volume − volume of tumor])

For a limited resection (< three segments)
Child-Pugh class A
Child-Pugh class B for a peripheral tumorectomy
Esophageal varices grade 2 maximum

---

hypertension is minor. The cause of the underlying cirrhosis also can be considered in evaluating the risk involved in a hepatectomy, which seems better tolerated in viral hepatitis B than other causes (hepatitis C, alcohol, steatohepatitis) [14]. The activity of the hepatitis, estimated by the serum transaminase levels, is an established risk factor [31,43]. Farges and colleagues [31] have shown that transaminases more than twice the normal level are associated with increased mortality after major hepatectomy in patients who have CLD. In the presence of active hepatitis, the resection may be preceded by antiviral treatment or abstinence from alcohol, according to the cause, until the transaminase levels normalize.

Table 1
Child-Pugh classification

Parameters	Score		
	1	2	3
Prothrombin time (%)	>50	40–50	<40
Bilirubin (μmol/L)	<25	25–40	>40
Albumin (g/L)	>35	28–35	<28
Ascites	Absent	Minimal	Significant
Encephalopathy	0	I–II	III–IV

Child-Pugh A: 5–6 points; Child-Pugh B: 7–9 points; Child-Pugh C: 9–15 points.

Biopsy of the nontumoral liver is recommended to evaluate the degree of fibrosis and any hepatitis activity. Quantification of the fibrosis by the METAVIR score (F0 to F4) is useful [44]. The operative risk is maximal in cases of established cirrhosis (F4), is elevated in cases of severe fibrosis (F3), and is low in cases of mild fibrosis (F2). In cases of minimal fibrosis (F1), the risk is close to that of a hepatectomy in normal liver. Biopsy soon may be replaced by noninvasive methods (eg, FibroTest, elastometry).

The estimation of residual liver volume after resection is essential for patient selection. It requires a precise analysis of the imaging taking into account the respective volumes of the total liver, resected liver, and the tumor. This analysis enables the calculation of the percentage resection of functional parenchyma ([volume of resected liver − volume of the tumor]/ volume of the total liver) and, more importantly, the percentage functional residual liver volume (volume of remaining liver/[volume of total liver − volume of the tumor]) [12,20].

When a major hepatectomy (three or more segments) is required, especially a right hepatectomy, the operative risk is elevated in the presence of cirrhosis. The estimation of the residual liver volume therefore becomes extremely important, and it is considered that a hepatectomy of more than 50% should not be performed on a cirrhotic liver. With a large tumor occupying the greater part of a lobe, a resection sacrifices little functional parenchyma, especially because a spontaneous contralateral hypertrophy is often present [29]. In this case, the resection can be performed safely (Fig. 6). In other cases, preoperative portal vein embolization plays an important role [12,20]. This method involves percutaneous embolization of the portal branches of the hemiliver to be resected with the aim of inducing

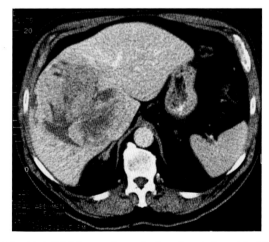

Fig. 6. A large right-sided HCC in a patient who has chronic hepatitis. The tumor occupies most of the right lobe, and left lobe hypertrophy has occurred. An extended right hepatectomy without prior portal vein embolization was performed.

hypertrophy of the future liver remnant (see Figs. 2–6). This method also has the advantage of evaluating the regenerative capacity of the liver and submits the liver to a stress test. If the portal embolization is not accompanied by contralateral hypertrophy, a major resection should be reconsidered. If hypertrophy is induced, the hepatectomy can be performed with a mortality rate less than 5%.

Today most authors agree that a portal vein embolization should be performed before a right hepatectomy in the cirrhotic liver. A left portal vein embolization also is possible but rarely is necessary, because the left liver rarely represents more the 40% of the total liver volume.

Surgical technique

A large incision is necessary to perform a safe resection. The incision consists of a bilateral subcostal incision with or without a median extension or, increasingly commonly, a J-shaped right subcostal incision avoiding an extension to the left.

Even though the extent of the resection and the type of clamping should be decided preoperatively, the initial surgical exploration is important and may lead to modifications of the surgical plan. This exploration evaluates the liver and the tumor and always should include intraoperative ultrasound [45]. The evaluation includes the consistency of the liver, the presence and type of cirrhosis (micro- or macronodular), the elasticity of the liver, and signs of portal hypertension. Ultrasonography is used to evaluate the tumor and its precise location and its relation to portal and hepatic venous structures and to search for vascular thromboses and other intrahepatic lesions. Ultrasonography is particularly important with impalpable tumors deep in a cirrhotic liver.

As with any hepatic resection, exposure of tumor in the transection line must be avoided, and a margin of at least 1 cm is recommended [46,47]. Once the indication for resection has been confirmed, three principles govern hepatic resection with CLD: parenchymal preservation, anatomic resection, and prevention of bleeding.

Parenchymal preservation and anatomic resection

Parenchymal preservation and anatomic resection, two principals that are apparently contradictory, are intimately linked and should be the guiding principles for resection of HCC with CLD. Unlike the healthy liver, in which the regenerative capacity allows resections of more than 60% of the hepatic parenchyma, resection in the presence of CLD requires preservation of parenchyma. The regenerative capacity is reduced by the hepatic fibrosis, especially when there is established cirrhosis, which incurs a risk of postoperative hepatic insufficiency. This concept is in apparent contradiction with that of the anatomic resection, which may require a greater parenchymal sacrifice than a simple tumorectomy or wedge resection. Parenchymal preservation requires precise analysis both preoperatively (imaging with volume studies) and intraoperatively (intraoperative ultrasound).

Although many recurrences after resection of a hepatocellular carcinoma are caused by the appearance of new nodules distant from the initial lesion (multicentric carcinogenesis in the setting of CLD), others are the result of intrahepatic dissemination of the tumor. HCC has a tendency for microscopic portal vascular invasion, the frequency of which increases with the size of the tumor. This portal invasion involves the adjacent portal branches leading to local metastatic spread. An anatomic resection removing the portal territory of the lesion therefore is the most logical treatment of hepatocellular carcinoma. Two recent retrospective studies have suggested that this theoretic advantage translates into significantly improved overall survival and disease-free survival [25,26]. Other studies, however, have not confirmed this advantage of an anatomic resection [48]. Therefore, if an anatomic resection remains the resection type of reference, parenchymal preservation may become a more important priority than anatomic resection in patients who have borderline hepatic function.

An anatomic resection is easily conceived when it involves a conventional hepatectomy: right hepatectomy, left hepatectomy or left-lateral sectionectomy. A major hepatectomy (three or more segments), however, should be considered only when the tumor is unsuitable for a more limited anatomic resection (see Fig. 5). With small, deep tumors, accommodation of the two principles (ie, both anatomic resection and parenchymal preservation) becomes more difficult and may require more complex resections, such as a central hepatectomy, also called "mesohepatectomy" (resection of segments 4, 5, and 8), a right anterior sectionectomy (bisegmentectomy, sections 5–8), a right posterior sectionectomy (bisegmentectomy, sections 6 and 7), or a nonsectional bisegmentectomy (bisegmentectomy, sections 5 and 6; and bisegmentectomy, sections 7 and 8) (Figs. 7–10) [15,49,50]. These anatomic resections are made possible by intraoperative ultrasound and selective vascular clamping, which allow the lines of transection to be defined by ischemia.

A peripheral tumor is an indication for a limited resection, either segmentectomy or subsegmentectomy. When the liver is very dysmorphic, and there is portal hypertension, it sometimes is preferable to settle for a nonanatomic wedge resection with a margin of at least 1 cm (tumorectomy) [46,47].

Prevention of bleeding

Numerous studies have shown that intraoperative bleeding and blood transfusions influence the prognosis for liver resections for cancer. This effect is seen both in operative morbidity and mortality and in long-term survival, bleeding and transfusions being associated with an increased frequency of tumor recurrence [10,11].

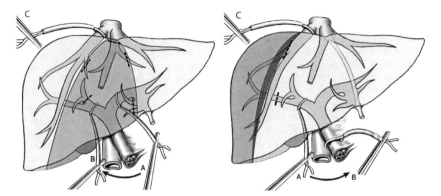

Fig. 7. Operative technique for central hepatectomy. (*Left panel*) Resection of segments 4, 5, and 8. For a central hepatectomy, alternate lobar clamping can be used for each transection (A for left transection followed by B for right transection) to reduce clamping time for each hemiliver. (*Right panel*) Posterior sectionectomy (resection of segments 6 and 7). For posterior sectionectomy, selective right lobar clamping (A) can be used and converted to a Pringle maneuver (B) if insufficient. For both operations, the right hepatic vein (C) can be clamped to occlude outflow, if necessary.

Limiting bleeding requires the use of vascular clamping, low central venous pressure anesthesia, the anterior approach for large tumors, and adequate methods of parenchymal transection.

The diseased liver is less tolerant of ischemia than the normal liver. Intermittent hepatic pedicle clamping (clamping for 15 minutes followed by unclamping for 5 minutes) is well tolerated by the cirrhotic liver and reduces bleeding effectively [10,11,51]. A prospective, randomized trial comparing intermittent clamping with continuous clamping demonstrated the advantages of intermittent clamping, particularly in the cirrhotic liver [51]. Intermittent clamping allows clamp times much longer than is possible with

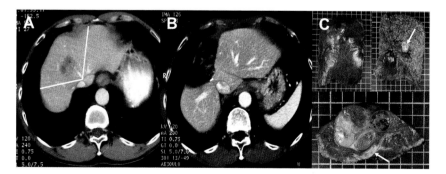

Fig. 8. Central HCC on a cirrhotic liver. (*A*) Tumor across segments 4 and 8. The principles of anatomic resection and parenchymal preservation can be accommodated by performing central hepatectomy (resections of segments 4, 5, and 8) as an alternative to extended right or left hepatectomy. (*B*) Follow-up CT. (*C*) Specimen. White arrows show the right anterior sectional pedicle.

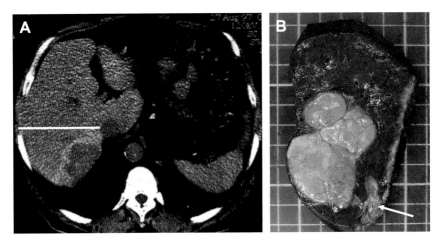

Fig. 9. (*A*) HCC in segment 7 of a cirrhotic liver. (*B*) Specimen of posterior sectionectomy (resection of segments 6 and 7). The arrow indicates the right posterior section pedicle.

continuous clamping, even in the diseased liver; clamp times longer than 90 minutes have been reported without deleterious effects [11]. This technique allows bleeding to be reduced and provides time for a meticulous and anatomic resection.

Another method aimed at reducing the ischemic injury to the liver during clamping is ischemic preconditioning, which consists of applying pedicular clamping for 10 minutes followed by unclamping for 10 minutes and then continuous clamping [52]. This method is effective in the healthy liver and for short clamp times (<30 minutes) but is less effective than intermittent

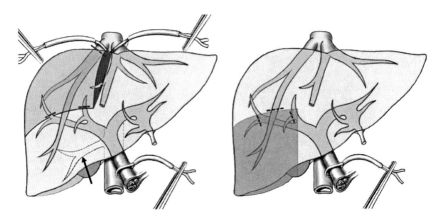

Fig. 10. Operative technique for bisegmentectomy. (*Left panel*) Bisegmentectomy of segments 7 and 8 includes resection of the right hepatic vein and requires the presence of a large right inferior accessory hepatic vein (*arrow*). (*Right panel*) Bisegmentectomy of segments 5 and 6.

clamping for long clamp times or in the diseased liver. It therefore is more applicable to surgery for metastases or benign lesions and rarely is applicable to resections for HCC.

Aside from clamping, the other essential element in the reduction of bleeding is low central venous pressure anesthesia maintained by limiting intraoperative fluid administration as much as possible, particularly before and during the phase of parenchymal transection [53]. This approach is effective in hepatectomies in both healthy and diseased livers but requires an experienced anesthetic team and an excellent collaboration between the surgical and anesthetic teams. The combination of intermittent pedicular clamping and low central venous pressure should avoid all massive bleeding and allow 80% of patients to be operated without requiring blood transfusion.

Total vascular exclusion of the liver is rarely necessary and is required only in cases involving the inferior vena cava. Total vascular exclusion seems to be less well tolerated in the diseased liver. Total vascular exclusion preserving the caval flow (clamping of the hepatic pedicle and the main hepatic veins) also may be used and has the advantage of making intermittent clamping possible [54].

Pedicular clamping is not always necessary, however. In cases of hemihepatectomy, initial section of the Glissonian pedicle outside the liver devascularizes and defines the lobe to be resected by the ischemia thus created. This method, combined with low central venous pressure, often is sufficient to perform a right or left hepatectomy without clamping and without bleeding. Nevertheless, in cases of even minimal bleeding, progression to clamping is recommended.

The selective control of the sectorial pedicles is very useful in performing complex anatomic resections [15]. A suprahilar approach allows the extrahepatic control of the right and left Glissonian pedicles so that alternating selective clamping can be used for central resections. This maneuver can be extended more distally on the right with control of the anterior and posterior sectorial pedicles. The selective clamping of these pedicles allows the exact anatomic definition of the sections by the zone of ischemia and thus allows formal anatomic resections.

Traditionally it has been recommended that, when a major hepatectomy is performed, the liver should be mobilized completely, with a dissection of the anterior surface of the inferior vena cava with control of the hepatic veins. This method is reliable and important in the training of surgeons. With a very large tumor of the right liver, however, mobilization is difficult, can cause bleeding, and can lead to tumor rupture or to the mobilization of endovascular tumor fragments. In these situations a hepatectomy via an anterior approach without initial mobilization of the liver has been proposed, and this approach represents an important advance [22]. This method reduces the risk of tumor rupture and bleeding during the maneuvers to mobilize the liver, limits the ischemia of the contralateral liver by removing the need for prolonged twisting of the liver, and may be associated with better oncologic results by reducing the number of tumor cells liberated into the circulation. For these reasons, certain authors now recommend wider use of this technique, even without a large tumor. A right hepatectomy by the anterior approach consists of dividing the right Glissonian pedicle and transecting the liver, from the front backward, with or without clamping, up to the retrohepatic vena cava. One then can divide the accessory hepatic veins followed by the right hepatic vein and the hepatocaval ligament and finish with the mobilization of the right liver, which now is excluded completely from the circulation. The anterior approach may be facilitated by a "hanging maneuver," as described by Belghiti [55], in which an umbilical tape is passed between the inferior vena cava and the liver. The entry point is the middle of the infrahepatic vena cava, and the exit point is between the terminations of the middle and right hepatic veins. This maneuver helps guide the transection plane and reduce bleeding, particularly at the end of the transection in front of the vena cava.

Numerous methods of transecting the liver have been proposed. The methods used most frequently include the clamp-fracture technique, the ultrasonic dissector, and the harmonic scalpel. Many authors recommend the use of the ultrasonic dissector, but two randomized studies investigating its use did not demonstrate its superiority [56,57]. All of the methods seem to be equivalent, the choice depending on availability and individual surgeon's preferences. Hemostasis is achieved with bipolar electrocautery, clips, and ties according to the size of the structures. Linear staplers also may be used on the Glissonian pedicles and the hepatic veins.

Closure and drainage

The risk of postoperative ascites mandates a watertight closure of the abdominal wall and skin because of the risk of an ascitic leak and infection of the ascites. For the same reason, it is recommended that abdominal drainage be avoided after hepatectomy in cirrhosis [58]. If drainage is deemed to be necessary, it should be under negative pressure and of small caliber [59].

Laparoscopic resections

Laparoscopic hepatic resection remains limited in its development, but it has generated a certain interest in the treatment of HCC in patients who have cirrhosis [60–66]. Laparoscopic hepatic resection can be considered in lesions smaller than 5 cm located in the peripheral segments of the liver (segments 2–6) (Fig. 11). Even though major resections have been performed laparoscopically, laparoscopic resections usually are minor resections: mono- or bi-segmentectomies, and in particular left lateral sectionectomies or tumorectomies (Fig. 12). The absence of large abdominal incisions seems to reduce morbidity, in particular postoperative ascites. This reduced

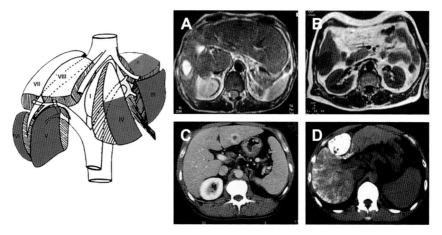

Fig. 11. (*Left panel*) Laparoscopic liver segments. (*Right panel A–D*) Examples of HCCs selected for laparoscopic resection.

morbidity allows the indications for resection to be extended to suitable peripheral tumors in patients who have ascites or moderate hepatic insufficiency in which a laparotomy generally would be contraindicated. Furthermore, reoperation is much easier after a laparoscopic resection than after a previous laparotomy. A subsequent liver transplantation can be performed without the added difficulties, particularly bleeding, created by a previous laparotomy.

Postoperative care

The morbidity rate for hepatic resections in the cirrhotic liver is in the order of 30% to 50%, and the complications may be severe [67,68]. The principal complication is postoperative hepatic insufficiency. The manifestations of postoperative hepatic insufficiency are jaundice, reduced coagulation factors (increased prothrombin time or international normalized ratio), ascites, and hepatic encephalopathy. Ascites is common even after minor resections in the cirrhotic liver. Abundant ascites can be complicated by leaking through the abdominal wall, infection, and respiratory compromise. The morbidity also includes respiratory complications, infection, and renal insufficiency, which themselves may be secondary to or causative factors for hepatic insufficiency.

For these reasons, hepatic resections in the cirrhotic liver require management in specialized centers. Measures should be taken to reduce these complications, including fluid and salt restriction, prophylactic antibiotics, nutritional support, and prudent drug management (analgesic and sedative medications, nephrotoxic medications). Early identification and management of complications is essential [69].

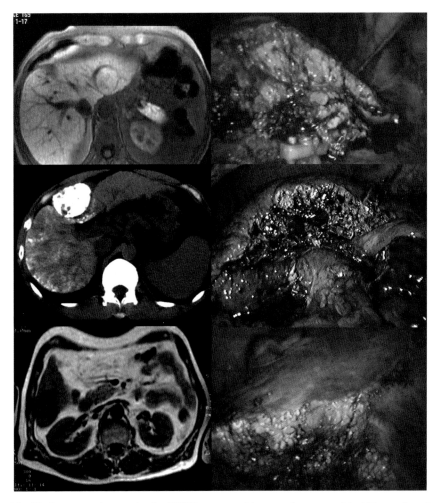

Fig. 12. Laparoscopic resection for HCC in segment 2 (*top panel*), segment 4 (*middle panel*), and segment 6 (*bottom panel*).

Results of hepatic resection for hepatocellular carcinoma with chronic liver disease

The results of the main Asian and Western series are summarized in Table 2 [8,10,14,23,43,70–77]. As discussed previously, operative mortality has improved greatly during the last 15 years. In the study by Poon and colleagues [10] comparing two consecutive periods, the hospital mortality decreased from 13% for the period 1989 to 1993 to 2.5% for the period 1994 to 1999. This study demonstrates that the criteria associated with improved survival are presentation at an asymptomatic stage, TNM stage, and the absence of blood transfusion. In the Japanese registry, which

LIVER RESECTION FOR HEPATOCELLULAR CARCINOMA

Table 2
Results of surgery with curative intent for hepatocellular carcinoma with chronic liver disease

Author	Year	Study period	N	Cirrhosis (%)	Diameter < 5 cm (%)	Operative mortality (%)	Survival (%)		
							1 year	3 years	5 years
Asian series									
Nagasue	1993	1980–1990	229	77	75	11	80	51	26
Kawasaki	1995	1990–1993	112	68	83	2	92	79	—
Chen	1997	1983–1994	382	45	40	4	71	52	46
Makuuchi	1998	1990–1997	352	—	—	<1	92	73	47
Poon	2001	1989–1993	136	50	29	13	68	47	36
		1994–1999	241	43	45	2.5	82	62	49
Shimozawa	2004	1987–2001	135	71	100	2	95	73	55
Western series									
Franco	1990	1983–1998	72	100	60	7	68	51	—
Vauthey	1995	1970–1992	106	33	17	6	—	—	41
Llovet	1999	1989–1997	77	100	75	NA	85	62	51
Fong	1999	1991–1998	154	65	24	4.5	81	54	37
Belghiti	2002	1990–1999	300	82	47	6	81	57	37
Ercolani	2003	1983–1999	224	100	81	3	83	63	42
Cha	2003	1990–2001	164	40	—	4	79	51	40
Author's series		1989–1999	98	80	51	11	65	51	44
		2000–2007	156	81	52	4	74	53	41

includes12,000 patients treated between 1990 and 1999, the operative mortality has decreased from 2.3% in 1990 and 1991 to 0.6% in 1998 and1999 [78].

The results in terms of long-term survival vary among series because of differing inclusion criteria. For patients who have favorable prognostic features (single tumor, Child-Pugh class A, absence of portal hypertension), survival rates of 50% to 70% have been reported. The largest series published to date is the Japanese registry with survival at 1, 3, and 5 years of 85%, 67%, and 50%, respectively [78]. Others have reported comparable results, without a notable difference between Asian and Western series [79].

Because of the persisting underlying liver disease, intrahepatic recurrences are common: 60% to 80% at 5 years in the literature [8,80]. The recurrences commonly occur at sites distant to the initial resection and are evidence of multicentric carcinogenesis. More rarely, a recurrence may develop close to the site of resection; this recurrence may be a metastatic extension of the initial lesion and therefore occurs early. Numerous prognostic factors that influence the survival after resection for HCC have been identified and are summarized in Table 3. These factors concern the state of the underlying liver, the pathologic features of the tumor, and the quality of the resection. Among these factors three principal ones are found commonly: the severity of the underlying liver disease, the size and number of lesions, and the presence or absence of micro- and macroscopic vascular invasion. In a multicentric American study, patients having a resection for a single tumor 5 cm or smaller had a survival at 5 years of 43%, compared with 32% for those who had a tumor larger than 5 cm [81]. The presence of multiple nodules usually is evidence of advanced disease and is associated with reduced survival and an increased rate of recurrence. In the Japanese registry, the 5-year survival was 57% for patients who had single tumors and 26% for patients who had three or more tumors [78]. The presence of macroscopic vascular invasion is the most unfavorable prognostic factor. In a recent Western multicentric study of 102 patients, resection in the presence of invasion of a portal branch or major vein was associated with survival at 1, 3, and 5 years of 47%, 17%, and 10% respectively [37]. Microscopic vascular invasion also has an independent prognostic value. In the study by Vauthey and colleagues [81] the 5-year survival in the absence of macroscopic and microscopic vascular invasion was 41% and 46%, respectively, and was 15% and 29%, respectively, in the presence of these criteria. There is a correlation between the size of the largest nodule and the presence of microscopic vascular invasion [82]. Microvascular invasion is present in 20% of cases with a tumor smaller than 2 cm, in 30% to 60% of cases with tumors between 2 and 5 cm, and 60% to 90% of cases with tumors larger than 5 cm [83].

Other criteria found in specific studies are tumor differentiation (Edmondson grade), the presence or absence of a peritumoral capsule, the presence or absence of blood transfusions during the procedure, and the

Table 3
Prognostic factors for survival after liver resection for hepatocellular carcinoma with chronic liver disease

Factor	Favorable	Unfavorable
Liver factors		
Child-Pugh class	A	B
Bilirubin	Normal	Elevated
Severity of fibrosis	No cirrhosis	Cirrhosis
Portal hypertension	Absent	Present
Hepatitis activity (transaminases)	Normal	>Two times normal
Tumor factors		
Size	<2–3 cm	>5 cm
Number	Single	Multiple, bilobar
Macroscopic vascular invasion	Absent	Present
Microscopic vascular invasion	Absent	Present
Differentiation	Well differentiated	Poorly differentiated
Satellite nodules	Absent	Present
Fibrous peritumoral capsule	Present and not breached	Absent or breached
Alpha-fetoprotein	Normal	>1000
Surgical factors		
Margin	>1 cm	<1 cm
Type of resection	Anatomic	Nonanatomic
Blood transfusion	Absent	Present

alpha-fetoprotein level. Molecular prognostic criteria (genetic expression) currently are under investigation [84,85].

Prevention, screening, and treatment of recurrences

Certain adjuvant strategies that aim to treat undetected intrahepatic micrometastases are chemoembolization, internal irradiation, and systemic chemotherapy. Other strategies aim to prevent the recurrence of de novo tumors by treatment of the hepatopathy (antiviral treatment, retinoids). Several randomized studies have been conducted in Asia. Systemic chemotherapy and chemoembolization have had no effect on recurrences [33]. Internal irradiation with Iodine-131–labeled lipiodol may have a beneficial effect, as suggested by one incomplete randomized trial and one nonrandomized French study [86–88]. Studies of immunotherapy (activated lymphocytes or alpha-interferon) or the administration of retinoids have suggested that these strategies might reduce the recurrence rate, but these strategies have not entered regular practice [89,90]. Antiviral treatment (interferon and ribavirin for hepatitis C, lamivudine and adefovir for hepatitis B) as primary prevention for HCC has been suggested and should be tested in secondary prevention [91,92]. The advent of targeted therapies, such as antiangiogenic drugs (sorafenib), may show promising results [93] and could lead to phase III studies for adjuvant treatment after resection of HCC.

The options for treatment of recurrences justify screening for them. This screening involves regular imaging by ultrasonography, CT scan, or MRI (every 3 months for the first year and every 6 months thereafter) and al-pha-fetoprotein level. The options for treatment of recurrences include re-peat resection, percutaneous destruction, and salvage transplantation [27,28,94,95]. Repeat resection is rarely performed; the published studies are few and include few patients. This option may be considered in cases of unifocal recurrence in patients who have compensated liver disease. Per-cutaneous ablation may be considered in cases of small unifocal recurrence. Salvage transplantation is theoretically the best option, although it is limited by the shortage of donors. It may be considered in cases conforming to the Milan criteria. Salvage transplantation occasionally can be offered to pa-tients who had previous resection for a tumor outside the Milan criteria, with the initial resection serving as a downstaging procedure. The Barcelona unit has proposed the pre-emptive transplantation of patients who have had a complete resection but have histologic criteria for an elevated recurrence rate (poorly differentiated, microscopic vascular invasion, satellite nodules) [96]. Resection may be considered as a method for selecting candidates for transplantation or even as a bridging treatment in patients on the waiting list who have a peripheral tumor that is easily resectable. The authors use laparoscopic resection in this situation [60].

Summary

Today, resection of HCC with curative intent has an important place in the treatment of HCC.

HCC without CLD is rare and normally is large and symptomatic at the time of diagnosis. A major hepatectomy is the reference treatment. It offers the best chances of survival and can be performed with a small operative risk.

HCC with CLD represents 90% of cases. Knowledge of the risk factors for HCC has lead to screening programs allowing these lesions to be iden-tified at an early stage. The possibilities for resection are limited by the un-derlying hepatopathy, which increases the operative risk and the risk of intrahepatic recurrence. Recent advances, however, have improved the tol-erance of these resections by better patient selection and surgical technique. Candidates for resection of HCC with CLD should have preserved hepatic function (Child-Pugh class A) without portal hypertension, and the resec-tion should not surpass 50% of the functional liver volume. The principles of resection of HCC with CLD include an anatomic resection, parenchymal preservation, and minimization of bleeding. Preoperative portal vein embo-lization increases the possibilities for a major hepatic resection in the pres-ence of CLD. For limited resections of peripheral lesions, the laparoscopic approach has given promising early results. All these advances allow the resection of HCC with CLD with mortality less than 5%, a transfusion rate less than 20%, and an overall survival at 5 years comparable to that of transplantation for early tumors (< 5 cm) and in the order of 50% for more advanced lesions. Intrahepatic recurrences are very common, nevertheless, because of the persistence of the underlying hepatopathy. Recurrences should be screened for and, when possible, treated by repeat resection, percutaneous destruction, or salvage liver transplantation.

References

[1] Llovet JM, Burroughs A, Bruix J. Hepatocellular carcinoma. Lancet 2003;362:1907–17.
[2] Bralet MP, Regimbeau JM, Pineau P, et al. Hepatocellular carcinoma occurring in nonfibrotic liver: epidemiologic and histopathologic analysis of 80 French cases. Hepatology 2000;32:200–4.
[3] Bismuth H, Chiche L, Castaing D. Surgical treatment of hepatocellular carcinomas in noncirrhotic liver: experience with 68 liver resections. World J Surg 1995;19:35–41.
[4] Mazzaferro V, Regalia E, Doci R, et al. Liver transplantation for the treatment of small hepatocellular carcinomas in patients with cirrhosis. N Engl J Med 1996;334:693–9.
[5] Tong MJ, Blatt LM, Kao VW. Surveillance for hepatocellular carcinoma in patients with chronic viral hepatitis in the United States of America. J Gastroenterol Hepatol 2001;16: 553–9.
[6] Bolondi L, Sofia S, Siringo S, et al. Surveillance programme of cirrhotic patients for early diagnosis and treatment of hepatocellular carcinoma: a cost effectiveness analysis. Gut 2001;48:251–9.
[7] Llovet JM, Fuster J, Bruix J. The Barcelona approach: diagnosis, staging, and treatment of hepatocellular carcinoma. Liver Transpl 2004;10:S115–20.
[8] Llovet JM, Fuster J, Bruix J. Intention-to-treat analysis of surgical treatment for early hepatocellular carcinoma: resection versus transplantation. Hepatology 1999;30:1434–40.
[9] Bismuth H, Chiche L, Adam R, et al. Liver resection versus transplantation for hepatocellular carcinoma in cirrhotic patients. Ann Surg 1993;218:145–51.
[10] Poon RT, Fan ST, Lo CM, et al. Improving survival results after resection of hepatocellular carcinoma: a prospective study of 377 patients over 10 years. Ann Surg 2001;234:63–70.
[11] Imamura H, Seyama Y, Kokudo N, et al. One thousand fifty-six hepatectomies without mortality in 8 years. Arch Surg 2003;138:1198–206.
[12] Azoulay D, Castaing D, Krissat J, et al. Percutaneous portal vein embolization increases the feasibility and safety of major liver resection for hepatocellular carcinoma in injured liver. Ann Surg 2000;232:665–72.
[13] Cha CH, Ruo L, Fong Y, et al. Resection of hepatocellular carcinoma in patients otherwise eligible for transplantation. Ann Surg 2003;238:315–21.
[14] Belghiti J, Regimbeau JM, Durand F, et al. Resection of hepatocellular carcinoma: a European experience on 328 cases. Hepatogastroenterology 2002;49:41–6.
[15] Chouillard E, Cherqui D, Tayar C, et al. Anatomical bi- and trisegmentectomies as alternatives to extensive liver resections. Ann Surg 2003;238:29–34.
[16] El-Serag HB, Davila JA. Is fibrolamellar carcinoma different from hepatocellular carcinoma? A US population-based study. Hepatology 2004;39:798–803.
[17] Bilimoria MM, Lauwers GY, Doherty DA, et al. Underlying liver disease, not tumor factors, predicts long-term survival after resection of hepatocellular carcinoma. Arch Surg 2001;136: 528–35.
[18] Kakar S, Burgart LJ, Batts KP, et al. Clinicopathologic features and survival in fibrolamellar carcinoma: comparison with conventional hepatocellular carcinoma with and without cirrhosis. Mod Pathol 2005;18:1417–23.

[19] Ng KK, Poon RT, Lo CM, et al. Impact of preoperative fine-needle aspiration cytologic examination on clinical outcome in patients with hepatocellular carcinoma in a tertiary referral center. Arch Surg 2004;139:193–200.

[20] Farges O, Belghiti J, Kianmanesh R, et al. Portal vein embolization before right hepatectomy: prospective clinical trial. Ann Surg 2003;237:208–17.

[21] Xia F, Poon RT, Fan ST, et al. Thoracoabdominal approach for right-sided hepatic resection for hepatocellular carcinoma. J Am Coll Surg 2003;196:418–27.

[22] Liu CL, Fan ST, Lo CM, et al. Anterior approach for major right hepatic resection for large hepatocellular carcinoma. Ann Surg 2000;232:25–31.

[23] Fong Y, Sun RL, Jarnagin W, et al. An analysis of 412 cases of hepatocellular carcinoma at a Western center. Ann Surg 1999;229:790–9.

[24] Caldwell SH, Crespo DM, Kang HS, et al. Obesity and hepatocellular carcinoma. Gastroenterology 2004;127:S97–103.

[25] Regimbeau JM, Kianmanesh R, Farges O, et al. Extent of liver resection influences the outcome in patients with cirrhosis and small hepatocellular carcinoma. Surgery 2002;131:311–7.

[26] Hasegawa K, Kokudo N, Imamura H, et al. Prognostic impact of anatomic resection for hepatocellular carcinoma. Ann Surg 2005;242:252–9.

[27] Minagawa M, Makuuchi M, Takayama T, et al. Selection criteria for repeat hepatectomy in patients with recurrent hepatocellular carcinoma. Ann Surg 2003;238:703–10.

[28] Poon RT, Fan ST, Lo CM, et al. Long-term survival and pattern of recurrence after resection of small hepatocellular carcinoma in patients with preserved liver function: implications for a strategy of salvage transplantation. Ann Surg 2002;235:373–82.

[29] Poon RT, Fan ST, Lo CM, et al. Extended hepatic resection for hepatocellular carcinoma in patients with cirrhosis: is it justified? Ann Surg 2002;236:602–11.

[30] Pawlik TM, Poon RT, Abdalla EK, et al. Critical appraisal of the clinical and pathologic predictors of survival after resection of large hepatocellular carcinoma. Arch Surg 2005;140:450–7.

[31] Farges O, Malassagne B, Flejou JF, et al. Risk of major liver resection in patients with underlying chronic liver disease: a reappraisal. Ann Surg 1999;229:210–5.

[32] Majno PE, Adam R, Bismuth H, et al. Influence of preoperative transarterial lipiodol chemoembolization on resection and transplantation for hepatocellular carcinoma in patients with cirrhosis. Ann Surg 1997;226:688–701.

[33] Schwartz JD, Schwartz M, Mandeli J, et al. Neoadjuvant and adjuvant therapy for resectable hepatocellular carcinoma: review of the randomised clinical trials. Lancet Oncol 2002;3:593–603.

[34] Aoki T, Imamura H, Hasegawa K, et al. Sequential preoperative arterial and portal venous embolizations in patients with hepatocellular carcinoma. Arch Surg 2004;139:766–74.

[35] Liu CL, Fan ST, Lo CM, et al. Hepatic resection for bilobar hepatocellular carcinoma: is it justified? Arch Surg 2003;138:100–4.

[36] Poon RT, Fan ST, Ng IO, et al. Prognosis after hepatic resection for stage IVA hepatocellular carcinoma: a need for reclassification. Ann Surg 2003;237:376–83.

[37] Pawlik TM, Poon RT, Abdalla EK, et al. Hepatectomy for hepatocellular carcinoma with major portal or hepatic vein invasion: results of a multicenter study. Surgery 2005;137:403–10.

[38] Minagawa M, Makuuchi M, Takayama T, et al. Selection criteria for hepatectomy in patients with hepatocellular carcinoma and portal vein tumor thrombus. Ann Surg 2001;233:379–84.

[39] Tantawi B, Cherqui D, Tran van Nhieu J, et al. Surgery for biliary obstruction by tumour thrombus in primary liver cancer. Br J Surg 1996;83:1522–5.

[40] Liu CL, Fan ST, Lo CM, et al. Management of spontaneous rupture of hepatocellular carcinoma: single-center experience. J Clin Oncol 2001;19:3725–32.

[41] Cherqui D, Panis Y, Rotman N, et al. Emergency liver resection for spontaneous rupture of hepatocellular carcinoma complicating cirrhosis. Br J Surg 1993;80:747–9.

[42] Bruix J, Castells A, Bosch J, et al. Surgical resection of hepatocellular carcinoma in cirrhotic patients: prognostic value of preoperative portal pressure. Gastroenterology 1996;111: 1018–22.

[43] Ercolani G, Grazi GL, Ravaioli M, et al. Liver resection for hepatocellular carcinoma on cirrhosis: univariate and multivariate analysis of risk factors for intrahepatic recurrence. Ann Surg 2003;237:536–43.

[44] Intraobserver and interobserver variations in liver biopsy interpretation in patients with chronic hepatitis C. The French METAVIR Cooperative Study Group. Hepatology 1994; 20:15–20.

[45] Makuuchi M, Hasegawa H, Yamazaki S, et al. The use of operative ultrasound as an aid to liver resection in patients with hepatocellular carcinoma. World J Surg 1987;11:615–21.

[46] Poon RT, Fan ST, Ng IO, et al. Significance of resection margin in hepatectomy for hepatocellular carcinoma: a critical reappraisal. Ann Surg 2000;231:544–51.

[47] Ochiai T, Takayama T, Inoue K, et al. Hepatic resection with and without surgical margins for hepatocellular carcinoma in patients with impaired liver function. Hepatogastroenterology 1999;46:1885–9.

[48] Kaibori M, Matsui Y, Hijikawa T, et al. Comparison of limited and anatomic hepatic resection for hepatocellular carcinoma with hepatitis C. Surgery 2006;139:385–94.

[49] Bismuth H. Surgical anatomy and anatomical surgery of the liver. World J Surg 1982;6:3–9.

[50] Makuuchi M, Hasegawa H, Yamazaki S, et al. Four new hepatectomy procedures for resection of the right hepatic vein and preservation of the inferior right hepatic vein. Surg Gynecol Obstet 1987;164:68–72.

[51] Belghiti J, Noun R, Malafosse R, et al. Continuous versus intermittent portal triad clamping for liver resection: a controlled study. Ann Surg 1999;229:369–75.

[52] Clavien PA, Selzner M, Rudiger HA, et al. A prospective randomized study in 100 consecutive patients undergoing major liver resection with versus without ischemic preconditioning. Ann Surg 2003;238:843–50.

[53] Wang WD, Liang LJ, Huang XQ, et al. Low central venous pressure reduces blood loss in hepatectomy. World J Gastroenterol 2006;14(12):935–9.

[54] Cherqui D, Malassagne B, Colau PI, et al. Hepatic vascular exclusion with preservation of the caval flow for liver resections. Ann Surg 1999;230:24–30.

[55] Belghiti J, Guevara OA, Noun R, et al. Liver hanging maneuver: a safe approach to right hepatectomy without liver mobilization. J Am Coll Surg 2001;193:109–11.

[56] Takayama T, Makuuchi M, Kubota K, et al. Randomized comparison of ultrasonic vs clamp transection of the liver. Arch Surg 2001;136:922–8.

[57] Lesurtel M, Selzner M, Petrowsky H, et al. How should transection of the liver be performed?: a prospective randomized study in 100 consecutive patients: comparing four different transection strategies. Ann Surg 2005;242:814–22.

[58] Liu CL, Fan ST, Lo CM, et al. Abdominal drainage after hepatic resection is contraindicated in patients with chronic liver diseases. Ann Surg 2004;239:194–201.

[59] Fuster J, Llovet JM, Garcia-Valdecasas JC, et al. Abdominal drainage after liver resection for hepatocellular carcinoma in cirrhotic patients: a randomized controlled study. Hepatogastroenterology 2004;51:536–40.

[60] Cherqui D, Laurent A, Tayar C, et al. Laparoscopic liver resection for peripheral hepatocellular carcinoma in patients with chronic liver disease: midterm results and perspectives. Ann Surg 2006;243:499–506.

[61] Champault A, Dagher I, Vons C, et al. Laparoscopic hepatic resection for hepatocellular carcinoma. Retrospective study of 12 patients. Gastroenterol Clin Biol 2005;29:969–73.

[62] Vibert E, Perniceni T, Levard H, et al. Laparoscopic liver resection. Br J Surg 2006;93:67–72.

[63] Teramoto K, Kawamura T, Takamatsu S, et al. Laparoscopic and thoracoscopic approaches for the treatment of hepatocellular carcinoma. Am J Surg 2005;189:474–8.

[64] Kaneko H, Takagi S, Otsuka Y, et al. Laparoscopic liver resection of hepatocellular carcinoma. Am J Surg 2005;189:190–4.

[65] Gigot JF, Glineur D, Santiago Azagra J, et al. Laparoscopic liver resection for malignant liver tumors: preliminary results of a multicenter European study. Ann Surg 2002;236:90–7.

[66] Montorsi M, Santambrogio R, Bianchi P, et al. Perspectives and drawbacks of minimally invasive surgery for hepatocellular carcinoma. Hepatogastroenterology 2002;49:56–61.

[67] Balzan S, Belghiti J, Farges O, et al. The "50-50 criteria" on postoperative day 5: an accurate predictor of liver failure and death after hepatectomy. Ann Surg 2005;242:824–8.

[68] Wei AC, Tung-Ping Poon R, Fan ST, et al. Risk factors for perioperative morbidity and mortality after extended hepatectomy for hepatocellular carcinoma. Br J Surg 2003;90: 33–41.

[69] Fan ST, Lo CM, Lai EC, et al. Perioperative nutritional support in patients undergoing hepatectomy for hepatocellular carcinoma. N Engl J Med 1994;331:1547–52.

[70] Nagasue N, Uchida M, Makino Y, et al. Incidence and factors associated with intrahepatic recurrence following resection of hepatocellular carcinoma. Gastroenterology 1993;105: 488–94.

[71] Kawasaki S, Makuuchi M, Miyagawa S, et al. Results of hepatic resection for hepatocellular carcinoma. World J Surg 1995;19:31–4.

[72] Chen MF, Jeng LB. Partial hepatic resection for hepatocellular carcinoma. J Gastroenterol Hepatol 1997;12:S329–34.

[73] Makuuchi M, Takayama T, Kubota K, et al. Hepatic resection for hepatocellular carcinoma—Japanese experience. Hepatogastroenterology 1998;45:s1267–74.

[74] Shimozawa N, Hanazaki K. Long term prognosis after hepatic resection for small hepatocellular carcinoma. J Am Coll Surg 2004;198:356–65.

[75] Franco D, Capussotti L, Smadja C, et al. Resection of hepatocellular carcinomas. Results in 72 European patients with cirrhosis. Gastroenterology 1990;98:733–8.

[76] Vauthey JN, Klimstra D, Franceschi D, et al. Factors affecting long-term outcome after hepatic resection for hepatocellular carcinoma. Am J Surg 1995;169:28–34.

[77] Cha C, Fong Y, Jarnagin WR, et al. Predictors and patterns of recurrence after resection of hepatocellular carcinoma. J Am Coll Surg 2003;197:753–8.

[78] Ikai I, Arii S, Kojiro M, et al. Reevaluation of prognostic factors for survival after liver resection in patients with hepatocellular carcinoma in a Japanese nationwide survey. Cancer 2004;101:796–802.

[79] Esnaola NF, Mirza N, Lauwers GY, et al. Comparison of clinicopathologic characteristics and outcomes after resection in patients with hepatocellular carcinoma treated in the United States, France, and Japan. Ann Surg 2003;238:711–9.

[80] Belghiti J, Panis Y, Farges O, et al. Intrahepatic recurrence after resection of hepatocellular carcinoma complicating cirrhosis. Ann Surg 1991;214:114–7.

[81] Vauthey JN, Lauwers GY, Esnaola NF, et al. Simplified staging for hepatocellular carcinoma. J Clin Oncol 2002;20:1527–36.

[82] Llovet JM, Schwartz M, Mazzaferro V. Resection and liver transplantation for hepatocellular carcinoma. Semin Liver Dis 2005;25:181–200.

[83] Pawlik TM, Delman KA, Vauthey JN, et al. Tumor size predicts vascular invasion and histologic grade: implications for selection of surgical treatment for hepatocellular carcinoma. Liver Transpl 2005;11:1086–92.

[84] Lee JS, Chu IS, Heo J, et al. Classification and prediction of survival in hepatocellular carcinoma by geneexpression profiling. Hepatology 2004;40:667–76.

[85] Iizuka N, Oka M, Yamada-Okabe H, et al. Oligonucleotide microarray for prediction of early intrahepatic recurrence of hepatocellular carcinoma after curative resection. Lancet 2003;361:923–9.

[86] Lau WY, Leung TW, Ho SK, et al. Adjuvant intra-arterial iodine-131-labelled lipiodol for respectable hepatocellular carcinoma: a prospective randomised trial. Lancet 1999;353: 797–801.

[87] Boucher E, Corbinais S, Rolland Y, et al. Adjuvant intra-arterial injection of iodine-131-labeled lipiodol after resection of hepatocellular carcinoma. Hepatology 2003;38:1237–41.

[88] Dupont-Bierre E, Compagnon P, Raoul JL, et al. Resection of hepatocellular carcinoma in noncirrhotic liver: analysis of risk factors for survival. J Am Coll Surg 2005;201:663–70.

[89] Takayama T, Sekine T, Makuuchi M, et al. Adoptive immunotherapy to lower postsurgical recurrence rates of hepatocellular carcinoma: a randomised trial. Lancet 2000;356:802–7.

[90] Muto Y, Moriwaki H, Ninomiya M, et al. Prevention of second primary tumors by an acyclic retinoid, polyprenoic acid, in patients with hepatocellular carcinoma. N Engl J Med 1996; 334:1561–7.

[91] Shiratori Y, Shiina S, Teratani T, et al. Interferon therapy after tumor ablation improves prognosis in patients with hepatocellular carcinoma associated with hepatitis C virus. Ann Intern Med 2003;138:299–306.

[92] Liaw YF, Sung JJ, Chow WC, et al. Lamivudine for patients with chronic hepatitis B and advanced liver disease. N Engl J Med 2004;351:1521–31.

[93] Pang RWC, Poon RTP. From molecular biology to targeted therapies for hepatocellular carcinoma: the future is now. Oncology 2007;72(Suppl 1):30–44.

[94] Nakajima Y, Ko S, Kanamura T, et al. Repeat liver resection for hepatocellular carcinoma. J Am Coll Surg 2001;192:339–44.

[95] Belghiti J, Cortes A, Abdalla EK, et al. Resection prior to liver transplantation for hepatocellular carcinoma. Ann Surg 2003;238:885–92.

[96] Sala M, Fuster J, Llovet JM, et al. High pathological risk of recurrence after surgical resection for hepatocellular carcinoma: an indication for salvage liver transplantation. Liver Transpl 2004;10:1294–300.

ELSEVIER
SAUNDERS

Surg Oncol Clin N Am
17 (2008) 635–648

SURGICAL
ONCOLOGY CLINICS
OF NORTH AMERICA

Management of Melanoma: A European Perspective

Alexander M.M. Eggermont, MD, PhD[a],*, Christiane Voit, MD[b]

[a]*Department of Surgical Oncology, Erasmus University Medical Center – Daniel den Hoed Cancer Center, 301 Groene Hilledijk, 3075 EA Rotterdam, the Netherlands*
[b]*Department of Dermatology, Charité, Humboldt University, Schumannstr 20/21, Berlin 10117, Germany*

Conservative surgical approach

In Europe, because of the outcomes of randomized, controlled trials during the last 3 decades, the adjuvant surgical procedures of wide excision margins (>2 cm), elective lymph node dissection (ELND), and prophylactic isolated limb perfusion (ILP) have disappeared from practice. Only sentinel node biopsy (SNB) is widely practiced, although it is increasingly being supplanted by the use of ultrasound, as discussed in detail below.

Excision margins

Breslow's demonstration in 1970 that prognosis is related to the thickness of the primary lesion challenged the then-prevailing view that a 5-cm-wide excision margin was necessary to treat primary cutaneous melanoma adequately [1]. Since then a number of randomized trials have investigated the relevance of width of excision. Four trials involved patients who had thin/intermediate melanomas (<2 mm). They compared margins of 1 cm versus 3 cm (World Health Organization [WHO]-10 Trial [2]) (N. Cascinelli, personal communication, 1995) and 2 cm versus 5 cm (French [3] and Swedish [4] Melanoma Study Group trials). A United States Intergroup Trial [5,6] randomly assigned patients who had 1- to 4-mm melanomas to undergo an excision of 2 cm or 4 cm. The results from all these trials were consistent: local recurrence rates, disease-free survival (DFS), and overall survival (OS) were virtually identical, irrespective of the width of excision.

---

* Corresponding author.
E-mail address: a.m.m.eggermont@erasmusmc.nl (A.M.M. Eggermont).

The lack of impact of width of excision on efficacy also applies to thick melanomas. A large, nonrandomized study suggested a 2-cm excision margin was safe in patients who had primaries thicker than 4 mm [7], and this finding has been confirmed by the results of a large, randomized trial from Scandinavia that was reported at the Sixth Melanoma World Conference in Vancouver in 2005 [8]. The study involved 936 patients who had melanomas thicker than 2 mm and compared 2-cm versus 4-cm margins of excision. There were no significant differences between the treatment arms in locoregional recurrences, DFS, or OS.

One large, randomized trial has given slightly discordant results. The United Kingdom Melanoma Study Group [9] compared excision margins of 1 cm versus 3 cm in 900 patients who had melanomas more than 2 mm thick. Outcome was inferior in the 1-cm arm, with significantly more locoregional metastases (local, in transit, regional lymph nodes; hazard ratio [HR], 1.26; $P = .05$) and a trend for worse DFS (HR, 1.21; $P = .06$). No differences in OS were observed, however (HR, 1.07; $P = .6$). The Scandinavian trial results avoid the argument about extending margins to 3 cm, because it found that 2-cm margins are as effective as 4-cm margins. All in all, it can be concluded that a 1-cm margin is adequate for melanomas less than 2 mm thick, and a 2-cm margin is safe for patients who have primary melanomas thicker than 2 mm.

Elective lymph node dissection

It is acknowledged that lymphatic spread usually occurs concurrently with hematogenous metastasis in most solid tumors, including melanoma, and that lymph node metastases are "indicators rather than governors of survival" [10]. Four randomized trials have evaluated the role of immediate ELND in relation to survival [11–14]. None of these four trials demonstrated a survival benefit for ELND, and as a result, ELND was largely abandoned. In one of these trials (WHO-14), however, a subset analysis suggested that in patients who have thick truncal melanomas and micrometastases in the dissected ELND specimen, ELND had a survival advantage compared with delayed dissection following clinically diagnosed relapse in the regional lymph nodes [14]. These data could be interpreted as supportive evidence for the concept of SNB as an ideal staging procedure with the hypothesis of a potential, albeit small, impact on survival because of complete lymph node dissection in patients who are sentinel node positive [15].

Sentinel node biopsy

Any sentinel node staging system is based on the hypothesis that melanoma lymphatic metastases follow an orderly progression through afferent lymphatic channels to sentinel lymph nodes before spreading into other regional, nonsentinel nodes [16]. Simultaneously, especially in the thicker melanomas, hematogenous spread occurs, and thus the axiom that lymph node metastases are indicators rather than governors still applies. There is good evidence to support the orderly progression of metastases at the level of the regional lymph node basin, and sentinel node status is the most powerful prognostic factor in patients who have melanoma. Studies have demonstrated 5-year survival rates of 93% to 89% for sentinel node–negative patients and of 67% to 64% for patients who have evidence of melanoma in the SNB specimen [15,17–19].

In a study by Doubrovsky and colleagues [18] SNB was shown to provide more accurate staging than ELND, although this result could have been affected by the use of superior histopathologic protocols to examine the lymph nodes in the patients undergoing SNB biopsy.

Sentinel node biopsy has no impact on survival

The survival impact of SNB and subsequent lymph node dissection for sentinel node–positive patients is still a matter of controversy. In a matched-control study by Doubrovsky and colleagues [18], patients who had undergone SNB had no survival advantage over those who underwent ELND. Other studies comparing outcomes in patients who underwent SNB versus those who underwent a therapeutic lymph node dissection (TLND) showed no improved survival calculated from the date of diagnosis of the primary melanoma [20,21]. Most importantly, the randomized, controlled Multicenter Selective Lymphadenectomy Trial-1 (MSLT-1) showed no survival benefit for the sentinel node–staged patients either in the whole population of 2001 randomized patients [22] or in the final analysis, in which only data from 63% of the patients (1269), the group "of greatest interest," were presented [23]. This group was a compilation of two subgroups who had melanomas 1.2 to 1.8 mm thick and less than 1.8 to 3.5 mm thick, respectively. Such statistical methodology is rather unconventional; furthermore, there is no evidence of a protocol-defined event-rate–driven analytic plan [23]. In the results published from 1269 patients, there was no difference in 5-year survival between those who did or did not undergo an SNB (87.1% versus 86.5%); a result that is consistent with the interim analysis that involved the entire study population [23]. The *New England Journal of Medicine* report also compared the survival of patients who underwent an SNB plus completion lymph node dissection (CLND) because of sentinel node positivity with the survival of patients who underwent a TLND in the wide excision–only group. This nonrandomized comparison analysis resulted in the authors' claiming a survival benefit for SNB of about 20%, with 5-year survival after SNB and CLND of 72.3% versus 52.4% for wide excision and TLND. Subgroup analyses are, by definition, exploratory, however, so the conclusion is only hypothesis building. Moreover the p-value that indicates statistical significance depends on the number of subgroup analyses performed and needs to be corrected accordingly. The authors assume that all SNB-positive patients progress to clinically detectable nodal relapse if they do not undergo immediate CLND and are prognostically identical to those who underwent wide excision alone with a later TLND for positive nodes. If this assumption were true, then the observed survival difference between the SNB and the wide excision–alone groups should have been detected in the overall population at a level of about 4%; in fact, the difference was only 0.5%.

SNB-positive patients represent a heterogeneous group with outcomes ranging from relatively good to very bad, whereas patients undergoing TLND who have macroscopic regional lymph nodes all have a poor prognosis reflecting more aggressive disease. These two groups of patients (CLND and TLND) cannot be compared directly. This argument is substantiated by recent findings regarding the importance of the size of micrometastases in the sentinel node.

Submicrometastases in sentinel nodes have a different prognosis

Van Akkooi and colleagues [24] recently published a series of patients from the Erasmus MC-Daniel den Hoed Cancer Center SNB database. They grouped SNB-positive patients according to the diameter of the clusters of tumor cells within the infiltrated lymph node (< 0.1 mm, 0.1–1 mm, > 1 mm). At a median follow-up of more than 3 years, 6% of SNB-positive patients had distant metastases smaller than 0.1 mm, 37% had distant metastases between 0.1 and 1 mm, and 71% had distant metastasizes larger than 1 mm ($P < .002$). This finding translated into a statistically significant difference in estimated 5-year survival, 94%, 73%, and 59%, respectively ($P < .04$). The 6% rate of distant metastatic events in the group with a minimal tumor burden was lower than that seen in the SNB-negative patient population in the Rotterdam sentinel node data base, and the survival of these two groups reflects this finding: patients who had minimal tumor burden had a better 5-year survival than the SNB-negative patients, although this difference was not statistically significant. Furthermore, not a single patient in the group with minimal tumor burden had additional positive nodes identified in the CLND specimens, in contrast to a 30% positivity rate in the CLND specimens from the patients who had micrometastases 0.1 to 1 mm or larger than 1 mm in diameter. Therefore, there is an identifiable group of SNB-positive patients who have an excellent prognosis, and they probably should be spared a CLND. These findings have been confirmed by reclassifying all positive sentinel nodes in the large data sets of Rotterdam, Berlin, and Warsaw [25]. These results question the claim of the MSLT-1 of a survival benefit for SNB-positive patients, because 22% of SNB-positive patients in the Rotterdam database were in the group that had minimal tumor burden and very good prognosis. How many patients belonged to this category in the MLST-1 study? Furthermore, SNB-positive patients and TLND-treated patients in the Rotterdam databases have very similar overall survival rates [20].

Rates of locoregional recurrence following sentinel node biopsy

Sentinel node staging, like any adjuvant surgical procedure, is more likely to impact locoregional control rates than OS. It has been suggested that there may be an increased rate of in-transit metastasis after SNB and CLND [26]. There are, however, important variations in the primary tumor characteristics, such as Breslow thickness and ulceration, in studies that found this correlation. More recent analyses of studies with larger patient numbers have demonstrated that there is no increase in the in-transit metastasis rate after SNB. There is an increased chance of an in-transit location being the site of first recurrence because the sentinel node procedure followed by CLND inevitably reduces the rate of nodal recurrences. The overall probability of in-transit disease remains unchanged, however, independent of whether early or delayed excision of nodal metastases is performed [27–30].

Sentinel node biopsy improves clinical trials

Sentinel node staging is very useful in the context of clinical trials. It can identify patients who are unlikely to relapse and are therefore are not suitable candidates for adjuvant studies. There are two main reasons for such unsuitability: first, an adjuvant trial may fail if too many patients who are unlikely to have an event are accrued. Second, many trials involve agents that have significant side effects, and a patient who has a very good prognosis is unlikely to benefit from any intervention. Therefore such patients should not be exposed to toxicities needlessly. Sentinel node staging also may be helpful in stratifying patients to create more homogeneous patient populations in randomized trials of adjuvant systemic therapy [31].

Emergence of ultrasound as alternative to sentinel node staging

The possibility remains that sentinel node staging followed by CLND may improve long-term disease control in the locoregional lymph node basin compared with the strategy of waiting for patients to relapse and undergo a TLND [20,21]. It is becoming increasingly apparent, however, that very small, nonpalpable lymph node metastases can be detected with regular ultrasound scans of the regional lymph nodes, and such patients then can be offered early intervention. This approach has an important potential advantage over SNB followed by CLND: it could reduce the number of unnecessary surgical procedures while increasing local disease control rates [32–34].

Moreover, ultrasound and fine-needle aspiration cytology of the regional node basin(s) of high-risk primary melanomas can identify the sentinel node and the presence of metastasis in the sentinel node, thus reducing significantly the need for surgical sentinel node procedures. In a series of 400 consecutive patients, Voit and colleagues [35,36] reported that in 50% to 65% of patients who had a positive sentinel node, this node could be detected by ultrasound. These developments will reduce further the number of surgical SNBs and increase the role of ultrasound in the management of patients who have melanoma.

Prophylactic isolated limb perfusion

In the 1980s and 1990s prophylactic ILP as an adjunct to the surgical management of patients at high risk of relapse received considerable attention in Europe because retrospective studies had suggested it was associated with improved outcomes. A large intergroup trial (European Organization for Research and Treatment of Cancer [EORTC] 18832/WHO-15) randomly assigned 832 patients who had primary melanoma at high risk of relapse to ILP or observation. ILP had a regional effect, reducing the rate of in-transit metastasis from 6.6% to 3.3% and regional lymph node relapse from 16.7% to 12.6%. These results were not statistically significant, however. Furthermore, there was no effect at all on distant relapse-free survival or OS [37]. Prophylactic ILP is no longer reimbursed in Europe and should no longer be used.

Therapeutic isolated limb perfusion

In contrast, therapeutic ILP for multiple in-transit metastases is practiced in many centers in Europe. Melphalan, especially when combined with tumor necrosis factor-alpha, is highly effective in patients who have multiple symptomatic or bulky in-transit metastases. With this combination complete remission rates are observed in about 70% of patients, even in those who have not responded to a previous ILP with melphalan alone [38,39].

Systemic adjuvant therapies

Chemotherapy, nonspecific immune stimulants, and vaccines

At least 25 randomized trials have been conducted in stage II–III melanoma evaluating chemotherapy, nonspecific immune stimulants such as Bacillus Calmette-Guerin, Corynebacterium parvum, levamisole, or combinations of these agents with dacarbazine. The trials almost invariably were underpowered and yielded negative results except for occasional incidental, nonrepeatable positive finding in trials involving small numbers of patients [40]. Seven large, randomized trials of allogeneic melanoma cell–based vaccines have been conducted, and not one has demonstrated a significant impact on survival. Only one trial came close to demonstrating a benefit for treatment, an Australia study that investigated an allogeneic tumor cell–based oncolysate [41]. In the United States, a trial of the Melacine vaccine in patients who had stage II disease showed no benefit for the total study population [42], but there seemed to be some activity in patients who had particular HLA types [43]. Unfortunately, a prospective study of the vaccine has never been conducted in patients who have the relevant HLA types. In 2006 negative results were reported for the two large, randomized trials of an allogeneic tumor cell–based vaccine Canvaxin in patients who had stage III or resected stage IV disease. Patients in the vaccine arms of these trials had worse outcomes than those in the control arms [44]. Canvaxin had shown great promise in historical case-control studies; the results of these two trials are powerful reminders of the unreliability of such methodology and that case-control studies can be used only for hypothesis-generating purposes [45].

A small phase III trial of the ganglioside GM2 did show a survival benefit for patients who had stage III disease, but this benefit was observed only in the subset of patients who were seronegative for ganglioside antibodies before trial entry [46]. This study led to the EORTC conducting a large phase III adjuvant trial of GM2 in patients who had stage II disease (18961); 1318 patients were accrued, of whom approximately 50% were staged by SNB. At the second interim analysis in 2007, it seemed that there was a detrimental outcome for survival in the vaccine arm, and this finding led to early stopping of the trial.

Interferon-alpha

Individual trial data

The use of high-dose interferon therapy is approved by both the Food and Drug Administration (FDA) in the United States and the European Medicines Agency (EMEA) in Europe for patients who have high-risk melanoma (stage IIB–III). High-dose interferon is used in the United States but is used in only a few European centers because there is doubt that its impact on OS justifies the toxicity and costs [40,47]. In Europe high-dose interferon or any adjuvant therapy, in the absence of solid evidence of an impact on survival, is not considered standard of care. Of importance is the recent communication by Gogas and colleagues [48], who demonstrated that 4 weeks of high-dose interferon, administered intravenously, is as effective as the classic Eastern Cooperative Oncology Group (ECOG) 1684 1-year schedule of high-dose interferon and is much better tolerated.

Intermediate doses of interferon were tested in the largest phase III trial to date (EORTC18952). The trial involved patients who had stage IIB–III disease. The results demonstrated a nonstatistically significant 7.2% increase in distant metastasis–free interval and a 5.4% increase in OS at 4.65 years of follow-up. This benefit, however, was seen only in patients treated for 25 months with 5 MU; there was no effect for 13 months of therapy at a dose of 10 MU [49]. The results suggest that duration of therapy may be more important than dose.

The question of treatment duration was addressed in the next EORTC trial (18991), in which patients were assigned randomly to 5 years of pegylated interferon α-2b (PEG-IFN) or observation. The outcome of this trial was reported at the 43rd Annual Meeting of the American Society of Clinical Oncology (ASCO) in Chicago in 2007 [50]. In this trial the dosing schedule was comparable to that for high-dose interferon. The PEG-IFN was administered for an induction period of 8 weeks at 6 µg/kg followed by long-term maintenance dosing of 3 µg/kg for 4 years and 10 months. This was a registration study, and the trial end point set by the regulatory authority was DFS, although the primary end point of the trial was distant metastasis–free survival with OS and toxicity as secondary end points. The report at ASCO revealed an outcome that is consistent with the other phase III trials of adjuvant interferon; namely, there was a significant effect on DFS and no significant impact on distant metastasis–free survival or OS. Interestingly, in patients who had only microscopic involvement of regional lymph nodes (SNB-positive patients), the impact on distant metastasis–free survival was statistically significant, whereas PEG-IFN therapy had no significant impact on this end point in patients who had palpable nodal involvement. The hazard ratios for patients who had microscopic nodal involvement were virtually identical to those observed in the 25-month treatment arm in EORTC18952. Thus a significant, or borderline significant, impact on early stage III disease has been observed in two consecutive EORTC trials involving 2644 patients, whereas there was no impact on outcome in patients who had palpable nodal involvement in either study. This observation is relevant in view of the current widespread practice of staging patients by SNB and supports the need for and value of sentinel node staging.

Reviews/meta-analyses

A systematic review of all trials [51], a meta-analysis of all trials [52], and a pooled data analysis of all high-dose interferon trials [53] demonstrated a consistent improvement in DFS but no statistically significant impact on OS. A meta-analysis based on data from individual patients reported at the 43rd Annual Meeting of ASCO in 2007 [54] confirms the consistently reported statistically significant benefit of high-dose interferon on DFS. It is also demonstrates, for the first time, a definite, statistically significant impact on OS. This impact, however, is extremely small: 3% absolute improvement. Moreover, this effect results in part from the inclusion of the trials ECOG1694 and ECOG2696, which have the ganglioside GM2 vaccine as comparator arm. The validity of including these trials recently has become very doubtful: the EORTC18961 trial (GM2 vaccine versus observation in 1312 patients who had stage II disease with tumors larger than 1.5 mm) had to be stopped because the second interim analysis indicated a detrimental effect in the vaccination arm. Another important finding from this individual patient data–based meta-analysis is that the benefits of interferon are observed across a wide range of doses and thus are not clearly dose related.

Low-dose interferon trials in stage II cancer

The impact of low-dose interferon in stage III may be somewhat less in stage II [54]. In stage II disease low-dose interferon therapy has been particularly successful; a consistent and significant effect on DFS was observed in the French [55], Austrian [56], and Scottish [57] studies, and the French trial even found a borderline significant effect on survival. Low-dose interferon therapy was approved as an adjuvant therapy for patients who had stage II disease by the EMEA in Europe but was rejected for this indication by the FDA in the United States. Meta-analysis confirms that low-dose interferon has an impact on DFS but no significant impact on OS. The significant impact of interferon in trials of patients who had stage II disease at a time when these patients were not sentinel node–staged corresponds very well with the observations in the EORTC18952 and 18991 trials, where the best benefit was observed in patients who had positive sentinel nodes.

Need for predictive factors: autoantibodies and adjuvant therapy?

Gogas and colleagues [58] recently have reported that patients treated with adjuvant interferon who developed autoantibodies against thyroglobulin, antinuclear factors, or cardiolipin had a significantly better outcome than patients who did not develop these signs of autoimmunity. That autoimmunity is associated with clinical benefits such as higher response rates and longer DFS and OS has been known for many years. The association applies to patients treated with immunotherapy but also may occur in patients given chemotherapy and sometimes without any therapy at all.

The development of markers that might predict which patients will mount a host immune response could be extremely important. They might be predictive factors and could be used to determine which patients should be treated with interferon and for how long. An evaluation of the presence or emergence of autoantibodies in patients who participated in the EORTC trial of adjuvant intermediate-dose interferon (18952) did not confirm Gogas' observations [59]. Also, a study in the ECOG2696 could not confirm autoantibodies as a strong independent prognostic factor [60], nor did antibodies have any prognostic value in the EORTC1899 trial of PEG-IFN in stage III melanoma [61]. In contrast, the serial determination of serum S100 levels was demonstrated to be a very powerful prognostic factor in an analysis of the EORTC18952 trial on intermediate doses of interferon in patients who had stage IIB–III disease, and its prognostic value was superior even to the number of positive regional lymph nodes [62].

Summary

The lack of effective drugs in stage IV melanoma is reflected by a lack of effective adjuvant therapies for patients who have stage II–III melanoma [63]. After decades of research, cytotoxics, immune stimulants, and vaccines have failed to have any clinically meaningful impact in the adjuvant setting. Interferon is the only drug that presently is considered for adjuvant therapy and is used with various schedules in Europe in both stage II and in stage III disease.

Interferon has a consistent impact on DFS, but the survival benefit is too small for it to be considered standard of care. The population of patients that can benefit from interferon needs to be identified by the new technologies of genomics and proteomics or by identifying novel biomarkers that can predict potential host immune responsiveness.

Novel targeted agents, antiangiogenics, and immune modulators are being investigated actively in the stage IV setting and some, such as bevacizumab and anti-CTLA4, already are being investigated for their potential as adjuvant therapies. Adjuvant trials of bevacizumab and anti-CTLA4 (EORTC18071) will commence in 2007/2008; results will not be known before 2011. PEG-IFN will be explored by EORTC (EORTC18081) in patients who have high-risk stage II disease.

Europe is extremely active in conducting phase III trials in the field of melanoma. It has played a major role in abandoning adjuvant surgical procedures and in the identification of adjuvant therapy regimens with interferon that have moderate activity in patients who have stage II and stage III melanoma. At present it takes the lead in exploring new agents in the adjuvant setting. It is hoped that these efforts will result in the identification of new and more active treatments for melanoma in the near future.

References

[1] Breslow A. Thickness, cross-sectional areas and depth of invasion in the prognosis of cutaneous melanoma. Ann Surg 1970;172(5):902–8.
[2] Veronesi U, Cascinelli N, Adamus J, et al. Thin stage I primary cutaneous malignant melanoma. Comparison of excision with margins of 1 or 3 cm [published erratum appears in N Engl J Med 1991 Jul 25;325(4):292]. N Engl J Med 1988;318:1159–62.
[3] Khayat D, Rixe O, Martin G, et al, French Group of Research on Malignant Melanoma. Surgical margins in cutaneous melanoma (2 cm versus 5 cm for lesions measuring less than 2.1-mm thick). Cancer 2004;97:1941–6.
[4] Cohn-Cedermark G, Rutqvist LE, Andersson R, et al. Long term results of a randomized study by the Swedish Melanoma Study Group on 2-cm versus 5-cm resection margins for patients with cutaneous melanoma with a tumor thickness of 0.8–2.0 mm. Cancer 2000; 89:1495–501.
[5] Balch CM, Urist MM, Karakousis CP, et al. Efficacy of 2-cm surgical margins for intermediate-thickness melanomas (1 to 4 mm). Results of a multi-institutional randomized surgical trial [see comments]. Ann Surg 1993;218:262–7 [discussion: 267–9].
[6] Balch CM, Soong SJ, Smith T, et al. Long-term results of a prospective surgical trial comparing 2 cm vs. 4 cm excision margins for 740 patients with 1–4 mm melanomas. Ann Surg Oncol 2001;8:101–8.
[7] Heaton KM, Sussman JJ, Gershenwald JE, et al. Surgical margins and prognostic factors in patients with thick (>4 mm) primary melanoma. Ann Surg Oncol 1998;5:322–8.

[8] Thomas JM, Newton-Bishop J, A'Hern R, et al, United Kingdom Melanoma Study Group; British Association of Plastic Surgeons; Scottish Cancer Therapy Network. Excision margins in high-risk malignant melanoma. N Engl J Med 2004;350(8):757–66.

[9] Ringborg U, Mansson Brahme E, Drzewiecki K, et al. Randomized trial of a resection margin of 2 cm versus 4 cm for cutaneous malignant melanoma with a tumor thickness of more than 2 mm [abstract 28]. In: Proceedings of the 6th World Melanoma Congress. Vancouver (BC, Canada), September 6–10, 2005.

[10] Eggermont AMM, Gore M. European approach to adjuvant treatments of intermediate- and high-risk malignant melanoma [review]. Semin Oncol 2002;29(4):382–8.

[11] Veronesi U, Adamus J, Bandiera DC, et al. Inefficacy of immediate node dissection in stage 1 melanoma of the limbs. N Engl J Med 1977;297:627–30.

[12] Sim FH, Taylor WF, Ivins JC, et al. A prospective randomized study of the efficacy of routine elective lymphadenectomy in management of malignant melanoma. Preliminary results. Cancer 1978;41:948–56.

[13] Balch CM, Soong S, Ross MI, et al. Long-term results of a multi-institutional randomized trial comparing prognostic factors and surgical results for intermediate thickness melanomas (1.0 to 4.0 mm). Intergroup Melanoma Surgical Trial. Ann Surg Oncol 2000;7:87–97.

[14] Cascinelli N, Morabito A, Santinami M, et al. Immediate or delayed dissection of regional nodes in patients with melanoma of the trunk: a randomised trial. WHO Melanoma Programme. Lancet 1998;351:793–6.

[15] Gershenwald JE, Thompson W, Mansfield PF, et al. Multi-institutional melanoma lymphatic mapping experience: the prognostic value of sentinel lymph node status in 612 stage I or II melanoma patients. J Clin Oncol 1999;17:976–83.

[16] Morton DL, Wen DR, Wong JH, et al. Technical details of intraoperative lymphatic mapping for early stage melanoma. Arch Surg 1992;127:392–9.

[17] Vuylsteke RJ, van Leeuwen PA, Statius Muller MG, et al. Clinical outcome of stage I/II melanoma patients after selective sentinel lymph node dissection: long-term follow-up results. J Clin Oncol 2003;21:1057–65.

[18] Doubrovsky A, De Wilt JH, Scolyer RA, et al. Sentinel node biopsy provides more accurate staging than elective lymph node dissection in patients with cutaneous melanoma. Ann Surg Oncol 2004;11:829–36.

[19] van Akkooi AC, de Wilt JH, Verhoef C, et al. High positive sentinel node identification rate by EORTC melanoma group protocol. Prognostic indicators of metastatic patterns after sentinel node biopsy in melanoma. Eur J Cancer 2006;42:372–80.

[20] van Akkooi AC, Bouwhuis MG, de Wilt JH, et al. Multivariable analysis comparing outcome after sentinel node biopsy or therapeutic lymph node dissection in patients with melanoma. Br J Surg 2007;94(10):1293–9.

[21] Koskivuo I, Talve L, Vihinen P, et al. Sentinel lymph node biopsy in cutaneous melanoma: a case-control study. Ann Surg Oncol 2007;14(12):3566–74.

[22] Morton DL, Thompson JF, Cochran AJ, et al. Interim results of the Multicenter Selective Lymphadenectomy Trial (MSLT-I) in clinical stage I melanoma. J Clin Oncol 2005;23: 7500. Available at: http://www.asco.org/ac/1,1003, _12-002511-00_18-0034-00_19-003013,00. asp. Accessed June 1, 2005.

[23] Morton DL, Thompson JF, Cochran AJ, et al, MSLT Group. Sentinel-node biopsy or nodal observation in melanoma. N Engl J Med 2006;355(13):1307–17.

[24] van Akkooi AC, de Wilt JH, Verhoef C, et al. Clinical relevance of melanoma micrometastases (<0.1 mm) in sentinel nodes: are these nodes to be considered negative? Ann Oncol 2006; 17(10):1578–85.

[25] van Akkooi AC, Nowecki ZI, Voit C, et al. Prognosis depends on micro-anatomic patterns of melanoma micrometastases within the sentinel node (SN). A multicenter study in 388 SN positive patients [abstract 7006]. Eur J Cancer Suppl 2007;5(4):397.

[26] Thomas JM, Clark MA. Selective lymphadenectomy in sentinel node-positive patients may increase the risk of local/in-transit recurrence in malignant melanoma. Eur J Surg Oncol 2004;30(6):686–91.

[27] Kretschmer L, Beckmann I, Thoms KM, et al. Sentinel lymphonodectomy does not increase the risk of loco-regional cutaneous metastases of malignant melanomas. Eur J Cancer 2005; 41:531–8.

[28] van Poll D, Thompson JF, Colman MH, et al. A sentinel node biopsy does not increase the incidence of in-transit metastasis in patients with primary cutaneous melanoma. Ann Surg Oncol 2005;12(8):597–608.

[29] Kang JC, Wanek LA, Essner R, et al. Sentinel lymphadenectomy does not increase the incidence of in-transit metastases in primary melanoma. J Clin Oncol 2005;23(21):4764–70.

[30] Pawlik TM, Ross MI, Thompson JF, et al. The risk of in-transit metastasis depends on tumor biology and not the surgical approach to regional lymph nodes. J Clin Oncol 2005;23: 4588–90.

[31] Eggermont AMM. Adjuvant therapy of malignant melanoma and the role of sentinel node mapping. Recent Results Cancer Res 2000;157:178–89.

[32] Voit C, Mayer T, Kron M, et al. Efficacy of ultrasound B-scan compared with physical examination in follow-up of melanoma patients. Cancer 2001;91:2409–16.

[33] Voit C, Schoengen A, Schwurzer-Voit M, et al. The role of ultrasound in detection and management of regional disease in melanoma patients. Semin Oncol 2002;29:353–60.

[34] Eggermont AMM. Reducing the need for sentinel node procedures by ultrasound examination of regional lymph nodes. Ann Surg Oncol 2005;12(1):3–5.

[35] Voit C, Kron M, Schafer G, et al. Ultrasound-guided fine needle aspiration cytology prior to sentinel lymph node biopsy in melanoma patients. Ann Surg Oncol 2006;12:1682–9.

[36] Voit CA, van Akkooi ACJ, Schaefer-Hesterberg G, et al. Reduction of need for operative sentinel node procedure in melanoma patients: fifty percent identification rate of sentinel node positivity by ultrasound (US)-guided fine needle aspiration cytology (FNAC) in 400 consecutive patients [abstract 3BA]. Eur J Cancer Suppl 2007;5(6):11.

[37] Koops HS, Vaglini M, Suciu S, et al. Prophylactic isolated limb perfusion for localized, high-risk limb melanoma: results of a multicenter randomized phase III trial. European Organization for Research and Treatment of Cancer Malignant Melanoma Cooperative Group Protocol 18832, the World Health Organization Melanoma Program Trial 15, and the North American Perfusion Group Southwest Oncology Group-8593. J Clin Oncol 1998;9:2906–12.

[38] Grünhagen DJ, Brunstein F, Graveland WJ, et al. One hundred consecutive isolated limb perfusions with TNF-alpha and melphalan in melanoma patients with multiple in-transit metastases. Ann Surg 2004;240:939–47.

[39] Grünhagen DJ, van Etten B, Brunstein F, et al. Efficacy of repeat isolated limb perfusions with tumor necrosis factor alpha and melphalan for multiple in-transit metastases in patients with prior isolated limb perfusion failure. Ann Surg Oncol 2005;12(8):597–608.

[40] Eggermont AM, Gore M. Randomized adjuvant therapy trials in melanoma: surgical and systemic. Semin Oncol 2007;34(6):509–15.

[41] Hersey P, Coates AS, McCarthy WH, et al. Adjuvant immunotherapy of patients with high-risk melanoma using vaccinia viral lysates of melanoma: results of a randomized trial. J Clin Oncol 2002;20(20):4181–90.

[42] Sondak VK, Liu PY, Tuthill RJ, et al. Adjuvant immunotherapy of resected, intermediate-thickness, node-negative melanoma with an allogeneic tumor vaccine: overall results of a randomized trial of the Southwest Oncology Group. J Clin Oncol 2002;20(8):2058–66.

[43] Sosman JA, Unger JM, Liu PY, et al. Southwest Oncology Group. Adjuvant immunotherapy of resected, intermediate-thickness, node-negative melanoma with an allogeneic tumor vaccine: impact of HLA class I antigen expression on outcome. J Clin Oncol 2002;20(8): 2067–75.

[44] Morton DL. Plenary presentation at the Annual Meeting of the Society of Surgical Oncology. Atlanta (GA), March 11–14, 2006.

[45] Hsueh EC, Essner R, Foshag LJ, et al. Prolonged survival after complete resection of disseminated melanoma and active immunotherapy with a therapeutic cancer vaccine. J Clin Oncol 2002;20(23):4549–54.

[46] Livingston PO, Wong GY, Adluri S, et al. Improved survival in stage III melanoma patients with GM2 antibodies: a randomized trial of adjuvant vaccination with GM2 ganglioside. J Clin Oncol 1994;5:1036–44.

[47] Eggermont AMM. Role of interferon in melanoma remains to be determined. Eur J Cancer 2001;37:2147–53.

[48] Gogas H, Dafni U, Bafaloukos D, et al. A randomized phase III trial of 1 month versus 1 year adjuvant high-dose interferon alfa-2b in patients with resected high risk melanoma [abstract]. J Clin Oncol 2007;25(Suppl):8505.

[49] Eggermont AM, Suciu S, MacKie R, et al. EORTC Melanoma Group. Post-surgery adjuvant therapy with intermediate doses of interferon alfa 2b versus observation in patients with stage IIb/III melanoma (EORTC 18952): randomised controlled trial. Lancet 2005; 366:1189–96.

[50] Eggermont AMM, Suciu S, Santinami M, et al. For the EORTC Melanoma Group. EORTC 18991: Long term adjuvant pegylated interferon-α2b (PEG-IFN) vs observation in resected stage iii melanoma: final results of a randomized phase 3 trial [abstract]. J Clin Oncol 2007; 25(Suppl):8504.

[51] Lens MB, Dawes M. Interferon alfa therapy for malignant melanoma: a systematic review of randomized controlled trials. J Clin Oncol 2002;20:1818–25.

[52] Wheatley K, Ives N, Hancock B, et al. Does adjuvant interferon-alpha provide a worthwhile benefit? A meta-analysis of the randomised trials. Cancer Treat Rev 2003;29: 241–52.

[53] Kirkwood JM, Manola J, Ibrahim J, et al. A pooled analysis of eastern cooperative oncology group and intergroup trials of adjuvant high-dose interferon for melanoma. Clin Cancer Res 2004;10:1670–7.

[54] Wheatley K, Ives N, Eggermont AM, et al. on behalf of the International Malignant Melanoma Collaborative Group. Interferon-α as adjuvant therapy for melanoma: an individual patient data meta-analysis of the randomised trials [abstract]. J Clin Oncol 2007;25(Suppl): 8526.

[55] Grob JJ, Dreno B, Chastang C, et al. Randomised trial of interferon a-2a as adjuvant therapy in resected primary melanoma thicker than 1.5 mm without clinically detectable node metastases. Lancet 1998;351:1905–10.

[56] Pehamberger H, Soyer HP, Steiner A, et al. Adjuvant interferon alpha 2-A treatment in resected primary stage II cutaneous melanoma. J Clin Oncol 1998;16:1425–9.

[57] Cameron DA, Cornbleet MC, MacKie RM, et al. Adjuvant interferon alpha in high risk melanoma: the Scottish study. Br J Cancer 2001;84:1146–9.

[58] Gogas H, Ioannovich J, Dafni U, et al. Prognostic significance of autoimmunity during treatment of melanoma with interferon. N Engl J Med 2006;354(7):709–18.

[59] Bouwhuis M, Suciu S, Kruit W, et al. Prognostic value of autoantibodies (auto-AB) in melanoma patients (pts) in the EORTC 18952 trial of adjuvant interferon (IFN) vs observation (Obs) [abstract]. J Clin Oncol 2007;25(Suppl):8507.

[60] Stuckert JJ II, Tarhini AA, Lee S, et al. Interferon alfa-induced autoimmunity and serum S100 levels as predictive and prognostic biomarkers in high-risk melanoma in the ECOG-intergroup phase II trial E2696 [abstract]. J Clin Oncol 2007;25(Suppl):8506.

[61] Bouwhuis M, Suciu S, Testori A, et al. Prognostic value of autoantibodies (auto-AB) in melanoma stage III patients in the EORTC 18991 phase III randomized trial comparing adjuvant pegylated interferon α2b (PEG-IFN) vs observation [abstract 3BA]. Eur J Cancer 2007;6(Suppl):5.

[62] Suciu S, Ghanem G, Kruit W, et al. Serum S-100B protein is a strong independent prognostic marker for distant-metastasis free survival (DMFS) in stage III melanoma patients: an evaluation of the EORTC 18952 trial comparing interferon (IFN) vs observation [abstract]. J Clin Oncol 2007;25(Suppl):8518.
[63] Eggermont AMM, Kirkwood JM. Re-evaluating the role of dacarbazine in metastatic melanoma: what have we learned in 30 years? Eur J Cancer 2004;40:1825–36.

ELSEVIER
SAUNDERS

Surg Oncol Clin N Am
17 (2008) 649–672

SURGICAL
ONCOLOGY CLINICS
OF NORTH AMERICA

Treatment of Soft Tissue Sarcoma: A European Approach

Fausto Badellino, MD[a], Salvatore Toma, MD, PhD[b],*

[a]Villa Serena, Piaza Leopardi 18, Genova, Italy
[b]Dipartimento di Oncologia, Biologia e Genetica, Università di Genova,
Largo Rosanna Benzi 10, 16132 Genova, Italy

Soft tissue sarcomas (STS) are very rare tumors. They represent less than 1% of all malignancies in adults, with an incidence of about 37 cases per million population per year. In children the incidence is higher, and STS (mainly rhabdomyosarcoma and fibrosarcoma) represent 6% to 7% of all childhood tumors. Sarcomas are responsible for about 2% of all tumor-related deaths each year. The low incidence is significant, given that mesenchymal tissue represents more than 50% of a person's total body weight [1].

No specific etiologic agents have been identified. Risk factors related to the development of sarcomas include

- Exposure to ionizing radiation
- Exposure to some chemical agents (phenoxyacetic acid, chlorophenols, vinyl chloride, arsenic, Thorotrast)
- HIV infection (Kaposi's sarcoma)
- Chronic lymphoedema of various origins, typically occurring after irradiation (lymphangiosarcoma)
- Use of immunosuppressive agents such as those used in renal transplantation or to treat other pathologic conditions
- Genetic alteration (eg, von Recklinghausen's disease [neurofibromatosis], tuberous sclerosis, Gardner syndrome, and Li-Fraumeni syndrome)

STS are more slightly common in males than in females, in a ratio of 1.4:1 [1]. There are more than 50 subtypes of STS. According to the American Cancer Society, the most common types are malignant fibrous histiocytoma (28%), liposarcoma (15%), leiomyosarcoma (12%), synovial sarcoma (10%), malignant peripheral nerve sheath tumors (6%), and

---

* Corresponding author. Via Camilla 20, 16146 Genova, Italy.
E-mail address: sandro_toma@virgilio.it (S. Toma).

1055-3207/08/$ - see front matter © 2008 Elsevier Inc. All rights reserved.
doi:10.1016/j.soc.2008.02.001   *surgonc.theclinics.com*

rhabdomyosarcoma (5%). All other types of STS occur in percentages of 3% or less [2]. The main histotypes of STS are listed in Table 1.

Clinical characteristics

STS can arise in any anatomic site but are observed most frequently in the body extremities (about 60%), trunk (15%–20%), retroperitoneum and abdomen (15%–25%), and cervicofacial area (5%–10%). The clinical picture also is extremely variable, ranging from a retroperitoneal mass found incidentally during a CT scan to a small lipoma-like lesion of the thorax to an enormous lesion involving the entire muscle compartment of a limb. Depending on the anatomic site involved and the relationship of the tumor with other organs and structures in surrounding areas, lesions can be completely asymptomatic or can manifest through a variety of symptoms. Therefore clinical outcome is highly variable. The clinical diagnosis often is delayed until the disease is locally advanced. Metastases are found in 50% of cases, mainly in the lung (30%–35%), liver (25%), bone (20%–23%), and brain (3%–5%). Metastases develop mainly through hematic paths; lymphatic spreading plays a secondary role, representing only 5% of cases [1,3].

Diagnosis

Diagnosis of suspected disease is made by various physicians: general practitioners, surgeons, radiologists, oncologists, specialists in various organs, or, often, by several specialists together. The histologic examination remains the basis for formulating the correct diagnosis and therapeutic program.

Few other human tumors require such clear communication between the pathologist and the treating physician. The physician must provide the pathologist with adequate tissue samples and also with a detailed clinical

Table 1
Main histotypes of soft tissue sarcoma

Tissue involved	Sarcoma
Fibrous tissue	Malignant fibrous histiocytoma Fibrosarcoma
Smooth muscle	Leiomyosarcoma
Skeletal muscle	Rhabdomyosarcoma
Adipose tissue	Liposarcoma
Peripheral nervous system	Neurofibrosarcoma
Blood and lymph vessels	Angiosarcoma
	Epithelioid hemangioendothelioma
	Hemangiopericytoma
	Kaposi's sarcoma
Other	Synovial sarcoma
	Alveolar soft part sarcoma
	Epithelioid sarcoma
	Unclassified sarcoma

history with exhaustive imaging documentation (radiographs, MR images, CT scans, positron emission tomography, and ultrasound, among others).

Therefore, once a diagnosis of sarcoma has been made, many aspects of the patient's history are known: (1) the patient's clinical features and his/her personal history, including details of first disease onset; (2) regional data of the disease (site, size, depth, adjacent organs, and vascular infiltrations); (3) possibility of metastasis; and (4) histologic type and grading. This information enables physicians to stage the tumor using either the TNM classification or Enneking's staging system [1,4].

Occasionally pathologists may need to use molecular biology or cytogenetic tests. From a prognostic point of view, many parameters are already known, but the lesion size, depth, location, and grading remain major parameters to consider when evaluating the risk of treatment failure [1,3]. Box 1 outlines the main prognostic factors of STS. Because of the rarity of STS, screening procedures are not feasible in the general population. It is important, however, to obtain an accurate patient history to uncover evidence of any possible genetic predisposition. In such cases, a more detailed clinical evaluation and genetic analysis are indicated.

Treatment

Surgery: diagnostic, curative, and reconstructive surgery

General considerations

In the past, the diagnosis of STS often was delayed and erroneous, and primary treatment was inadequate. In STS affecting the limbs, amputation

---

Box 1. Main prognostic factors of soft tissue sarcoma

Favorable prognostic factors
- Size < 5 cm
- Superficial location with respect to the muscular fascia
- Localization to limbs
- Distal location on a limb
- Absence of invasion of vessels, bones, and nerves
- Low tumor grade

Unfavorable prognostic factors
- Size > 5 cm
- Deep location with respect to the muscular fascia
- Localization to trunk, retroperitoneum, or head and neck
- Proximal location on a limb
- Invasion of vessels, bones, and nerves
- High tumor grade

was the most frequently used surgical procedure and was applied at different levels, according to tumor involvement. If the tumor involved the root of the limb or had spread to shoulder or pelvis, interscapulothoracic and hindquarter disarticulations were treatments of choice, and hemipelvectomy was performed in extreme cases.

For the past 20 to 25 years, multimodal treatments and the development of reconstructive surgery have made amputation necessary in only about 10% of cases [1]. Instead, depending on the size and depth of the tumor, it is now possible to perform various types of excisions or extracompartmental resections, but the muscles and fasciae surrounding the tumor mass must be healthy.

"Buttectomy" is the procedure performed for sarcoma of the gluteal area. If the tumor involves regional vascular structures and/or is infiltrating their walls, conservation surgery also is indicated to resect arterial and venous segments and to replace them with vascular prostheses.

If the size of sarcoma is less than 5 cm (and if the tumor is superficial), conservative surgery is a feasible treatment. In all other cases multimodal therapy is indicated, that is, surgery plus pre- and/or postoperative radiation therapy and chemotherapy. The surgical procedure used also depends on the findings of the preoperative biopsy.

An inadequate surgical biopsy can be considered almost a resection with positive margins (R1 or R2), and the risk of a local recurrence is high (69%–80%) [5]. After amputation the risk of recurrence is low (10%–15%), but the likelihood of distant metastases is great (30%–40%).

Hoekstra and colleagues [5] have described a surgical approach they call "interval surgery": "a procedure by induction treatment with chemotherapy and/or radiation for a solid tumor, followed by surgery." In STS the goal of the combined treatment strategy is to improve the limb salvage rate, local tumor control, and/or survival. Interval surgery is used in the treatment of bone sarcomas, extraosseous Ewing's sarcoma, primitive neuroectodermal tumor, and rhabdomyosarcoma. There is limited experience with interval surgery for STS with isolated limb perfusion, neoadjuvant chemotherapy, and preoperative radiation.

An important European study on melphalan and tumor necrosis factor-alpha (TNF-α) in patients who had locally advanced sarcoma reported an objective response in 76% of cases. Amputation was avoided in 71% of patients [6].

Specific landmarks

The preliminary discussion in the previous sections has shown the complexity of the topic and has outlined the anatomic and surgical considerations involved in selecting the best possible treatment. The following discussion delineates the surgical procedures indicated for particular tumor sites and for the reconstruction of the soft tissue and vascular tract (if resected). It also discusses the use of arterial chemotherapy (perfusion and/or infusion), sarcomas with particular biologic features, lymph node mapping, and rehabilitation barriers and procedures.

Surgery also includes multimodal and combined treatments. Therefore it is important to understand any difficulties and/or side effects of chemotherapy and radiation, both intraoperative and postoperative, that might affect surgical procedures.

For a complete understanding of the surgical techniques indicated in STS, it may be useful to define the term "compartment." The anatomic compartment is an anatomic area defined by natural barriers. An intracompartmental tumor is located completely within a natural anatomic compartment. An extracompartmental tumor extends beyond the barriers of the anatomic compartment.

According to the TNM classification of STS by American Joint Committee on Cancer (AJCC) and by the Union International Contre le Cancer (UICC), STS are staged in by size ($</>$ 5 cm) and by their connection with superficial fasciae (above, beneath, or superficial to the fascia, with invasion of or through the fascia itself) [2,7].

From a clinical and surgical point of view, it is very important to achieve negative margins with an adequate and safe peritumoral layer.

The tumor resection is described as "intralesional" if the tumor is excised inside its capsule or pseudocapsula or is fragmented. It is said to be "marginal" if the resected tumor is covered only by capsule or pseudocapsula. The tumor resection is "wide" if it is surrounded entirely by healthy tissue; it is "radical" if the tumor is removed by en bloc resection of intact compartments.

In some of the sites in which STS occur (eg, anterior sites in the extremities), a compartment resection interferes with anatomic function. In the buttock and in the medial and posteriors compartments of the thigh, an extracompartmental resection is possible and safe [2,8].

Another important issue is revascularization when, to save a limb, some arterial and venous segments enclosed by the tumor are resected. The use of tracts of vein or of synthetic grafts provides a good blood supply and prevents regional edema, which in some cases can be severe and progressive [9,10].

Retroperitoneal sarcoma often is diagnosed late, when the tumor mass is large. The surgical procedure for retroperitoneal sarcoma always involves en bloc resection of some abdominal organs and of other retroperitoneal structures.

The most frequently diagnosed sarcomas are liposarcoma, followed by leiomyosarcoma and by malignant fibrous histiocytoma. These tumors are associated with a high risk of malignant cell deposits persisting in the tumor bed after surgery, causing local recurrences. Therefore these tumors should be treated with adjuvant radiation and/or chemotherapy.

Today, with few exceptions, conservative surgery is a part of the combined therapy for both (1) highly aggressive STS [11] and (2) tumors suspected of being malignant [12].

An exemplar of the first group, clear cell sarcoma is a highly malignant STS characterized by poor prognosis with a high rate of local recurrences and distant metastases involving the lymph nodes. This aggressive behavior also is seen in tumors larger than 5 cm.

The desmoid tumor is paradigmatic of the second group. Its behavior is enigmatic, with frequent local recurrences. It can recur spontaneously and without correlation to the state of the margins. Because of its unpredictable behavior and because the margin condition is not related to local recurrences, it has been argued that desmoid tumors should be considered fully fledged tumors and that surgical treatment should be aggressive. This issue has no unequivocal answer. A valid approach would be monitoring the rate of growth, which is considered an indirect marker of the biologic aggressiveness of this tumor. The lymphatic system is not frequently involved in STS, but lymph node mapping and sentinel node biopsy are recommended in cases of advanced STS and in high-grade, aggressive tumors (eg, synovial sarcoma) [13].

Neoadjuvant and adjuvant treatments preceding or following conservative surgery also are important. One must consider both the clinical outcome (ie, local control, progression-free interval, and overall survival) and the postsurgical complications caused by systemic and regional radiation and chemotherapy (arterial perfusion and infusion).

In the past, few side effects have been observed [14] because of the ability to control complications and the application of the famous "modified Eilber protocol" [15]. Myocutaneous flaps [16] and vascular reconstructions [17] also involve minor morbidity. If a wound is infected, waiting is very hazardous, and it is mandatory to amputate without delay [18].

The timing of these combined treatments must be planned and well organized, because an accidental delay in radiation following surgery may reduce the local control of the disease significantly [19].

Treatment of local recurrences

Surgery also plays a major role in the treatment of local recurrences, which generally manifest as single or multiple nodules at the site of surgical scarring or radiation. A correct re-resection, with negative margins around the operative specimen, is of great importance to avoid the risk of further recurrences. Such re-resections must be evaluated and individualized to obtain local control [6,20].

The effect of local relapse on survival remains uncertain, and some authors associate local relapse with decreased survival [21]. The timing of the radiation in relation to surgery, the extent of surgery required, the extent of apparently normal tissue around the tumor bed that is included in the irradiated volume, and the best dose and fractionation schedule remain unresolved issues. There have been no systematic reviews or randomized trials of extremity STS in adult patients.

There is no evidence that the international practice of irradiating large volumes of normal tissue is necessary. The randomized trial on postoperative radiation given to adult patients who had extremity STS was designed to address this question. (The first patient was randomized in August, 2007).

Most patients who develop a local recurrence need aggressive treatment and may be considered for trials of adjuvant systemic therapy. For distant metastases, surgery can be successful in treating secondary tumors of the skin, lymphatic system, and lung.

Surgery of lung metastasis

In the 1990s a series of international publications reported on surgery in the treatment of lung metastasis. A retrospective study of 255 patients by the European Organization for Research and Treatment of Cancer (EORTC) Soft Tissue and Sarcoma Group reported 3-year and 5-year overall post-metastasectomy survival rates of 54% and 38% respectively, suggesting that such treatment can be considered a first-line choice if preoperative evaluation indicates that complete clearance of the metastasis is possible [22]. Such results were confirmed later by several studies at the Memorial Sloan-Kettering Cancer Center (MSKCC) (New York, New York) [23].

The next step was to assess when chemotherapy could be effective in patients undergoing metastasectomy. A European retrospective study at the Department of Surgery, Istituto Portugues de Oncologia Francisco Gentil (Lisbon, Portugal) analyzed prognostic factors in 85 patients who had undergone resection of pulmonary metastasis. In a multivariate analysis, only metastasis dimension and involvement of surgical margins were found to be independent factors associated with survival. Adjuvant chemotherapy was associated with survival only at univariate analysis [24].

A study conducted at the MSKCC of the effects of perioperative chemotherapy in patients undergoing pulmonary resection for metastatic STS of the extremities suggests that systemic chemotherapy has minimal, if any, long-term impact on outcome for these patients [25].

Rehabilitation after surgery

Another important topic related to surgical procedures in the treatment of STS is rehabilitation addressing medical, oncologic, psychologic, and environmental problems [26]. Early and multidisciplinary rehabilitation is crucial to prevent and treat complications that often arise from conservation surgery and adjuvant treatments. Rehabilitation also must deal with the functional disabilities caused by amputations and repeated operations. Special procedures (eg, rotationplasty) are performed in pediatric surgery. In all patients, the immediate use of a prosthesis after the amputation is desirable, whenever possible.

Coordinated efforts by the surgeon, physiotherapist, and prosthetist are essential to guarantee better results and a better quality of life. After surgery STS can become a chronic disease, with prolonged survival rates, if function is satisfactory and good cosmesis is used.

In conclusion, surgery plays multiple roles in diagnostic and therapeutic procedures, involving biopsies, amputations, conservative resections (more or less extended), interaction with neoadjuvant and adjuvant chemotherapy and radiation, arterial infusion and perfusion, and vascular, soft tissue, and skin reconstruction.

In the future, multimodal treatment strategies probably will modify the role of primary surgery in the treatment of STS.

Radiotherapy

The two principal methods of radiation are external-beam radiotherapy and brachytherapy, but no randomized trial has compared these two approaches. External-beam radiotherapy is highly effective in preventing local recurrences in patients who have STS and who are at risk for local failure.

A dose of 40 Gy generally is used in presurgery radiation. For tumors of the limb (> 5 cm) and for high-grade malignancies radiation is recommended after surgery, sometimes in association with presurgical radiation, because it allows preservation of the limb and drastically reduces the likelihood of local failure by less than 15%. In fact, randomized trials have demonstrated the effectiveness of radiation in reducing local recurrence in both high-grade and low-grade tumors [1]. Whether pre- or postsurgical radiation is more effective has long been debated; actually, both approaches can be beneficial [27–29]. Box 2 summarizes the advantages and disadvantages of adjuvant and neoadjuvant radiation.

There is no evidence from randomized trials that local control influences survival. Quality of life and limb function, however, depend on achieving a good local control and on radiation dose and technique [30,31].

When radiation was given by brachytherapy, positive effects were not achieved in low-grade tumors [32]. In patients who had STS of the extremities or superficial trunk, a randomized trial demonstrated that the overall morbidity associated with adjuvant brachytherapy was not significantly higher than that of surgery alone [33].

Radiotherapy also is appropriate in resected STS with positive margins. In such cases better local control is obtained with doses higher than 64 Gy and in superficial locations on the extremities [34,35].

There also is good evidence that radiation therapy improves the rate of local control in retroperitoneal STS. In this case preoperative external-beam radiotherapy may be preferred instead of intraoperative radiation, which improves local control but also increases toxicity [36].

The Department of Oncology of Karolinska Hospital (Stockholm, Sweden) recently conducted an overview of radiation therapy in STS based on data from five randomized trials and other studies involving 4579 patients [37]. In summary, the reviewers found:

- Histologic grade, tumor size, and age are the main factors involved in tumor-related death.

- The location (superficial versus deep) and the anatomic site are important prognostic factors.
- Adjuvant radiotherapy improves the local control rate (90%) in combination with conservative surgery in STS of extremities and trunk with negative, marginal, or minimal microscopic positive surgical margins.
- In intralesional surgery, radiotherapy improves outcome.
- For other anatomic sites, such as retroperitoneum, head and neck, breast, and uterus, there are only weak indications for adjuvant radiation.
- Data on whether pre- or postoperative radiation is superior for the local control of primary advanced tumors are still insufficient.

Box 2. Advantages and disadvantages of adjuvant and neoadjuvant radiotherapy in soft tissue sarcoma

Neoadjuvant radiotherapy
Advantages
  - Permits radiation of smaller volumes
  - Total dose lower than with adjuvant radiotherapy
  - Reduces tumor dissemination during surgery
  - Can makes surgery easier
  - Permits the preservation of the limb and improves local control
  - Reduces the percentage of local failure
Disadvantages
  - Complications and side effects are increased
  - Overall survival is not improved
  - Patients may refuse surgery after radiotherapy
  - Interpretation of histology can be more difficult after surgery

Adjuvant radiotherapy
Advantages
  - Minor risk of injury complications
  - Reduces recurrences
  - Improves local control
  - No delay in surgery because of complications from radiotherapy
Disadvantages
  - Requires treatment of larger volumes
  - Does not diminish the incidence of distant metastasis
  - Does not improve overall survival

Radiotherapy and hyperthermia

The combination of radiotherapy and hyperthermia sometimes is used as local adjuvant treatment. Despite the satisfactory local regional control, its application still is considered experimental, and it is used primarily for high-risk STS [38,39].

Chemotherapy

STS always have been considered somewhat chemoresistant, and chemotherapy has played an increasing role in advanced and/or metastatic disease, for many years. The drugs most commonly used are doxorubicin (or epirubicin, which is less cardiotoxic), ifosfamide, cyclophosphamide, dacarbazine, actinomycin, methotrexate, and cisplatin.

On the other hand, chemotherapy can be said to have played an increasing role in the different phases of disease, both alone and in association with radiation.

Adjuvant chemotherapy

Large tumors (> 5 cm in diameter) and/or high-grade malignancies (grade 2 or higher) carry a high risk of recurrence and of distant metastasis, particularly in the lung (up to 58%) [40]. For this reason, trials on the efficacy of postoperative (adjuvant) chemotherapy have been conducted for many years. The role of adjuvant chemotherapy was analyzed in the STS Meta-Analysis Collaboration's meta-analysis of 14 trials of chemotherapeutic regimens using doxorubicin and was found to improve the local recurrence–free interval (6%), the distant relapse–free interval (10%), and recurrence-free survival (10%) from 45% to 55% at 10 years, but its effect on overall survival was only a trend. There was a higher benefit for tumors localized to the extremities, with a significant increase in survival rate (7%) [41–43]. After this meta-analysis, three more randomized studies were undertaken to clarify the still-controversial results concerning adjuvant chemotherapy. These studies, with a wide interstudy variability, failed to demonstrate an improvement in survival [44–46].

Preoperative chemotherapy

Beginning in the 1970s in the United States and the 1980s in Europe, studies have been conducted to evaluate the advantages of preoperative (or neoadjuvant) chemotherapy, which in theory would lead to the rapid and measurable volumetric reduction of primitive tumor, would measure in vivo chemosensitivity to the prescribed drugs, and would act immediately on possible occult micrometastases. The studies are few, and the number of subjects is low. Nevertheless, the results seem to demonstrate the same advantages observed with postoperative chemotherapy. Such studies refer to sarcoma of extremities treated by either intra-arterial or intravenous chemotherapy or by isolated arterial infusion [47,48].

As Pisters [49] noted, " it is important to bear in mind that one of every two patients will live at least 5 years without pre- or postoperative chemotherapy." Therefore, in terms of locoregional failure or disease-free survival, pre- and postoperative chemotherapy do not seem at present to offer any advantages over local treatment with surgery plus radiation [50]. More recent retrospective analyses of the role of chemotherapy for stage III sarcomas deriving from the experience gained at the MSKCC and at the MD Anderson Cancer Center (Houston, Texas) have yielded interesting results [51,52]. The clinical benefits associated with doxorubicin-based chemotherapy seem not to be sustained beyond 1 year, suggesting caution in the interpretation of adjuvant chemotherapy trials [46]. The MSKCC investigators retrospectively compared the treatment of primary high-grade sarcomas with neoadjuvant chemotherapy (doxorubicin, ifosfamide, and Mesna) or with surgery alone. There was a significant improvement in disease-specific survival in patients who had sarcomas larger than 10 cm in the group treated with chemotherapy [52].

Of particular interest is the recent phase II study on neoadjuvant chemotherapy (Mesna, doxorubicin, ifosfamide, and dacarbazine [modified MAID]) and interdigitated radiation (44 Gy) in high-risk STS of the extremities and body wall conducted by a multi-institutional intergroup in the United States [53]. According to the authors, this study substantially confirms the feasibility of this complex therapeutic scheme, with a partial response rate of only 22% and with an estimated 3-year rates of disease-free survival, distant disease–free survival, and overall survival of 56.6%, 64%, and 75.1%, respectively; significant toxicity was shown, however. A randomized phase II study by the EORTC was performed using doxorubicin, 50 g/m^2, versus local therapy alone. The results did not demonstrate any differences between the two groups: 66% in the no-chemotherapy arm versus 65% for the control arm [47].

Chemoradiation

A possible synergistic effect of combined radiation and chemotherapy has been investigated in many tumors, including STS. The first encouraging results date back to the early 1980s [54,55], when researchers in the United States demonstrated that sequential radiation and chemotherapy (with doxorubicin) could reduce the number of amputations in cases of locally advanced STS selected for the surgery. Combined therapy has been investigated continually for almost 20 years, and studies have confirmed the drastic reduction in the number of amputations, the reduction of recurrences, and the possibility of achieving complete response. Furthermore, studies have confirmed that intra-arterial and intravenous chemotherapy are equally effective [56].

The first clinical trials on the concomitant use of radiation and chemotherapy in sarcoma were conducted in the United States in the 1980s. These trials investigated the possible synergy of action between chemotherapy and radiation, using low doses of doxorubicin in continuous infusion and concomitant low doses of radiation in the management of nonoperable STS [57,58]. In the light of these preliminary data, the authors' group at the National Institute for Cancer Research (Genoa, Italy) enrolled a first cohort of STS patients who had advanced/metastatic STS to test the feasibility and activity of an outpatient regimen of doxorubicin, 12 mg/m^2/d for 5 days, administered by continuous infusion and concomitant radiotherapy (150 cGy for the trunk or 200 cGy for the limbs) in repeated cycles every 3 weeks. Clinical results were very good in terms of toxicity and efficacy [59]. Therefore the therapeutic scheme was accelerated, with cycles repeated every 2 weeks and support of granulocyte colony-stimulating factor at days 6 through 12. The authors' group treated 115 consecutive patients, all with biopsy-proven and measurable locally advanced unresectable, recurrent, and/or metastatic STS of any primary tumor site and grade (excluding Ewings' sarcoma and osteogenic sarcoma), using this accelerated schedule [60]. This therapeutic approach confirmed the low toxicity and manageability of the regimen in an outpatient setting and was associated with very high percentage of objective response (67%) and complete response (11%). The median survival was 29 months, and some patients survived for more than 50 months.

On the other hand, the approach in the United States continues to use sequences of chemotherapy and radiation therapy at the maximum tolerated doses or even to use combinations of different drugs followed by preoperative radiation, with appreciable results in terms of survival.

The initial protocol of Eilber and colleagues [56], opportunely modified (doxorubicin, 30 mg/d for 3 days, and sequential radiation, 300 cGy/d for 10 days) is still the standard protocol in Canada and has proved successful in the local control of the disease and in minimizing complications in STS of both limbs and trunk.

Recently the Radiation Therapy Oncology Group in the United States concluded a phase II study based on a previous single-institution pilot study of neoadjuvant chemotherapy and radiation in the management of high-risk STS of the extremities and body wall [48]. Treatment consisted of three cycles of neoadjuvant chemotherapy (modified MAID), interdigitated preoperative radiation (44 Gy administered in split courses), and three postoperative cycles (again, modified MAID). The authors concluded that this combined-modality treatment can be delivered successfully in a multi-institutional setting, but the toxicity seems to be significant. In fact only 79% of the 64 patients in this study completed preoperative chemotherapy, and only 59% completed all planned chemotherapy, which also entailed significant toxicity: 3 patients (5%) experienced fatal-grade toxicity, another 53 patients (83%) experienced grade 4 hematologic toxicity, and 19% experienced grade 4 nonhematologic toxicity.

Chemotherapy in advanced or metastatic soft tissue sarcoma

The prognosis of patients who have advanced metastatic STS remains poor, with 5-year disease-free survival at less than 10%. Only few chemotherapeutic agents have been shown to be active, mainly doxorubicin and ifosfamide, with a response rate around 20%.

Systemic chemotherapy differs, depending on whether it is used in patients who have nonoperable locally advanced disease or in patients who have metastatic disease with or without locally advanced disease [57]. In the first case, it is still hoped that chemotherapy may induce a volumetric reduction of the tumor so the tumor can be treated locally by surgery or radiation. Aggressive chemotherapy, generally various doses of doxorubicin and ifosfamide in combination, should be used in this type of STS; the toxicity is justified by the goal. In STS associated with metastatic disease, however, chemotherapy is considered a merely palliative treatment, because only a small percentage of patients will experience any effect on survival [58]. Because treatment is palliative in this phase of the disease, it is extremely important to consider the toxicity of the selected therapy.

A systematic review and meta-analysis of ifosfamide-based combination chemotherapy was published by the Division of Medical Oncology of Ottawa Hospital in Canada [59]. This review suggested a detailed practice guideline: the addition of ifosfamide to standard first-line doxorubicin-containing regimens is not recommended over single-agent doxorubicin, but it may induce sensitive clinical improvement and even lead to tumor resection. Therefore the use of ifosfamide in combination with doxorubicin is reasonable only in selected patients, and the dose of ifosfamide should not exceed 7.5 g/m^2 (either as a split bolus or by continuous infusion).

Among other drugs, gemcitabine and docetaxel alone show modest activity, but they show more interesting results in combination. In fact, a recent phase II study comparing gemcitabine plus docetaxel versus gemcitabine alone in metastatic STS proved that this drug combination achieved a 16% objective response, versus 8% with gemcitabine alone, and with an overall survival of 17.9 months for the combination versus 11.5 months for gemcitabine alone [60]. These scores confirmed the results obtained in a retrospective study previously published by the Groupe Sarcome Francais reporting an objective response of 18.4% and a median survival of 12.1 months [61].

Hyperthermia

The increased therapeutic efficacy of chemotherapy when associated with hyperthermia has been the rationale for its use in the treatment of high-grade sarcoma that carries a high risk of local and distant recurrence. Hyperthermia is proposed most frequently as a combination treatment, especially with radiation and/or chemotherapy [39].

Recently, at the American Society of Clinical Oncology (ASCO) meeting in 2007, the European Cooperative Research Group [62] presented the results of a randomized study in high-grade STS of the extremities, the body wall, and the abdomen treated with chemotherapy (etoposide, ifosfamide, and doxorubicin) or the same chemotherapy regimen combined with regional hyperthermia. At a median follow-up of 24.9 months, regional hyperthermia plus chemotherapy yielded a statistically significant improvement in tumor response (28.7% versus 12.6%), disease-free survival (median, 31.7 months versus 16.2 months) and local progression (median survival, 45.3 months versus 23.7 months). At present, hyperthermia remains an experimental approach.

Chemotherapy perfusion

Limb perfusion in STS of the extremities is a practice dating back to the 1970s [63]. It has never been proved that it is superior to conventional treatment with melphalan or TNF-α or the combination of the two drugs. The use of this method is widespread in Europe [6,64]. At the ASCO meeting 2007 the Institut Gustave Roussy presented a final report of a prior randomized phase II trial comparing hyperthermia isolated limb perfusion with melphalan and with four different doses of TNF-alpha. The study concluded that the 1-mg dose of TNF-α was as effective as the standard 4-mg dose when measuring response rates and patient outcomes and avoided systemic toxicity [65].

Therapeutic approach for unusual anatomic sites

In addition to the limbs and trunk, other anatomic sites are, less frequently, affected by sarcoma; they also are less investigated. These sites are the retroperitoneum, breast, head and neck, and abdomen. There is modest international experience for these STS; therefore the treatment reflects the experience acquired with STS of limbs and trunk. In these cases, radical surgery, often associated with radiation (and also intraoperative radiation for retroperitoneal STS) is the treatment of choice, because it is difficult to achieve radical resection at these sites [1,6,66].

Follow-up

In general the follow-up assessments should focus on the status of the primary tumor and the evaluation of distant metastases, mainly in the lung. Every patient who has localized resectable STS should have a clinical examination every 3 to 6 months for the first 2 years. The patient also should have a chest CT scan every 6 months for 3 years and then annually. Patients who have high-grade tumors need more frequent surveillance to exclude local and systemic relapse. Table 2 presents suggested guidelines for the treatment and follow-up of STS according to stage.

Table 2
Suggested guidelienes for treating soft tissue sarcoma according to stage

TNM Stage	Treatment	Comments	Follow-up
I T1a–b, N0, M0	Surgery alone when margins are > 1 cm or the fascia plane is intact or adjuvant radiation when margins are ≤ 1 cm	Because of the low metastatic potential of these tumors, chemotherapy usually is not given	Chest radiograph and physical examination every 6–12 months for 2–3 years and then annually
I T2a–b, N0, M0	Wide surgery with or without neoadjuvant or adjuvant radiation	Because of the low metastatic potential of these tumors, chemotherapy usually is not indicated	Chest radiograph and physical examination every 6–12 months for 2–3 years and then annually
IIB, IIC, III	Surgery with or without neoadjuvant or adjuvant radiation and with or without neoadjuvant or adjuvant chemotherapy	High-grade, no lymph node or distant metastases	CT scan every 3–4 months for 3 years, then every 6–12 months for the next 2 years, and annually thereafter
IV	Surgical resection of the primary tumor with radiation therapy If the tumor is unresectable, high-dose radiation therapy may be used, often associated with chemotherapy for patients eligible for clinical trials; amputation when necessary	Metastatic involvement of regional lymph nodes (in some subtype of STS) and/or spread to distant organs	CT scan and other imaging tests every 3–4 months; frequent physical examinations

New therapeutic strategies

Overall survival is dramatically low in advanced or metastatic STS. Therefore new therapeutic approaches are necessary. Consistent improvements have been achieved in understanding the molecular biology and pathogenesis of STS. It is likely that such knowledge may be incorporated rapidly in clinical practice and provide a targeted therapy to be used along with the available cytotoxic regimens for these tumors. Among the emerging therapies are antiangiogenetic therapy, immunomodulant drugs, Bcl-2 antisense therapy, and others [67–69].

New drugs include exatecan (DX-8951f), a totally synthetic analogue of the topoisomerase I inhibitor Camptothecin, that is less toxic than Camptothecin, topotecan, or irinotecan. A phase II study by the EORTC Soft

Tissue and Bone Sarcoma Group reported a stable disease in 60% of pre-treated patients who had leiomyosarcoma and in 53% of pretreated patients who had non-leiomyosarcoma tumors [70]. The same investigators studied a new DNA minor groove binder in patients who had advanced or inoper-able STS and gastrointestinal tumor who had not responded to first-line therapy. They reported two partial responses, with an acceptable level of toxicity, among 43 recruited patients [71].

In patients who had refractory STS, bendamustine, a new bifunctional alkylating agent, was evaluated in a noncomparative multicenter phase II study by the German Sarcoma Group. Investigators reported a good toxicity profile but only a 3% partial response rate and 31% rate of stable disease [72].

Proton beam therapy is used increasingly in radiotherapy and also is used in the treatment of STS. It reduces the treated volume, thus permitting the administration of a higher radiation dose to the tumor and reduced toxicity. The Center for Radiation Therapy in Switzerland recently published its experience on tumors located in proximity to critical structures, such as the spinal cord, optic system, bowel, and kidney. Although the number of patients is small, the results seem to show the efficacy of protein beam ther-apy in this patient population [73].

Summary

Until 20 years ago there was little knowledge of STS, and few studies had been conducted because of its rarity. STS was considered a disease that was difficult to diagnosis and treat. These tumors, considered radiation- and che-moresistant and inoperable, seemed to always be incurable. Clinically there were, and still are, frequent errors and delays in diagnosis and no consistent treatment practice.

The principal clinical and organizational problems that must be addressed to achieve appropriate management of patients who have STS are

The high frequency of late diagnosis
The difficult histologic classification
The great variability in cases and in diagnostic and therapeutic practices
The use of frequently inappropriate initial surgery
The relatively low efficacy of treatments for the most advanced disease

The consequences of late or wrong diagnosis and of inappropriate treat-ment are very relevant. Many patients applying to a specialist center for STS have received previous inappropriate treatment. Often they have to undergo further surgery, including amputation. On the other hand, the most recent diagnostic, pathologic, and radiologic advances, and, above all, a thorough multidisciplinary clinical approach have made it possible to confront STS with more extensive and exhaustive knowledge: bioptic techniques, standardized surgical procedures, defined staging, and knowledge about prognostic factors that is essential to therapeutic planning (eg, the lesion's size, grading, and depth) have contributed considerably to improved survival.

Although surgery remains the cornerstone for treating localized STS, the importance of radiation in association with surgery in the local control of STS has been increasingly recognized. A recent report on outcomes of 8249 cases by the Florida Cancer Data System [3] emphasizes that tumor site and stage are prognostic factors independent from histologic subtype and confirms that surgical resection and radiation are unique among treatment modalities in being associated with a significant survival benefit. Of course, radiation also remains of primary importance in unresected STS. In this case, higher radiation doses (between 63 and 68 Gy) yield superior tumor control and survival [74].

It also is necessary to remember that preoperative treatments such as radiation, chemotherapy, chemoradiation, and isolated limb perfusion are increasingly reducing the number of amputations in locally advanced disease, as well as allowing less extensive local surgery [1,6].

The role of adjuvant chemotherapy is still controversial, although it is obviously important. Only a few studies have shown that chemotherapy has a positive effect on the local control of STS, particularly in reducing mortality in STS of the limbs and in high-grade malignancy. At the ASCO meeting in 2007, the EORTC presented an interim analysis of the largest study of adjuvant chemotherapy with doxorubicin and ifosfamide ever undertaken in STS: there was no survival advantage or improvement on local disease control [75]. Therefore the use and timing of adjuvant chemotherapy or adjuvant chemoradiotherapy remains controversial. The appropriate target population generally is accepted as UICC/AJCC stage III extremity or trunk sarcomas (ie, > 5 cm, grade 3–4, located deep to the superficial fascia, with no evidence of metastasis). After definitive local treatment, the 5-year disease-free and overall survival rates in this population are approximately 52% and 56% [76].

One more important advance in therapeutic knowledge has been the common recognition that metastatic disease also can be cured: metastatic pulmonary STS can be treated, and the presence of lung metastasis does not preclude treatment of the primary tumor. Long-term observation of patients who had metastases enabled researchers to select a group of patients who can be considered long-term survivors. One main prognostic parameter seems to be complete response to chemotherapy after radical resection. Unfortunately the drugs at the clinician's disposal are substantially two: doxorubicin and ifosfamide. Treatment with ifosfamide doses higher than 9 g/m^2 seems encouraging, but the real impact on survival is not known. Therefore doxorubicin, 75 mg/m^2 every 21 days, remains the first-line standard treatment unless radical surgery results in a significant objective response or complete response. In these cases, more complex chemotherapy schedules, such as the combination of doxorubicin and ifosfamide, may be justified [77].

Table 3
Ongoing randomized clinical trials in locally advanced and or metastatic soft tissue sarcomas
in European and non-European countries

Country	Phase	Date of activation	Number of subjects	Purpose
Europe EORTC	III	07/11/1997 (closed on 03/20/2007)	340	To determine local progression-free survival of patients who have high-risk STS treated with neoadjuvant etoposide, ifosfamide
Europe EORTC	III	08/04/2003	450	To compare the progression-free and overall survival of patients who have locally advanced or metastatic STS treated with doxorubicin with or without ifosfamide and pegfilgrastim as first-line therapy
Canada	II	May 2003	41	To study preoperative intensity-modulated radiation therapy for lower limb STS
Europe (United Kingdom)	III	01/11/2003 (closed on 03/31/2008)	450	To study whether the combination of ifosfamide and doxorubicin is better than doxorubicin alone in the treatment of advanced sarcoma
Europe (Germany and France)	II	August 2004	117	To determine whether oral continuous (metronomic) therapy with trofosfamide has similar progression-free survival at 6 months as intravenous treatment with doxorubicin.
United States, Canada, Israel	III	August 2005	200	To provide access to treatment with trabectedin to patients who have relapsed or who are refractory to/intolerant of standard therapy
India	—	January 2006; (will close in December 2014)	500	To evaluate the impact on overall survival of an intensive follow-up protocol (as practiced today at Tata Memorial Hospital) versus a more cost-effective follow-up protocol in patients operated for extremity sarcoma

Table 3 (*continued*)

Country	Phase	Date of activation	Number of subjects	Purpose
Europe (United Kingdom)	III	01/02/2006 (will close on 01/02/2009)	400	To reduce the size of the radiotherapy treatment area and expose less normal tissue to treatment
Europe (United Kingdom)	III	August 2007 (will close on 02/15/2011)	400	To evaluate the impact of postoperative radiotherapy on changes in volume, on morbidity, and limb functionality in adult patients who have extremity STS

Data from www.clinicaltrials.gov.

Because the 5-year survival rate for locally advanced and/or metastatic disease is less than 10%, research has been oriented to improving knowledge concerning new chemotherapeutic drugs or to developing innovative biologic approaches to improve survival in this cohort of patients.

Individual tumor subtypes are under investigation, inaugurating for STS a new era of targeted therapy similar to that observed for other solid tumors. Targeted therapy could be adjuvant to conventional drugs, although, for the moment, it has been little success in treating STS [78]. Ultimately it must be emphasized that the best therapeutic results have been obtained in patients treated by interdisciplinary working groups and, above all, in centers of recognized specialization [79–81].

Many international researchers agree with the need for better coordination among the various oncologic centers specializing in the treatment of sarcomas. Researchers in Europe share these objectives. Some French authors, in particular, have devised multidisciplinary co-operative strategies and cancer networks to optimize the treatment of patients who have STS [82].

Among several research and coordinate groups for the study of STS in Europe are the

British Sarcoma Group
European Organization Research and Treatment of Cancer Soft Tissue and Bone Sarcoma Group
French Sarcoma Group
Italian Sarcoma Group
Scandinavian Sarcoma Group
Spanish Group for Research on Sarcomas

Table 3 lists some ongoing randomized clinical trials in advanced STS found at the Web site www.clinicaltrials.gov. These clinical trials mostly address advanced or metastatic STS, because it is, unfortunately, the most widespread clinical presentation of STS in the main oncologic centers both in Europe and in non-European countries.

In Europe studies seem mainly to be concerned with the effects of chemotherapy (doxorubicin and ifosfamide) on STS. In Great Britain studies seem to address the effects of radiation treatment on volume reduction and the morbidity of such treatment in clinical practice. Research studies in the United States seem to be more interested in investigating the use of new drugs. Of great interest, from a practical point of view, is the Indian clinical trial on the effects of intensity of follow-up on survival.

With pride, the authors would like to remind the reader of Eilber's words at the ASCO meeting in 2007 (unpublished data): "Investigators in the United States could learn from the cooperative abilities of our European Colleagues, whose studies are attempting to answer questions and validate new treatments."

Acknowledgments

The authors thank Drs. Fabio Rizzo and Cristina Poli for their help in the preparation of this article.

References

[1] Pisters PWT, O'Sullivan B. Soft tissue sarcoma. In: Pollock RE, Doroshow JH, Khayat D, editors. Union International Contre le Cancer: manual of clinical oncology. 8th edition. Hoboken (NJ): John Wiley & Sons inc.; 2004. p. 649–69.

[2] Wittekind CH, Gheene FL, Hutter RVP, editors. Union International Contre le Cancer TNM atlas. 5th edition. Berlin: Springer; 2004.

[3] Gutierrez JC, Perez EA, Franceschi D, et al. Outcomes for soft-tissue sarcoma in 8249 cases from a large state cancer registry. J Surg Res 2007;141(1):105–14.

[4] Enneking WF, Spanier SS, Goodman MA. A system for the surgical staging of musculoskeletal sarcoma 1980. Clin Orthop Relat Res 2003;(415):4–18.

[5] Hoekstra HJ, Thijssens K, van Ginkel RJ. Role of surgery as primary treatment and as intervention in the multidisciplinary treatment of soft tissue sarcoma. Ann Oncol 2004; 15(Suppl 4:iv):181–6.

[6] Eggermont AM, Schraffordt Koops H, Lienard D, et al. Isolated limb perfusion with high-dose tumor necrosis factor-alpha in combination with interferon-gamma and melphalan for nonresectable extremity soft tissue sarcomas: a multicenter trial. J Clin Oncol 1996;14(10): 2653–65.

[7] Sobin LH, Wittekind CH, editors. TNM classification of malignant tumours (Union International Contre le Cancer). 6th edition. New York: John Wiley & Sons inc.; 2002.

[8] Kulaylat MN, King B, Karakousis CP. Posterior compartment resection of the thigh for soft-tissue sarcomas. J Surg Oncol 1999;71(4):243–5.

[9] Adelani MA, Holt GE, Dittus RS, et al. Revascularization after segmental resection of lower extremity soft tissue sarcomas. J Surg Oncol 2007;95(6):455–60.

[10] McKay A, Motamedi M, Temple W, et al. Vascular reconstruction with the superficial femoral vein following major oncologic resection. J Surg Oncol 2007;96(2):151–9.

[11] Malchau SS, Hayden J, Hornicek F, et al. Clear cell sarcoma of soft tissues. J Surg Oncol 2007;95(6):519–22.

[12] Zippel DB, Temple WJ. When is a neoplasm not a neoplasm? When it is a desmoid. J Surg Oncol 2007;95(3):190–1.

[13] Tunn PU, Andreou D, Illing H, et al. Sentinel node biopsy in synovial sarcoma. Eur J Surg Oncol 2007; [epub ahead of print].

[14] Temple WJ, Temple CL, Arthur K, et al. Prospective cohort study of neoadjuvant treatment in conservative surgery of soft tissue sarcomas. Ann Surg Oncol 1997;4(7):586–90.

[15] Mack LA, Crowe PJ, Yang JL, et al. Preoperative chemoradiotherapy (modified Eilber protocol) provides maximum local control and minimal morbidity in patients with soft tissue sarcoma. Ann Surg Oncol 2005;12(8):646–53.

[16] Temple CL, Ross DC, Magi E, et al. Preoperative chemoradiation and flap reconstruction provide high local control and low wound complication rates for patients undergoing limb salvage surgery for upper extremity tumors. J Surg Oncol 2007;95(2):135–41.

[17] Mack LA, Temple WJ, DeHaas WG, et al. Soft tissue tumors a challenge for local control and reconstruction: a prospective cohort analysis. J Surg Oncol 2004;86(3):147–51.

[18] Wanebo HJ, Temple WJ, Popp MB, et al. Preoperative regional therapy for extremity sarcoma. A tricenter update. Cancer 1995;75(9):2299–306.

[19] Schwartz DL, Einck J, Hunt K, et al. The effect of delayed postoperative irradiation on local control of soft tissue sarcomas of the extremity and torso. Int J Radiat Oncol Biol Phys 2002; 52(5):1352–9.

[20] Moureau-Zabotto L, Thomas L, Bui BN, et al. Management of soft tissue sarcomas (STS) in first isolated local recurrence: a retrospective study of 83 cases. Radiother Oncol 2004;73(3): 313–9.

[21] Stotter AT, A'Hern RP, Fisher C, et al. The influence of local recurrence of extremity soft tissue sarcoma on metastasis and survival. Cancer 1990;65(5):1119–29.

[22] van Geel AN, Pastorino U, Jauch KW, et al. Surgical treatment of lung metastases: the European organization for research and treatment of cancer-soft tissue and bone sarcoma group study of 255 patients. Cancer 1996;77(4):675–82.

[23] Billingsley KG, Burt ME, Jara E, et al. Pulmonary metastases from soft tissue sarcoma: analysis of patterns of diseases and postmetastasis survival. Ann Surg 1999;229(5):602–10 [discussion: 610–2].

[24] Abecasis N, Cortez F, Bettencourt A, et al. Surgical treatment of lung metastases: prognostic factors for long-term survival. J Surg Oncol 1999;72(4):193–8.

[25] Canter RJ, Qin LX, Downey RJ, et al. Perioperative chemotherapy in patients undergoing pulmonary resection for metastatic soft-tissue sarcoma of the extremity: a retrospective analysis. Cancer 2007;110(9):2050–60.

[26] Custodio CM. Barriers to rehabilitation of patients with extremity sarcomas. J Surg Oncol 2007;95(5):393–9.

[27] Yang JC, Chang AE, Baker AR, et al. Randomized prospective study of the benefit of adjuvant radiation therapy in the treatment of soft tissue sarcomas of the extremity. J Clin Oncol 1998;16(1):197–203.

[28] Pollack A, Zagars GK, Goswitz MS, et al. Preoperative vs. postoperative radiotherapy in the treatment of soft tissue sarcomas: a matter of presentation. Int J Radiat Oncol Biol Phys 1998;42(3):563–72.

[29] Robinson MH, Keus RB, Shasha D, et al. Is pre-operative radiotherapy superior to postoperative radiotherapy in the treatment of soft tissue sarcoma? Eur J Cancer 1998;34(9): 1309–16.

[30] Davis AM, O'Sullivan B, Bell RS, et al. Function and health status outcomes in a randomized trial comparing preoperative and postoperative radiotherapy in extremity soft tissue sarcoma. J Clin Oncol 2002;20(22):4472–7.

[31] Davis AM, O'Sullivan B, Turcotte R, et al. Canadian sarcoma group; NCI Canada clinical trial group randomized trial. Late radiation morbidity following randomization to preoperative versus postoperative radiotherapy in extremity soft tissue sarcoma. Radiother Oncol 2005;75(1):48–53.

[32] Harrison LB, Franzese F, Gaynor JJ, et al. Long-term results of a prospective randomized trial of adjuvant brachytherapy in the management of completely resected soft tissue sarcoma of the extremity and superficial trunk. Int J Radiat Oncol Biol Phys 1993;27:259–65.

[33] Alektiar KM, Zelefsky MJ, Brennan MF. Morbidity of adjuvant brachytherapy in soft tissue sarcoma of the extremity and superficial trunk. Int J Radiat Oncol Biol Phys 2000;47(5): 1273–9.

[34] Alektiar KM, Velasco J, Zelefsky MJ, et al. Adjuvant radiotherapy for margin-positive high-grade soft tissue sarcoma of the extremity. Int J Radiat Oncol Biol Phys 2000;48(4):1051–8.

[35] Delaney TF, Kepka L, Goldberg SI, et al. Radiation therapy for control of soft-tissue sarcomas resected with positive margins. Int J Radiat Oncol Biol Phys 2007;67(5):1460–9.

[36] Pawlik TM, Ahuja N, Herman JM. The role of radiation in retroperitoneal sarcomas: a surgical perspective. Curr Opin Oncol 2007;19(4):359–66.

[37] Strander H, Turesson I, Cavallin-Stahl E. A systematic overview of radiation therapy effects in soft tissue sarcomas. Acta Oncol 2003;42(5–6):516–31.

[38] Prosnitz LR, Maguire P, Anderson JM, et al. The treatment of high-grade soft tissue sarcomas with preoperative thermoradiotherapy. Int J Radiat Oncol Biol Phys 1999;45(4): 941–9.

[39] Issels RD, Schlemmer M, Lindner LH. The role of hyperthermia in combined treatment in the management of soft tissue sarcoma. Curr Oncol Rep 2006;8(4):305–9.

[40] Spiro IJ, Gebhardt MC, Jennings LC, et al. Prognostic factors for local control of sarcomas of the soft tissues managed by radiation and surgery. Semin Oncol 1997;24(5):540–6.

[41] Tierney JF, Mosseri V, Stewart LA, et al. Adjuvant chemotherapy for soft-tissue sarcoma: review and meta-analysis of the published results of randomised clinical trials. Br J Cancer 1995;72(2):469–75.

[42] Bramwell VHC. Adjuvant chemotherapy for adult soft tissue sarcoma: is there a standard of care? J Clin Oncol 2001;19(5):1235–7.

[43] Adjuvant chemotherapy for localised resectable soft-tissue sarcoma of adults: meta-analysis of individual data. Sarcoma meta-analysis collaboration. Lancet 1997;350(9092):1647–54.

[44] Kotz R, Brodowicz T, Zielinski C, et al. Intensified adjuvant IFADIC chemotherapy for adult soft tissue sarcoma: a prospective randomized feasibility trial. Sarcoma 2000;4(10): 151–60.

[45] Frustaci S, Gherlinzoni F, De Paoli A, et al. Adjuvant chemotherapy for adult soft tissue sarcomas of the extremities and girdles: results of the Italian randomized cooperative trial. J Clin Oncol 2001;19(5):1238–47.

[46] Petrioli R, Coratti A, Correale P, et al. Adjuvant epirubicin with or without ifosfamide for adult soft-tissue sarcoma. Am J Clin Oncol 2002;25(5):468–73.

[47] Gortzak E, Azzarelli A, Buesa J, et al. E.O.R.T.C. Soft tissue bone sarcoma group and the National Cancer Institute of Canada Clinical Trials Group/Canadian Sarcoma Group. A randomised phase II study on neo-adjuvant chemotherapy for 'high-risk' adult soft-tissue sarcoma. Eur J Cancer 2001;37(9):1096–103.

[48] Antman KH. Adjuvant therapy of sarcomas of soft tissue. Semin Oncol 1997;24(5):556–60.

[49] Pisters PWT. Preoperative chemotherapy and split-course radiation therapy for patients with localized soft tissue sarcomas: home run, base hit, or strike out? J Clin Orthop 2006; 24(4):549–51.

[50] O'Sullivan B, Davis AM, Turcotte R, et al. Preoperative versus postoperative radiotherapy in soft-tissue sarcoma of the limbs: a randomised trial. Lancet 2002;359(9325):2235–41.

[51] Cormier JN, Huang X, Xing Y, et al. Cohort analysis of patients with localized, high-risk, extremity soft tissue sarcoma treated at two cancer centers: chemotherapy-associated outcomes. J Clin Oncol 2004;22(22):4567–74.

[52] Grobmyer SR, Maki RG, Demetri GD, et al. Neo-adjuvant chemotherapy for primary high-grade extremity soft tissue sarcoma. Ann Oncol 2004;15(11):1667–72.

[53] Kraybill WG, Harris J, Spiro IJ, et al. Phase II study of neoadjuvant chemotherapy and radiation therapy in the management of high-risk, high-grade, soft tissue sarcomas of the

extremities and body wall: radiation therapy oncology group trial 9514. J Clin Oncol 2006;
24(4):619–25.

[54] Eilber FR, Morton DL, Eckardt J, et al. Limb salvage for skeletal and soft tissue sarcomas.
Multidisciplinary preoperative therapy. Cancer 1984;53(12):2579–84.

[55] Eilber FR, Guiliano AE, Huth J, et al. High-grade soft-tissue sarcomas of the extremity:
UCLA experience with limb salvage. Prog Clin Biol Res 1985;201:59–74.

[56] Eilber F, Eckardt J, Rosen G, et al. Preoperative therapy for soft tissue sarcoma [review].
Hematol Oncol Clin North Am 1995;9(4):817–23.

[57] Sordillo PP, Magill GB, Schauer PK, et al. Preliminary trial of combination therapy with
Adriamycin and radiation in sarcomas and other malignant tumors. J Surg Oncol 1982;
21(1):23–6.

[58] Rosenthal CJ, Rotman M. Pilot study of interaction of radiation therapy with doxorubicin
by continuous infusion. NCI Monogr 1988;(6):285–90.

[59] Toma S, Palumbo R, Sogno G, et al. Concomitant radiation-doxorubicin administration in
locally advanced and/or metastatic soft tissue sarcomas: preliminary results. Anticancer Res
1991;11(6):2085–9.

[60] Toma S, Canavese G, Grimaldi A, et al. Concomitant chemo-radiotherapy in the treatment
of locally advanced and/or metastatic soft tissue sarcomas: experience of the National
Cancer Institute of Genoa. Oncol Rep 2003;10(3):641–7.

[61] Bay JO, Ray-Coquard I, Fayette J, et al. Groupe sarcome Français. Docetaxel and gemcitabine combination in 133 advanced soft-tissue sarcomas: a retrospective analysis. Int J Cancer
2006;119(3):706–11.

[62] Issels RD, Lindner LH, Wust P, et al. Regional hyperthermia (RHT) improves response
and survival when combined with systemic chemotherapy in the management of locally
advanced, high grade soft tissue sarcomas (STS) of the extremities, the body wall and
the abdomen: a phase III randomised pros [abstract]. J Clin Oncol 2007;25(18S):10009.

[63] Krementz ET, Carter RD, Sutherland CM, et al. Chemotherapy of sarcomas of the limbs by
regional perfusion. Ann Surg 1977;185(5):555–64.

[64] Bonvalot S, Laplanche A, Lejeune F, et al. Limb salvage with isolated perfusion for soft
tissue sarcoma: could less TNF-alpha be better? Ann Oncol 2005;16(7):1061–8, Epub 2005
Jun 1.

[65] Bedard V, Vataire A, Desouche C, et al. A prospective database of 100 patients with locally
soft tissue sarcoma (STS) treated by isolated limb perfusion with melphalan and TNFα 1mg
[abstract]. J Clin Oncol 2007;25(18S):10010. ASCO Annual Meeting Proceedings part I
(June 20 Supplement).

[66] Perez EA, Gutierrez JC, Moffat FL Jr, et al. Retroperitoneal and truncal sarcomas: prognosis depends upon type not location. Ann Surg Oncol 2007;14(3):1114–22.

[67] Mocellin S, Rossi CR, Brandes A, et al. Adult soft tissue sarcomas: conventional therapies
and molecularly targeted approaches. Cancer Treat Rev 2006;32(1):9–27.

[68] Kasper B, Gil T, D'Hondt V, et al. Novel treatment strategies for soft tissue sarcoma. Crit
Rev Oncol Hematol 2007;62(1):9–15.

[69] Yang JL, Crowe PJ. Targeted therapies in adult soft tissue sarcomas. J Surg Oncol 2007;
95(3):183–4.

[70] Reichardt P, Nielsen OS, Bauer S, et al. EORTC Soft Tissue and Bone Sarcoma Group.
Exatecan in pretreated adult patients with advanced soft tissue sarcoma: results of a phase
II–study of the EORTC soft tissue and bone sarcoma group. Eur J Cancer 2007;43(6):
1017–22.

[71] Leahy M, Ray-Coquard I, Verweij J, et al. European Organisation for Research and Treatment of Cancer Soft Tissue and Bone Sarcoma Group. Brostallicin, an agent with potential
activity in metastatic soft tissue sarcoma: a phase II study from the European Organisation
for Research and Treatment of Cancer Soft Tissue and Bone Sarcoma Group. Eur J Cancer
2007;43(2):308–15.

[72] Hartmann JT, Mayer F, Schleicher J, et al. German Sarcoma Group. Bendamustine hydrochloride in patients with refractory soft tissue sarcoma: a noncomparative multicenter phase 2 study of the German Sarcoma Group (AIO-001). Cancer 2007;110(4):861–6.

[73] Weber DC, Rutz HP, Bolsi A, et al. Spot scanning proton therapy in the curative treatment of adult patients with sarcoma: the Paul Scherrer Institute experience. Int J Radiat Oncol Biol Phys 2007;69(3):865–71.

[74] Kepka L, DeLaney TF, Suit HD, et al. Results of radiation therapy for unresected soft-tissue sarcomas. Int J Radiat Oncol Biol Phys 2005;63(3):852–9.

[75] Woll PJ, van Glabbke M, Hohenberger P, et al. Adjuvant chemotherapy (CT) with doxorubicin and ifosfamide in resected soft tissue sarcoma (STS): interim analysis of a randomised phase III trial [abstract]. J Clin Oncol 2007;25:10008.

[76] Bramwell V. When to consider adjuvant/neoadjuvant therapy for adult soft-tissue sarcoma. Oncology (Williston Park) 2007;21(4):511–4.

[77] Souhami RL, Tannok I, Hoenberger P, et al. Oxford textbook of oncology. 2nd edition. New York: Oxford University Press; 2001.

[78] Ma BB, Bristow RG, Kim J, et al. Combined-modality treatment of solid tumors using radiotherapy and molecular targeted agents. J Clin Oncol 2003;21(14):2760–76.

[79] Rydholm A. Improving the management of soft tissue sarcoma. Diagnosis and treatment should be given in specialist centres. BMJ 1998;317(7151):93–4.

[80] Rydholm A. Centralization of soft tissue sarcoma. The southern Sweden experience. Acta Orthop Scand Suppl 1997;273:4–8.

[81] Gutierrez JC, Perez EA, Moffat FL, et al. Should soft tissue sarcomas be treated at high-volume centers? An analysis of 4205 patients. Ann Surg 2007;245(6):952–8.

[82] Ray-Coquard I, Thiesse P, Ranchère-Vince D, et al. Conformity to clinical practice guidelines, multidisciplinary management and outcome of treatment for soft tissue. Ann Oncol 2004;15(2):307–15.

ELSEVIER
SAUNDERS

Surg Oncol Clin N Am
17 (2008) 673–699

SURGICAL
ONCOLOGY CLINICS
OF NORTH AMERICA

Sentinel Lymph Node Biopsy in Breast Cancer

Lucio Fortunato, MD[a],*, Alessandra Mascaro, MD[a],
Mostafa Amini, MD[b], Massimo Farina, MD[a],
Carlo Eugenio Vitelli, MD[a]

[a]*Department of Surgery, San Giovanni- Addolorata Hospital,
Via Amba- Aradam 4, Rome 00184, Italy*
[b]*Department of Pathology, San Giovanni- Addolorata Hospital,
Via Amba- Aradam 4, Rome 00184, Italy*

No other single cancer site has witnessed such a tremendous change and improvement in clinical management as breast cancer in the last 2 decades. Around the world, hundreds of thousand of women who have breast cancer have been treated with the removal of the primary tumor and a simple biopsy of the first draining lymph node. Only a few years ago, they would have been subjected to the physical and psychologic devastation of mastectomy and total axillary clearance.

Thanks are owed to Veronesi and colleagues [1] for demonstrating, in an era of surgical aggressiveness, that quadrantectomy and mastectomy are equivalent in terms of survival. This understanding has opened a completely new approach for patients who have breast cancer, in which the key word is "conservation" instead of "the more radical the excision, the better." This revolutionary strategy has helped many women to accept their disease in a more active way, while maintaining a good locoregional control.

Conservation of the axillary lymph nodes, however, has been impractical for many years, and attempts to avoid any staging procedure in the axilla have been largely unsuccessful, even for small tumors. Whether or not the removal of such lymph nodes has a therapeutic benefit, their involvement by cancer cells represents an important prognostic factor for survival in

This work was supported by the Fondazione Prometeus, ONLUS, for development and research in oncology.

* Corresponding author.

E-mail address: lfortunato@tiscali.it (L. Fortunato).

breast cancer patients [2,3], and consequently information about axillary lymph node status is still sought.

Although the term "sentinel lymph node" (SLN) had been coined earlier [4], Cabanas [5] introduced the concept for penile carcinomas in 1977. In 1992 Morton and colleagues [6] demonstrated the possibility of applying this procedure for melanoma, and in 1994 Giuliano and colleagues [7] reported it for breast cancer patients. The technique of injecting a blue dye soon was followed by the use of a radiocolloid and a handheld gamma probe [8]. Since then, the procedure has become a standard of care in many centers, as reflected by the increasing number of studies published in the literature. Fig. 1 gives the results of a PUBMED search using the terms "Sentinel lymph node" AND "breast cancer."

Much of what is known today regarding SLN biopsy in breast cancer does not result from randomized trials. The procedure has been accepted quickly by most dedicated surgeons around the world on the basis of a growing body of evidence that SLN is effective. Often, patients' demands have overcome the caution that surgeons usually demonstrate before abandoning a well-tested procedure, such as axillary node dissection. In some cases, randomized trials have been closed prematurely because of accrual problems, either because randomization was not acceptable to patients or because surgeons, after acquiring sufficient experience with SLN biopsy, were unwilling to allow their patients to participate. This situation may not be surprising if the procedure is considered a diagnostic tool; for example, clinicians usually do not wait for randomized trials to indicate that a radiologic technique is good enough to detect cancer in any part of the body.

Many aspects of SLN biopsy are still unclear, however, and the variability of techniques, methods of examination, and even applications risks weakening the effectiveness of the procedure.

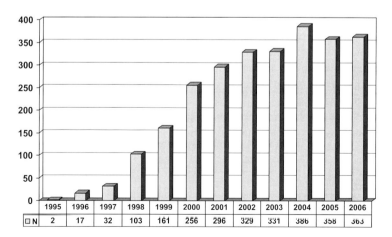

Fig. 1. Number of articles published on sentinel lymph node biopsy and breast cancer.

What is known

Identification of the sentinel lymph node and type of injection

Sentinel lymph node biopsy is relatively easy and reproducible in experienced hands, and generally no more that 20 to 50 cases are needed for a surgeon to acquire the necessary experience to perform the procedure and to reduce the failure rate to an acceptable 5% [9,10]. More importantly, the number of cases performed each month by a given surgeon seems to affect the ability to identify the sentinel node, and the cut off seems to be around 5 to 10 cases per month [10]. In experienced hands, only older patient age seems to affect significantly the ability to identify the SLN [11].

It is now clear that the entire breast has a major lymphatic efferent pathway, starting from a rich periareolar plexus and connected to the SLN [12]. It is well documented that if blue dye and radiocolloid are injected in different quadrants of the same breast, both tracers drain to the same SLN in 93% of cases [13]. Two prospective, randomized trials [14,15] and one multicentric study of 3961 patients [16] have demonstrated that an intradermal or periareolar injection allows a higher incidence of localization of SLN than a peritumoral injection, while decreasing time to identification of the SLN. Therefore many groups, including the authors' group, have switched to one of these two approaches. The periareolar route has the additional advantage of simplicity because it can be used for nonpalpable and multicentric tumors and can minimize the shine-through effect, particularly for tumors in the upper external quadrants, because the site of injection is far from the axilla. Intradermal injection, however, has been associated with an increased number of SLNs harvested and with a greater possibility of retrieving four or more SLNs [17].

Surgeons continue to debate the advantages of using a combination of radiocolloid and blue dye, and in some centers the use of blue dye alone is considered equivalent to radiocolloid, although the learning curve can be quite lengthy, and the technique can involve a decreased success rate [18]. In a recent retrospective review of 1187 patients treated by high-volume ($\geq$ 100 cases) or low-volume ($<$ 100 cases) surgeons, SLN were identified more efficiently by the former group [19]. This difference was minimal, however, after radiocolloid injection (96% versus 94%), but it was substantial after injection of blue dye (92.9% versus 78.5%). The authors suggest that surgeons use both tracers during their initial experiences with SLN biopsy, because the topographic guidance of the gamma probe and the visual intraoperative identification of colored lymphatic structures may be additive tools. With experience, a declining marginal benefit from the blue dye has been reported [20]; most groups tend to simplify the procedure by using the radiocolloid alone, but the choice of tracer is matter of personal preference.

Therefore, site of injection, type of injection, and the tracer used seem to be less important for SLN identification, provided each group sets up a specific protocol to optimize the collaboration and participation of surgeons

and nuclear medicine specialists involved in this procedure. Identification of
the SLN depends mostly on the surgeon's experience, regardless of the technique used.

False-negative rate

SLN biopsy is now considered an adequate axillary staging procedure for
patients who have breast cancer. Many concerns were raised in the past
because SLN biopsy can result in some false-negative cases. A recent
meta-analysis of 69 trials found the rate of false negatives to be about 7%
of the node-positive patients [21], although in multicentric studies recruiting
a large number of surgeons early in their experience with SLN biopsy this
incidence can be as high as 10% [22]. Although multiple studies have documented that identification rates can be improved over time and with increased individual experience, there have been concerns that false-negative
cases, although rare, may not follow the same trend. In two studies, however, the false-negative rate dropped from a range of 9% to 15% to a range
of 2% to 4% after the first 20 to 30 cases performed [18,23]. Removal of palpable suspicious nodes, or preoperative identification of such cases by ultrasound, may decrease the false-negative rate further [24]; the authors
routinely digitally explore the axilla from the SLN incision to rule out the
presence of enlarged or hard nodes. Additionally, the potential false-negative rate is lower when multiple SLN's are removed instead of only one
[25]. The chance of missing a positive node may also depend on factors other
than the surgeon's experience. Evidently, the smaller the risk of harboring
a metastatic lymph node, the smaller is the risk of a false negative. One
study employing a Bayesian nomogram on 213,292 women from the Surveillance, Epidemiology, and End Results (SEER) database has shown that this
possibility may be as low as 1% for pT1a or pT1b disease but is several
times higher for larger tumors [26].

Interestingly, the theoretic possibility of leaving a number of metastatic
lymph nodes behind does not seem to translate to clinically apparent axillary local recurrences to date, with most groups reporting a rate of 0.1%
to 0.3% at 3 to 5 years' follow-up [27,28]. Three randomized trials [29–31]
have attempted to determine whether this very small risk adversely affects
breast cancer survival, but, given the very low rates of reported recurrence,
the results almost certainly will be negative. Nevertheless, clinicians must
inform patients that false negatives are reported universally in the literature,
and the risk, albeit small, is real. Therefore, patients who undergo this procedure need to be enrolled in follow-up programs with routine postoperative
physical and ultrasound examinations.

Morbidity

It is well recognized that axillary node dissection carries a significant risk
for a number of sequelae, some of which may be long term. Arm

lymphedema, which is experienced in varying degrees by 15% to 30% of patients, is of most concern to women, but tenderness, paresthesia, chronic pain, and decreased range of shoulder motion can be present and can affect quality of life [32]. Although these sequelae could be accepted as a reasonable "price to pay" in an era in which patients were generally diagnosed with palpable or advanced tumors, patients now diagnosed with very small tumors in screening mammographic programs find them harder to accept. The probability of these patients harboring axillary node metastases is in the range of 10% to 15%. These patients have a good chance of being cured of cancer with minimal disfiguration, and they often do not need adjuvant systemic therapies other than hormonal.

Results from a large, prospective multicentric trial including 5327 patients have documented a very low incidence of complications after SLN biopsy performed by a wide range of surgeons in both academic and community settings [33]. Complications included wound infection and hematoma, each in 1% of cases, seroma in 7% of patients, paresthesia in 8% of patients, and a decreased upper extremity range of motion in 4% of patients.

A number of prospective studies [34–36] and three randomized trials [37–39] have consistently demonstrated less morbidity after SLN biopsy than after axillary dissection, even after a prolonged follow-up, although with time the differences tend to diminish. In the Axillary Lymphatic Mapping Against Nodal Axillary Clearance (ALMANAC) trial, which included 1031 patients from 11 centers in the United Kingdom randomly assigned to SLN biopsy (with axillary dissection only in positive cases) or standard axillary treatment (which included four-node sampling, popular in the United Kingdom, in 25% of cases), primary end points were arm morbidity and quality of life [39]. The risk of lymphedema or sensory loss was reduced by two thirds in the SLN group (absolute rates, 11% versus 31%), and the length of hospital stay, time to resumption to normal activities, and patient-recorded quality of life were significantly better in the SLN group.

Intraoperative examination

Intraoperative examination is desirable because it may identify positive cases and may avoid an unpleasant and sometimes stressful return of the patient to the operating room. It also expedites the surgical process and may allow a more timely initiation of adjuvant therapies. Intraoperative identification of metastases in the SLN allows concurrent axillary node dissection and may be a money-saving approach for the health system [40,41]. The cost effectiveness of intraoperative assessment of SLNs, especially for larger tumors, was recently evidenced by a study that applied a decision-analysis model [42].

The value of intraoperative identification of SLN metastases relies on the present belief that further dissection is warranted in most positive cases. Nevertheless, not all cases may be equivalent, and prospective, randomized trials are under way to clarify this issue [43–45]. At present, the presence of isolated tumor cells should not be considered in further treatment planning, and this information should be reserved for clinical and experimental studies. Consequently, even micrometastases are often an isolated event, and the presence of further metastases in non–SLNs is verifiable in a small minority of cases. Therefore, the pathologist's true task at the intraoperative examination of SLN is to rule out macrometastases. Intraoperative examination seems fairly reliable in this respect. In the authors' recent experience, fewer than 1 in 10 patients has currently returned to the operating room for completion lymphadenectomy. Positive findings are identified in 2 out of 10 patients, who therefore undergo concomitant axillary dissection (L. Fortunato, personal communication, 2007).

Several methods of intraoperative examination have been described. These methods include frozen section and imprint cytology [46], scrape cytology [47], immunohistochemistry staining [48,49], and an exhaustive method of serial intraoperative sectioning described by Veronesi's group [50]. The last is appealing, because the entire lymph node is step analyzed during the operation, but the human and financial resources required are not readily available in most centers. Whether intraoperative examination of the entire SLN by frozen section, even with extensive step sectioning, carries the risk of decreasing the ability to recognize occult nodal metastases because of several technical problems has not been studied and needs thorough evaluation.

Several studies have shown frozen section and imprint cytology to have relatively equivalent sensitivities [40,46,51–53]. The latter has the advantage of preserving tissue for step analysis of the lymph node, whereas at least 25% of the material may be lost during frozen section [46]. Currently, many groups prefer cytology for intraoperative examination because it is simple and inexpensive, and a recent meta-analysis of 31 studies found that it identifies more than 80% of macrometastases and 20% of micrometastases [54]. Accordingly, the sensitivity of intraoperative examination has been reported to be higher for larger tumors, because the proportion of macrometastases increases in these patients. Although in one report the sensitivity of intraoperative examination for T2 tumors was almost double that for T1a tumors, the actual benefit of intraoperative examination in avoiding a second operation in patients who have T1a tumors may be as little as 4% [55]. This finding has been confirmed by the authors' experience [40]. Although the usefulness of intraoperative examination for patients who have T2 tumors seems clear, the clinical benefit of intraoperative examination for smaller tumors may be questionable and needs to be better elucidated. It is the authors' current practice to refrain from routine intraoperative examination for T1a and T1b tumors because of the very low yield, but they do use it selectively in particular clinical situations.

Histology also can affect the false-negative rate of intraoperative examination of the SLN. The diagnosis of nodal metastases can be more problematic in lobular cancers than in ductal cancers because of their geographic distribution and their cell morphology [56]. Ductal metastases are found more frequently in the marginal sinus of the SLN. Lobular metastases are found more often within the subcapsular region or the medullary sinus. Furthermore, lymph node metastases from lobular carcinoma are more difficult to identify because of their low-grade cytomorphology, because of their tendency to have a single-cell pattern, and because individual cells can resemble lymphocytes.

Enhanced pathology

No other aspect of SLN biopsy has generated as much confusion and even controversy as the pathologic evaluation of the retrieved nodes. This situation is demonstrated by the striking differences among national and international guidelines on handling SLNs published in the literature thus far (Table 1). Furthermore, a survey by the European Working Group for Breast Screening Pathology reported that 240 pathologists replying to a questionnaire described 123 different pathology protocols [65]. Even the most commonly used method, slicing the SLN at six levels at 150-micron intervals, was used by only eight departments. Twelve percent of departments investigated only one level, and some engaged in a labor-intensive protocol resulting in more than 100 levels. Immunohistochemistry was not used by 29% of departments.

This heterogeneity in the routine work-up of the SLN has several important drawbacks. It limits the comparison of results published by different groups, and even surgical treatment strategies may be altered by discordant pathology protocols and results, as shown by recent research on this subject in four different hospitals in The Netherlands [66].

Enhanced pathology remains a strategic cornerstone for SLN evaluation. Micrometastases (< 2 mm in diameter) or isolated tumor cells (< 0.2 mm, usually diagnosed by immunohistochemistry) are diagnosed far more commonly now than in the pre-SLN era. This concept has been known since the

Table 1
National and international guidelines on handling sentinel lymph nodes

Country	Intraoperative examination	Step sections	IHC
United States/CAP [57]	TP	no	no
United States/Philadelphia [58]	TP or FS	three levels	no
European Working Group [59]	TP or FS	200 microns	no
Italy (Forza Operativa Natzionale Cancro della Mamella) [60]	FS	50 microns	yes
United Kingdom [61]	no	no	no
Germany [62]	TP or FS	500 microns	no
Austria [63]	FS	200 microns	yes
Australia [64]	—	four levels	yes

Abbreviations: CAP, College of American Pathologist; FS, frozen section; IHC, immunohistochemistry; TP, touch preparation.

beginning of the SLN experience, when the group at the John Wayne Cancer Center demonstrated a 13% increase in node-positive cases in the SLN group compared with matched historical controls staged by axillary dissection [67]. Several large studies have confirmed this finding. In a group of 2150 breast cancer patients, micrometastases and isolated tumor cells were found in 6.8%, and 4.9% of cases, respectively, after step sectioning of the sentinel node [68]. Similarly, in a large retrospective review of 1440 patients by the Rome Breast Cancer Study Group, micrometastases and isolated tumor cells were found in 7.6% and 4.5% of cases, respectively [69], confirming that enhanced pathology can diagnose "occult" nodal disease in more than 1 in 10 patients.

Few comparisons have been made of the different methods of step sectioning SLN in patients who have breast cancer. In one study of 246 patients, multiple sections every 50 to 100 microns detected more micrometastases than sections at a 250-micron interval [70]. In another study in which SLN were analyzed at five different levels, the addition of the last two levels increased the detection rate by 4% and 2%, respectively [71]. Ten-level step sectioning of SLN at 40-micron intervals has been reported to confer little advantage (3%) after the first two sections [72]. Another report found no advantage to six versus three levels of investigation [73].

The authors studied 891 comparable patients at two different hospitals participating in the Rome Breast Cancer Study Group and analyzed the yield of two different protocols. One protocol entailed SLN sectioning at three levels at 100-micron intervals. The other protocol called for 15 levels at 50-micron intervals. Immunohistochemistry was used in all three levels at one center and in five levels at the other. No statistically significant difference could be detected in each T category in the ability of methods to detect either micrometastases or isolated tumor cells (S. Drago, personal communication, 2007). The costs of the "labor-intensive" and "limited" protocol have been estimated at 65 and 35 euros per SLN, respectively, raising questions about whether an exhaustive pathologic evaluation of the SLN is necessary or cost effective.

The authors have also retrospectively studied 448 consecutive breast cancer patients whose SLNs were analyzed with step sectioning at three levels. Among them, the retrieved material of 151 patients initially defined as node negative has been further step sectioned at two additional levels from the paraffin-embedded specimens. Additional micrometastases and isolated tumor cells were diagnosed in 0.7% and in 0.9% of cases, respectively, but no additional macrometastases were found (L. Fortunato, personal communication, 2007). Therefore, although it is clear that "the more you cut, the more you get," it seems reasonably evident that after a certain limit, the additional yield of serial sections of the SLN and the extensive use of immunohistochemistry is very small, particularly in certain situations. With the rapidly expanding knowledge and experience in this field, the need to perform 10 or 15 sections with immunostaining of the SLN for a 5-mm low-grade tumor can be questioned. Perhaps the indications for this extensive search should be more restricted.

The authors' group recently has proposed a simple, practical standardized protocol, with slicing at three levels at 100-micron intervals and double staining with both hematoxylin and eosin (H&E) and immunohistochemistry (MNF 116) (Fig. 2) [74]. This protocol has allowed the group's pathologists to increase the diagnosis of additional nodal disease by nearly two thirds compared with standard, single-section analysis of the lymph nodes

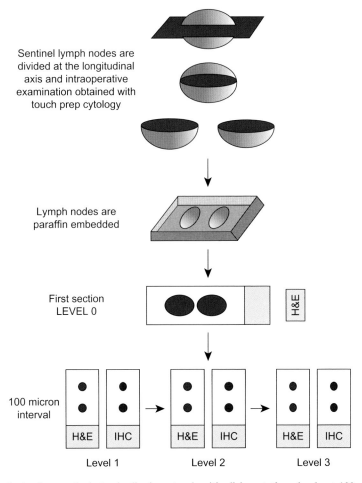

Fig. 2. A simple, practical standardized protocol, with slicing at three levels at 100-micron intervals and double staining with both hematoxylin-eosin and immunohistochemistry, that has allowed the pathologists in the authors' group to diagnose additional nodal disease with an increment of nearly two thirds compared with standard, single-section analysis of the lymph nodes stained with hematoxylin-eosin. (*Adapted from* Fortunato L, Amini M, Costarelli L, et al. A standardized sentinel lymph node enhanced pathology protocol (SEPP) in patients with breast cancer. J Surg Oncol 2007;96(6):471; with permission.)

stained with H&E. The majority of this additional yield, however, has been limited to the recognition of isolated tumor cells; micrometastases have been noted in approximately one third of these cases.

Predicting involvement of non–sentinel lymph nodes

The current standard of care after a positive SLN biopsy remains a completion axillary lymph node dissection. Reasons used to justify axillary node dissection under these circumstances include achieving locoregional control, improved survival, and staging purposes (the number of pathologically involved nodes is the most powerful predictor of prognosis) [75–77]. As evidenced in a recent overview of 69 studies [21], however, metastases are present in "non-sentinel" nodes in approximately 50% of such cases. With the practice of universally performing a complete node clearance in this setting, many patients undergo an unnecessary operation. Confusion is compounded, because a recent meta-analysis of 25 studies disclosed that the identification of even "low-volume" SLN metastases (eg, micrometastases or isolated tumor cells) is associated with a 10% to 15% risk of non-SLN metastases [78].

Several clinicopathologic features have been associated with a patent's likelihood of harboring additional axillary disease after a positive SLN biopsy. Individual reports have reached different conclusions about utility of some of these factors, and none of them, when used alone, is sufficiently powerful to identify patients at very low risk of additional disease who could be spared an additional operation [79]. A few factors play a major role (eg, the size of primary tumor, the size of SLN metastases, the number or proportion of positive SLNs, and lymphovascular invasion) [25,78,80–83], and it is relatively easy to identify a small subgroup of patients who have all these favorable characteristics (ie, very small tumors and only one micrometastasis in the SLN) who could be managed with observation. For other patients, these factors need to be integrated in a more complex scoring system that can provide more useful information. Of course, any scoring system is an arbitrary tool, because the concept of "risk" may vary from patient to patient. Therefore, the purpose of such system is to provide the basis for a thorough discussion between the patient and the surgeon regarding treatment options and the risks and benefits of the procedure.

Four scoring systems have been described so far in the literature. In three of them, developed at MD Anderson Cancer Center [84], at the Hopital Tenon in Paris [85], and at the University of Louisville [81], three to five independent risk factors were identified and assigned a point value resulting in a score.

The Memorial Sloan Kettering Cancer Center group, instead, has developed a nomogram that includes eight characteristics (primary tumor diameter, grade, lymphovascular invasion, hormone receptor status, multifocality, number of positive and retrieved SLNs, method of detection, and use of frozen section) with a calculation of the percentage of risk [80]. The nomogram is available on line at www.mskcc.org and has been validated by six different groups in independent data sets including 2808 patients overall [86]. Whether the nomogram is applicable in particular situations (eg, in patients who have micrometastases in the SLN) has been questioned [86]. The use of this nomogram has been associated with a declining rate of completion axillary dissection after a positive SLN biopsy [87]. In one report, patients selected for axillary conservation despite a positive SLN biopsy were likely to be older patients, patients who had breast-conservation surgery, or patients who had more favorable tumors. In these patients the median calculated risk of axillary residual disease was below 10%, and the rate of axillary recurrence was 2% at 30 months [87].

It is unfortunate that a clinical trial (American College of Surgeons Oncology Group [ACOSOG] Z-10011) designed to answer the specific question of the value of axillary node dissection in cases of positive SLN biopsy has been closed prematurely because of slow accrual. Therefore this question remains open. The randomized European Organization for the Research and Treatment of Cancer trial 10981-22023, the After Mapping of the Axilla: Radiotherapy or Surgery (AMAROS) trial, is underway to clarify whether axillary radiotherapy, as used for treatment of the breast parenchyma to clear potential foci of multicentric disease, may have a role in these cases. This trial involves 2500 patients and compares axillary dissection and radiotherapy for locoregional control after a positive SLN biopsy [88].

Once the decision is made to treat the axilla, do all patients who have SLN involvement need the same operation? This issue is particularly interesting, because only a small percentage of such patients have N2 disease, and therefore a more limited dissection may be indicated, particularly when SLN involvement is limited. This possibility has been proposed by a recent review of 467 patients from the University of Kentucky. All patients who had SLN metastases 5 mm or smaller had three or fewer positive nodes, and 95% of cases were SLN positive only [89]. Extracapsular extension in the SLN, albeit rare, seems to be a particularly sensitive discriminating tool in this regard, because it is present in 41% of patients who have N2 or N3 disease but in only 16% of patients who have N1a disease. Therefore, patients who have small SLN metastases may be selected for a more limited completion dissection (eg, restricted to level one) to reduce the morbidity of the operation.

Prognostic significance of micrometastases

The incidence of micrometastases in the SLN is increasing rapidly (17% per annum since 1997) as reported by a recent analysis of the SEER database of 175,000 patients between 1990 and 2002 [90]. This increase probably results from a combination of factors, including the widespread use of mammographic screening and the resulting diagnosis of smaller tumors and the implementation of SLN biopsy with recognition of minimal node involvement by step sectioning.

The prognostic significance of such micrometastases is unknown at present. In the most important retrospective study, conducted by the International (Ludwig) Breast Cancer Study Group, 9% of 921 patients who had negative axillary lymph nodes on routine H&E single-section analysis were found to be node positive on serial sectioning [91]. In some, but not in all, groups these women had a significantly poorer 5-year disease-free and overall survival. Recent data seem to confirm the hypothesis that micrometastases are indeed a marker of poorer prognosis. In a review of the published literature in 1997, Dowlatshahi [92] analyzed all large and long-term studies and confirmed a statistically significant decrement in survival associated with the presence of axillary node micrometastases. The group at Memorial Sloan Kettering Cancer Center has used serial sections and immunohistochemistry to re-evaluate all axillary lymph nodes from 373 patients operated in the 1970s who were deemed to be node negative by routine histopathology [93]. The presence of any detectable micrometastatic disease was associated with worse disease-free and overall survival. In a review of 1959 cases treated at the European Institute of Oncology from 1997 to 2000, Colleoni and colleagues [94] have found that minimal involvement (micrometastases or isolated tumor cells) of a single lymph node correlated with decreased disease-free survival and doubled the risk of distant metastases.

Despite these findings, the clinical significance of micrometastases is not yet well understood. Several multicenter randomized trials, such as the International Breast Cancer Study Group 23-01 [95], the National Surgical Adjuvant Breast and Bowel Project B32 [30], and the ACOSOG Z0010 [96], are designed to study this issue, and their results will contribute to a better understanding.

The role of sentinel lymph node biopsy in special circumstances

Ductal carcinoma in situ

Management of ductal carcinoma in situ (DCIS) is clinically relevant, because its incidence is increasing and today it comprises 20% to 25% of newly diagnosed cases of breast cancer. Traditionally, axillary node metastases were identified by conventional histology in fewer than 2% of patients whose surgical specimen was interpreted as containing DCIS only, probably because the presence of invasive cancer was unrecognized [97]. Enhanced pathology of the SLN has increased the yield of positive SLN findings in case of DCIS in a recent review of 2196 cases [98], although in most cases this increment involved micrometastases or isolated tumor cells found at immunohistochemistry. Studies of patients who had "pure" DCIS undergoing SLN biopsy have confirmed an extremely low rate of axillary node involvement [99,100]. Unfortunately, these cases are relatively difficult to identify, because microinvasion can be missed even with an extensive histologic search and immunostaining and because a preoperative diagnosis is not always feasible. Therefore, at present the role of SLN biopsy under these circumstances is limited to those high-risk lesions, including palpable disease, extensive disease requiring mastectomy, or the presence of necrosis or high tumor grade, because in these cases the upstaging of DCIS to invasive cancer is more frequent [101]. This group, representing up to 22% of all patients who have DCIS, has been associated with a 9% incidence of SLN involvement in a multicentric review of 470 cases [102]. In such cases, SLN biopsy may a helpful tool for identifying patients who have microinvasion (and who may have a worse prognosis), for whom a different treatment protocol might be more appropriate.

In DCIS with diagnosed microinvasion, the incidence of axillary metastases has been reported to range from 7% to 10% in small series [103–108]. In the experience of the Rome Breast Cancer Study Group, there was a trend toward a higher incidence of nodal SLN metastases in these "microinvasive" tumors than in the group with pT1a disease [109]. SLN biopsy may represent an optimal compromise in this scenario, because it recognizes the need to minimize surgery and the desire to stage patients appropriately.

Furthermore, SLN biopsy may be selected after DCIS diagnosis by microbiopsy to avoid a second operation in case either microinvasion or an infiltrating cancer is diagnosed at final histology.

It is not yet clear whether a completion axillary node dissection should be performed or additional systemic therapy should be considered when SLN involvement is found after diagnosis of DCIS. In one report only 4% of such patients were found to have additional disease by routine H&E analysis of the dissected lymph nodes [102]. A review of 21 series collected 29 such patients undergoing axillary dissection after a positive SLN finding, and no patient was diagnosed with additional metastases [98].

Tumor diameter

The accuracy of SLN biopsy is not affected by the type of diagnostic biopsy, by the interval between initial biopsy and definitive surgery, by the location of the primary tumor, or by the type of definitive surgery (quadrantectomy or mastectomy). Initially, SLN biopsy was limited to patients who had small, unicentric cancers because clinicians feared that larger tumors might obstruct or alter lymphatic drainage, leading to false-negative results. Node involvement is present in 50% of T2 cancers, however, and even in T3 tumors axillary lymph nodes are negative in approximately 20% of cases [110]. Therefore, SLN biopsy in these situations may spare an unnecessary lymphadenectomy in a substantial number of cases.

Although some reports still express caution regarding the higher incidence of false-negative findings for T2 tumors [111], many studies have demonstrated that the accuracy of SLN biopsy in patients who have T2 or T3 breast tumors is comparable to that in patients who have smaller tumors (Table 2).

Table 2
Sentinel lymph nodes for large breast cancers

Authors	Year	N	SLN Identification rate (%)	Positive SLN (%)	False-negative rate (%)
Bedrosian et al [112]	2000	103	103/103 (100)	61/103 (59)	1/62 (2)
Olson et al [113]	2000	59	53/59 (91)	35/53 (66)	1/36 (3)
Chung et al [114]	2001	41	41/41 (100)	30/41 (73)	1/31 (3)
Wong et al [110]	2001	589	551/589 (93)	282/551 (51)	28/310 (9)
Lelievre et al [115]	2006	152	148/152 (97)	102/152 (67)	4/106 (4)
Schule et al [116]	2007	109	103/109 (94)	67/103 (65)	9/76 (12)
TOTAL	—	1015	968/1015 (95)	562/968 (58)	41/603 (7)

Abbreviation: SLN, sentinel lymph node.

Therefore, tumor size no longer is a contraindication to SLN biopsy in patients who have a clinically negative axilla.

Sentinel lymph node biopsy for multicentric disease

Multicentric breast cancer has been considered a contraindication for SLN biopsy in the past. Because this entity may occur in up to 10% of cases, this issue is quite important. There is now ample evidence from single-center reports and from one multi-institutional validation study in Europe that SLN biopsy can be applied in these cases with good results, because the SLN represents the whole breast, regardless of tumor location in the parenchyma (Table 3).

In the largest report to date, from the Austrian Sentinel Node Study Group, a retrospective comparison between 142 patients who had multicentric cancers and 3216 patients who had unicentric cancers showed no difference in detection and false-negative rates [122]. Therefore, the authors believe that SLN should be considered standard of care for these tumors.

Table 3
Sentinel lymph node biopsy for multicentric or multifocal disease

Author	Year	N	SLN identification rate (%)	Percent accuracy	Positive SLN (%)	False-negative rate (%)
Schrenk et al [117]	2001	19	19/19 (100)	100	10/19 (53)	0/10
Fernandez et al [118]	2002	53	52/53 (98)	100	18/52 (35)	0/18
Kumar et al [119]	2003	59	55/59 (93)	100	19/55 (34)	0/19
Tousimis et al [120]	2003	70	67/70 (96)	96	38/67 (54)	3/41 (8)
Goyal et al [121]	2004	75	71/75 (95)	96	31/71 (44)	3/34 9
Knauer et al [122]	2006	150	130/150 (91)	97	79/130 (61)	3/82 (4)
Ferrari et al [123]	2006	31	31/31 (100)	97	13/31 (42)	1/14 (8)
Gentilini et al [124]	2006	42	42/42 (100)	100	21/42 (50)	NR
D'Eredita et al [125]	2007	30	30/30 (100)	94	16/30 (53)	1/19 (6)
TOTAL	—	529	497/529 (94)	—	245/497 (49)	11/237 (5)

Abbreviations: NR, not reported; SLN, sentinel lymph nodes.

Both multiple Technitium-99 injections and a single intradermal injection over the largest lesion have been described. However, a single periareolar injection of the tracer has been proposed as a means to simplify this technical aspect, and there is evidence that this technique leads to the identification of a single, representative SLN [123].

Neoadjuvant chemotherapy

An area of particular interest is the use of SLN biopsy in patients undergoing neoadjuvant chemotherapy, because the number of patients choosing this option is increasing. There are several studies on this subject, most with a small number of patients, including some patients who had clinically positive axillae before treatment. This practice has been criticized because of wide variation in reported false-negative cases, ranging from 0% to 25% (Table 4).

Table 4
Sentinel lymph node biopsy after neoadjuvant chemotherapy

Author	Year	N	Tumor Diameter in cm	Identification rate (%)	Positive SLN (%)	False-negative rate (%)
Breslin et al [126]	2000	51	5	43/51 (84)	22/43 (51)	3/22 (13)
Tafra et al [127]	2001	29	—	27/29 (93)	15/29 (52)	0
Fernandez et al [128]	2001	40	—	34/40 (85)	16/34 (47)	4/18 (22)
Julian et al [129]	2002	34	<4	31/34 (91)	12/31 (39)	0
Stearns et al [130]	2002	34	>5	29/34 (85)	13/29 (45)	3/13 (23)
Brady et al [131]	2002	14	—	13/14 (93)	10/13 (77)	0
Schwartz et al [132]	2003	21	>3	21/21 (100)	11/21 (53)	1/11 (9)
Piato et al [133]	2003	42	<5	41/42 (98)	25/41 (61)	3/25 (12)
Reitsamer et al [134]	2003	30	4	26/30 (87)	14/26 (54)	1/15 (7)
Kang et al [135]	2004	54	>3	39/54 (72)	27/39 (69)	3/27 (11)
Lang et al [136]	2004	53	—	50/53 (94)	23/50 (43)	1/23 (4)
Shimazu et al [137]	2004	47	—	44/47 (94)	29/44 (67)	4/33 (12)
Balch et al [138]	2004	32	—	31/32 (97)	18/31 (58)	1/19 (5)
Aihara et al [139]	2004	20	—	17/20 (85)	12/17 (71)	1/12 (8)
Mamounas et al [140]	2005	428	—	343/428 (85)	125/343 (36)	15/125 (12)
Tausch et al [141]	2006	167	3	144/167 (85)	70/144 (48)	6/70 (8)
Shen et al [142]	2007	69	4	64/69 (93)	31/64 (48)	10/40 (25)
Newman et al [143]	2007	54	3	53/54 (98)	36/53 (68)	3/39 (8)
Kinoshita [144]	2007	104	5	97/104 (93)	36/97 (35)	4/40 (10)
TOTAL	—	1323	—	1147/1323 (87)	545/1147 (47)	63/516 (12)

Abbreviation: SLN, sentinel lymph node.

Fundamental concerns regarding the feasibility and accuracy of SLN biopsy in this context are related to the possible alterations of intramammary lymphatic patterns after chemotherapy and to the possibility that the effect of chemotherapy on axillary metastases is not necessarily uniform or predictable. A recent meta-analysis of 21 studies has reached different conclusions, however [145], and the authors' review of 1323 patients reported so far in the literature shows an identification rate of 87% and a false-negative rate of 12% (see Table 4). Therefore, although larger multicenter studies would be necessary to reach definitive conclusions, SLN may be feasible in this clinical scenario if one is willing to accept higher non-identification and false-negative rates.

An alternative approach, preferred by the authors' group, is to consider SLN biopsy before the beginning of neoadjuvant chemotherapy. This approach has several advantages: staging is secured before any eventual downstaging caused by systemic therapy; comparison between groups consequently becomes more meaningful, particularly if we need to compare treatments; and a negative result allows a simple quadrantectomy/mastectomy to be performed at the end of the systemic therapy. Exact knowledge of the SLN status may be particularly important if an immediate breast reconstruction is planned, because diagnosis of micrometastases is almost certainly deferred, but the option of re-accessing the axilla after breast reconstruction may be problematic and unwarranted.

With an initially positive SLN biopsy, patients traditionally have been considered for delayed lymph node dissection at the time of definitive breast surgery. The group at the University of Michigan has described the results of a repeated SLN biopsy after chemotherapy in 54 such patients [143]. They reported a false-negative rate of 8%. The strategy of a repeat SLN biopsy has the potential to spare an additional axillary clearance in about one third of such cases.

Repeat sentinel lymph node biopsy for recurrent breast cancer

Because approximately 10% of breast cancer patients are expected to experience an ipsilateral recurrence 10 to 15 years after their initial treatment [146], their management is a very relevant issue. Although patients who have ipsilateral recurrence of breast cancer are at increased risk of systemic relapse, their prognosis is not uniformly bad, and approximately two thirds of patients are alive at 5 years [147]. Until recently, these patients were not candidates for any additional axillary re-evaluation. A few recent studies, however, have suggested that a repeat SLN can be offered after a previous SLN biopsy, or even after an axillary node dissection, because this approach can help stratify the risk of systemic disease, assist in decisions regarding adjuvant therapies, and alter clinical management in up to one third of cases [148]. Furthermore, many patients who have DCIS diagnosed initially by a core biopsy are evaluated initially with SLN biopsy. Some of these cases present later with an invasive recurrence; a second SLN evaluation is appealing in such clinical situations to spare an axillary dissection.

Data presented in Table 5 seem to indicate that, in case of recurrent breast cancer, a repeat SLN biopsy is significantly more successful after a previous SLN biopsy than after a previous axillary node dissection. In the latter scenario, a SLN can be identified in only half the cases. An aberrant pattern of flow directed to the parasternal, interpectoral, or supraclavicular region or to the contralateral axilla is fairly common (occurring in 24% of cases in the authors' review), particularly after a previous axillary node dissection. Regional nodal metastases are not common in these circumstances: in the authors' review of the literature, they were identified in approximately 17% of cases.

Preoperative identification of node involvement by ultrasound

By now there should be little doubt that SLN is the preferred staging procedure for virtually all patients who have breast cancer, with rare exceptions. Many patients who have clinically nonpalpable lymph nodes may indeed harbor macrometastases, however. Preoperative axillary ultrasound may identify these cases and alter management strategy, because they clearly

Table 5
Sentinel lymph node biopsy for recurrent breast cancer

Author	Year	N	Success after previous SLND (%)	Success after previous ALND (%)	Total success rate (%)	Extra-axillary localization of SLN (%)	Positive SLN (%)
Sood et al [149]	2004	4	—	4/4	4/4 (100)	2/4	0/4
Agarwal et al [150]	2005	2	—	2/2	2/2 (100)	2/2	1/2 (50)
Newman et al [151]	2006	8	0/1	7/7	7/8 (87)	10/10	0/7
Roumen et al [148]	2006	12	2/2	8/10	10/12 (83)	7/12	4/10 (40)
Taback et al [152]	2006	15	5/6	6/9	11/15 (73)	8/15	3/11 (27)
Intra et al [153]	2007	65	65/65	—	63/65 (97)	5/63	7/63 (11)
Port et al [154]	2007	117	40/54	24/63	64/117 (55)	2/64	10/64 (64)
Barone et al [155]	2007	19	6/7	0/12	16/19 (84)	NS	2/16 (12)
Axelsson et al [156]	2007	46	—	22/46	22/46 (45)	13/46	7/22 (32)
TOTAL	—	288	118/135 (87)	73/153 (54)	199/288 (69)	51/216 (24)	34/199 (17)

Abbreviations: ALND, axillary lymph node dissection; NS, not specified; SLN, sentinel lymph node; SLND, sentinel lymph node dissection.

would not benefit from SLN biopsy. A careful study of the hilum and cortical regions may give rise to a sonographic pattern of doubtful or suspicious nodal status, a finding that may be present in 23% of cases [157]. Ultrasound-guided biopsy of nonpalpable axillary nodes was proposed a decade ago [158], and it may have a major clinical impact by identifying more than 40% of patients who have axillary node metastases [157]. This approach has been reported to predict the final node pathology in up to 92% of patients [157], but the actual benefit may vary according to the T status of the patient, because ultrasound plus fine-needle aspiration may detect lymph node metastases preoperatively in 6% of patients who have T1 disease, 20% to 25% of patients who have T2 disease, and in 50% to 70% of patients who have T3 disease [159,160]. Therefore, this method can be cost effective, particularly for tumors larger than 2 cm in diameter, because these patients may undergo a one-stage procedure and be prepared to undergo concomitant axillary node dissection at the time of quadrantectomy or may be counseled to undergo neoadjuvant therapies. After adoption of this strategy, the need of SLN biopsy may decrease by 14% to 20%, as reported by two studies from The Netherlands [161,162].

Internal mammary sentinel lymph node biopsy

Although prospective, randomized trials have not demonstrated a therapeutic benefit of removing internal mammary lymph nodes in patients who have breast cancer [163], it is well known that involvement of this chain is associated with worse prognosis. Furthermore, medial and inferior tumors have been reported to drain more commonly to internal mammary lymph nodes [164], although this drainage has not been taken in consideration routinely in the last decades. Indeed, the internal mammary lymph nodes are an important pathway, draining lymphatics from the deep breast lobules along the pectoral fascia and intercostal muscles [165].

Several studied have shown that SLN biopsy of the internal mammary lymph nodes is feasible, although it requires mapping through a deep intraparenchymal or peritumoral injection, because the identification of internal mammary lymph nodes is almost impossible after an intradermal injection [166,167]. The procedure more commonly involves a direct exposure of the second or third intercostal space and division of the intercostal muscle fibers and is associated with the rare possibility of breach of the pleural cavity [168]. This possibility has raised concerns regarding the acceptability of this procedure if there is no definitive demonstration of a survival benefit.

Studies have shown that internal mammary SLNs can be identified in 8% to 17% of patients who have breast cancer and, among them, positive findings at final pathology are reported in 15% of these patients [166,168–170]. Therefore, even though the identification of internal mammary lymph nodes may affect the management of an individual patient, and reportedly could benefit 7% to 15% of patients in whom a positive histologic finding was identified in the internal mammary lymph nodes, a change in management in the whole group is unlikely. In these cases adjuvant radiotherapy or systemic therapy may be offered, and clinical trials would be needed to determine whether such treatment improves survival.

Summary

Breast cancer today is at the forefront of basic research applied to the clinical field, engaging each of the many clinical practitioners involved in the multidisciplinary team working with patients who have breast cancer. If diagnosed early, breast cancer is one of the most curable solid cancers.

SLN biopsy decreases morbidity, allows detailed pathologic analysis, reveals "occult" disease, and enables more precise staging. Several issues remain to be clarified, however. Among them, a better understanding of how to evaluate the retrieved node seems more urgent.

The authors hope that next time the *Surgical Oncology Clinics of North America* devotes an article to this subject it will be possible to show further improvements and to declare that at least some subgroups of patients who have breast cancer can always be cured. This goal would be a tribute to all women around the world who participate in randomized trials or clinical studies, and contribute in such a compassionate way to the understanding of this disease.

References

[1] Veronesi U, Cascinelli N, Mariani L, et al. Twenty-year follow-up of a randomized study comparing breast-conserving surgery with radical mastectomy for early breast cancer. N Engl J Med 2002;347:1227–32.

[2] Harris JR, Lippman ME, Veronesi U, et al. Breast cancer. N Engl J Med 1992;327:473–80.

[3] Fisher B, Bauer M, Wickerham DL, et al. Relation of number of positive axillary nodes to the prognosis of patients with primary breast cancer: an NSABP update. Cancer 1983;52: 1551–7.

[4] Gould EA, Winship T, Philbin PH, et al. Observations on a "sentinel node" in cancer of the parotid. Cancer 1960;13:77–8.

[5] Cabanas RM. An approach for the treatment of penile carcinoma. Cancer 1997;39: 456–66.

[6] Morton DL, Wen DR, Wong JH, et al. Technical details of intraoperative lymphatic mapping for early stage melanoma. Arch Surg 1992;127:392–9.

[7] Giuliano AE, Kirgan DM, Guenther JM, et al. Lymphatic mapping and sentinel lymphadenectomy for breast cancer. Ann Surg 1994;220:391–8.

[8] Albertini JJ, Lyman GH, Cox C, et al. Lymphatic mapping and sentinel node biopsy in the patient with breast cancer. JAMA 1996;276:1818–22.

[9] Tafra L. The learning curve and sentinel node biopsy. Am J Surg 2001;182:347–50.

[10] Cox CE, Salud CJ, Cantor A, et al. Learning curves for breast cancer sentinel lymph node mapping based on surgical volume analysis. J Am Coll Surg 2001;192:9–16.

[11] Chagpar AB, Martin RC, Scoggins CR, et al. Factors predicting failure to identify a sentinel lymph node in breast cancer. Surgery 2005;138:56–63.

[12] Kern KA. Lymphoscintigraphic anatomy of sentinel lymphatic channels after subareolar injection of technetium 99 sulfur colloid. J Am Coll Surg 2001;193:601–8.

[13] Nathanson SD, Wachna DL, Gilman D, et al. Pathways of lymphatic drainage from the breast. Ann Surg Oncol 2001;8:837–43.

[14] Povoski SP, Olsen JO, Young DC, et al. Prospective randomized clinical trial comparing intradermal, intraparenchymal, and subareolar injection routes for sentinel lymph node mapping and biopsy in breast cancer. Ann Surg Oncol 2006;13:1412–21.

[15] Rodier JF, Velten M, Wilt M, et al. Prospective multicentric randomized study comparing periareolar and peritumoral injection of radiotracer and blue dye for the detection of sentinel lymph node in breast sparing procedure: FRANSENODE trial. J Clin Oncol 2007;25:3664–9.

[16] Chagpar A, Martin RC, Chao C, et al. Validation of subareolar and periareolar injection techniques for breast sentinel lymph node biopsy. Arch Surg 2004;139:614–20.

[17] Chagpar AB, Carlson DJ, Laidley AL, et al. Factors influencing the number of sentinel lymph nodes identified in patients with breast cancer. Am J Surg 2007;194:860–4.

[18] McMasters KM, Wong SL, Chao C, et al. Defining the optimal surgeon experience for breast cancer sentinel lymph node (SLN) biopsy. A model for implementation of new surgical technique. Ann Surg 2001;234:292–300.

[19] Nathanson SD, Grogan JK, DeBruyn D, et al. Breast cancer lymph node identification rates: influence of radiocolloid mapping, case volume, and the place of the procedure. Ann Surg Oncol 2007;14:1629–37.

[20] Derossis AM, Fey J, Young H, et al. A trend analysis of the relative value of the blue dye and isotope localization in 2000 consecutive cases of sentinel node biopsy for breast cancer. J Am Coll Surg 2001;193:473–8.

[21] Kim T, Giuliano AE, Lyman GH. Lymphatic mapping and sentinel lymph node biopsy in early-stage breast carcinoma. Cancer 2006;106:4–16.

[22] Krag DN, Anderson SJ, Julian TB, et al. Technical outcomes of sentinel-lymph-node resection and conventional axillary-lymph-node dissection in patients with clinically node-negative breast cancer: results from the NSABP B-32 randomised phase III trial. Lancet Oncol 2007;8:881–8.

[23] Tafra L, Lannin DR, Swanson MS, et al. Multicenter trial of sentinel lymph node biopsy for breast cancer using both technetium sulfur colloid and isosulfan blue. Ann Surg 2001; 233:51–9.

[24] Cody HS, Hill ADK, Tran KN, et al. Credentialing for breast lymphatic mapping: how many cases are enough? Ann Surg 1999;229:723–8.

[25] Veronesi U, Paganelli G, Viale G, et al. Sentinel lymph-node biopsy as a staging procedure in breast cancer: update of a randomised controlled study. Lancet Oncol 2006;7: 983–90.

[26] Barone JE, Tucker JB, Perez JM, et al. Evidence-based medicine applied to sentinel lymph node biopsy in patients with breast cancer. Am Surg 2005;71:66–70.

[27] Naik AM, Fey J, Gemignani M, et al. The risk of axillary relapse after sentinel lymph node biopsy for breast cancer is comparable with that of axillary lymph node dissection: a follow-up study of 4008 procedures. Ann Surg 2004;240:462–8.

[28] Veronesi U, Galimberti V, Mariani L, et al. Sentinel node biopsy in breast cancer: early results in 953 patients with negative sentinel node biopsy and no axillary dissection. Eur J Cancer 2005;41:231–7.

[29] Veronesi U, Paganelli G, Viale G. A randomized comparison of sentinel-node biopsy with routine axillary dissection in breast cancer. N Engl J Med 2003;349:546–53.

[30] Krag DN, Julian TB, Harlow SP, et al. NSABP-32: phase III randomized trial comparing axillary resection with sentinel lymph node dissection. A description of the trial. Ann Surg Oncol 2004;11(Suppl 3):208S–10S.

[31] Clarke D, Khonji NI, Mansel RE. Sentinel node biopsy in breast cancer: ALMANAC trial. World J Surg 2001;25:819–22.

[32] Sakorafas GH, Perso G, Cataliotti L, et al. Lymphedema following axillary lymph node dissection for breast cancer. Surg Oncol 2006;15:153–65.

[33] Wilke LG, McCall LM, Posther KE, et al. Surgical complications associated with sentinel lymph node biopsy: results from a prospective international cooperative group trial. Ann Surg Oncol 2006;13:491–500.

[34] Burak WE, Hollenbeck ST, Zervos EE, et al. Sentinel lymph node biopsy results in less post-operatibe morbidity compared with axillary lymph node dissection for breast cancer. Am J Surg 2002;183:23–7.

[35] Schulze T, Markwardt J, Schlag P, et al. Long-term morbidity of patients with early breast cancer after sentinel lymph node biopsy compared to axillary lymph node dissection. J Surg Oncol 2006;93:109–19.

[36] Baron RH, Fey JV, Borgen PI, et al. Eighteen sensation after breast cancer surgery: a 5-year comparison of sentinel lymph node biopsy and axillary lymph node dissection. Ann Surg Oncol 2007;14:1653–61.

[37] Del Bianco P, Zavagno G, Burelli P, et al. Morbidity comparison of sentinel lymph node biopsy versus conventional axillary node dissection for breast cancer patients: results of the sentinella-GIVOM Italian randomised clinical trial. EJSO 2007; [Epub ahead of print].

[38] Purushotam AD, Upponi S, Klevesath MB, et al. Morbidity after sentinel lymph node biopsy in primary breast cancer. Results from a randomized controlled trial. J Clin Oncol 2005;23:4312–21.

[39] Fleissig A, Fallowfield LJ, Langridge CI, et al. Post-operative arm morbidity and quality of life. Results of the ALMANAC randomized trial comparing sentinel node biopsy with standard axillary treatment in the management of patients with early breast cancer. Breast Cancer Res Treat 2006;95:279–93.

[40] Fortunato L, Amini M, Farina M, et al. Intraoperative examination of sentinel nodes in breast cancer: Is the glass half full or half empty? Ann Surg Oncol 2004;11:1005–10.

[41] Attebery ML, Sielig BA, Ciocca R, et al. Touch prep cytology as a preferred approach for sentinel lymph nodes in breast cancer. Breast J 2007;13:106–7.

[42] Jeruss JS, Hunt KK, Xing Y, et al. Is intraoperative touch imprint cytology of sentinel lymph nodes in patients with breast cancer cost effective? Cancer 2006;107:2328–36.

[43] Wilke LG, Giuliano A. Sentinel lymph node biopsy in patients with early stage breast cancer: status of the National Clinical Trials. Surg Clin North Am 2003;83:901–10.

[44] Grube BJ, Giuliano AE. Observation of the breast cancer patient with a tumor-positive sentinel node: implications of the ACOSOG Z0011 trial. Semin Surg Oncol 2001;20:230–7.

[45] Harlow SP, Krag DN. Sentinel lymph node—why study it: implications of the B-32 study. Semin Surg Oncol 2001;20:224–9.

[46] van Diest PJ, Torrenga H, Borgstein PJ, et al. Reliability of intraoperative frozen section and imprint cytological investigation of sentinel lymph nodes in breast cancer. Histopathology 1999;35:14–8.

[47] Smidt ML, Besseling R, Wauters CA, et al. Intraoperative scrape cytology of the sentinel lymph node in patients with breast cancer. Br J Surg 2002;89:1290–3.

[48] Salem AA, Douglas-Jones AG, Sweetland HM, et al. Intraoperative evaluation of axillary sentinel lymph nodes using touch imprint cytology and immunohistochemistry: a protocol of rapid immunostaining of touch imprints. EJSO 2003;29:25–8.

[49] Nahrig JM, Richter T, Kuhn W, et al. Intraoperative examination of sentinel lymph nodes by ultrarapid immunohistochemistry. Breast J 2003;9:277–81.

[50] Veronesi U, Zurrida S, Mazzarol G, et al. Extensive frozen section examination of axillary sentinel nodes to determine selective axillary dissection. World J Surg 2001;25:806–8.

[51] Motomura K, Inaji H, Komoike Y, et al. Intraoperative sentinel lymph node examination by imprint cytology and frozen sectioning during breast surgery. Br J Surg 2000;87:597–601.

[52] Menes TS, Tatter PI, Mizrachi H, et al. Touch preparation or frozen section of sentinel lymph node metastases from breast cancer. Ann Surg Oncol 2003;10:1166–70.

[53] Aihara T, Munakata S, Morino H, et al. Comparison of frozen section and touch imprint cytology for evaluation of sentinel lymph node metastasis in breast cancer. Ann Surg Oncol 2004;11:747–50.

[54] Tew K, Irwig L, Matthews A, et al. Meta-analysis of sentinel node imprint cytology in breast cancer. Br J Surg 2005;92:1068–80.

[55] Weiser MR, Montgomery LL, Susnik B, et al. Is routine intraoperative frozen-section examination of sentinel lymph nodes in breast cancer worthwhile? Ann Surg Oncol 2000; 45:185–90.

[56] Shiver SA, Creager AJ, Geisinger K, et al. Intraoperative analysis of sentinel lymph nodes by imprint cytology for cancer of the breast. Am J Surg 2002;184:424–7.

[57] Fitzgibbons PL, Connolly JL, Page DL. Updated protocol for the examination of specimens from patients with carcinomas of the breast. Cancer Committee. Arch Pathol Lab Med 2000;12:1027–33.

[58] Schwartz GF, Giuliano AE, Veronesi U. Consensus Conference Committee. Proceedings of the Consensus Conference on the Role of Sentinel Lymph Node Biopsy in Carcinoma of the Breast April 19-22, 2001, Philadelphia, Pennsylvania. Hum Pathol 2002; 33:579–89.

[59] Perry N, Broeders M, de Wolf C, et al. European guidelines for quality assurance in breast cancer screening and diagnosis. 4th edition. Luxembourg (Luxembourg): European Communities; 2006.

[60] Forza Operativa Nazionale Cancro della Mammella (FONCAM). Linee guida sul linfonodo sentinella nel cancro della mammella. Available at: http://www.societaitalianasenologia.it/pdf%20nuovo/anatomia%20patologica.pdf. Accessed December 1, 2007.

[61] Pathology reporting on breast disease. NHS cancer screening programmes. Sheffield (UK): NHSBSP publication 58; 2005. Available at: http://www.cancerscreening.nhs.uk/breast screen/publications/nhsbsp58-low-resolution.pdf. Accessed December 1, 2007.

[62] Kuehn T, Bembenek A, Decker T, et al. A concept for the clinical implementation of sentinel lymph node biopsy in patients with breast carcinoma with special regards to quality assurance. Cancer 2005;103:451–61.

[63] Sentinel-Lymphknotenbiopsien. Available at: http://www.pathology.at/sentinel.htm. Accessed December 1, 2007.

[64] Australian Cancer Network Breast Pathology Working Party. The pathology reporting of breast cancer. A guide for pathologists, surgeons, radiologists and oncologists. 2nd edition. ACN Publication n 7. Sidney (Australia). Australian Cancer Network. 2001. Available at: http://www.cancer.org.au/documents/The_Pathology_reporting-of-breast-cancer-2001.pdf. Accessed December 1, 2007.

[65] Cserni G, Amendoeira I, Apostolikas N, et al. Discrepancies in current practice of pathological evaluation of sentinel lymph nodes in breast cancer. Results of a questionnaire-based survey by the European Working Group for Breast Screening Pathology. J Clin Pathol 2005;57:695–701.

[66] Bolster MJ, Bult P, Schapers RFM, et al. Differences in sentinel lymph node pathology protocols lead to differences in surgical strategy in breast cancer patients. Ann Surg Oncol 2006;13:1466–73.

[67] Giuliano AE, Dale PS, Turner RR, et al. Improved axillary staging of breast cancer with sentinel lymphadenectomy. Ann Surg 1995;180:700–4.

[68] van Rijk MC, Deterse JL, Nieweg OE, et al. Additional axillary metastases and stage migration in breast cancer patients with micrometastases or submicrometastases in sentinel lymph nodes. Cancer 2006;107:467–71.

[69] Fortunato L, Drago S, Vitelli CE, et al. Il linfonodo sentinella nel cancro della mammella: results of the Rome Breast Cancer Study Group. Chir Ital 2006;58:689–96.

[70] Cserni G. Complete sectioning of axillary sentinel nodes in patients with breast cancer. Analysis of two different step sectioning and immunohistochemistry protocols in 246 patients. J Clin Pathol 2002;55:926–31.

[71] Torrenga H, Rahusen FD, Meijer S, et al. Sentinel node investigation in breast cancer: detailed analysis of the yield from step sectioning and immunohistochemistry. J Clin Pathol 2001;54:550–2.

[72] Turner RR, Ollila DW, Stern S, et al. Optimal histopathologic examination of the sentinel lymph node for breast carcinoma staging. Am J Surg Pathol 1999;23:263–7.

[73] Freneaux P, Nos C, Vincent-Salomon A, et al. Histological detection of minimal metastatic involvement in axillary sentinel nodes: a rational basis for a sensitive methodology usable in daily practice. Mod Pathol 2002;15:641–6.

[74] Fortunato L, Amini M, Costarelli L, et al. A standardized sentinel lymph node enhanced pathology protocol (SEPP) in patients with breast cancer. J Surg Oncol 2007;96:470–3.

[75] Joslyn SA, Konety BR. Effect of axillary lymphadenectomy on breast cancer survival. Breast Cancer Res Treat 2005;91:11–8.

[76] Orr RK. The impact of prophylactic axillary node dissection on breast cancer survival: a Bayesian meta-analysis. Ann Surg Oncol 1999;6:109–16.

[77] Carter CL, Allen C, Henson DC, et al. Relation of tumor size, lymph node status and survival in 24740 breast cancer cases. Cancer 1989;63:181–7.

[78] Cserni G, Gregori D, Merletti F, et al. Meta-analysis of non-sentinel node metastases associated with micrometastatic sentinel nodes in breast cancer. Br J Cancer 2004;91:1245–52.

[79] Fortunato L, Amini M, Farina M, et al. Sentinel lymph node metastases in patients with breast cancer: axillary dissection or observation? Osp Ital Chir 2005;13:693–7.

[80] Van Zee K, Manasseh DME, Bevilacqua JLB, et al. A nomogram for predicting the likelihood of additional nodal metastases in breast cancer patients with a positive sentinel node biopsy. Ann Surg Oncol 2003;10:1140–51.

[81] Chagpar AB, Scoggins CR, Martin RC. Prediction of sentinel lymph node-only disease in women with invasive cancer. Am J Surg 2006;192:882–7.

[82] Bolster MJ, Peer PG, Bult P, et al. Risk factors for non-sentinel lymph node metastases in patients with breast cancer: the outcome of a multi-institutional study. Ann Surg Oncol 2006;14:181–9.

[83] Turner RR, Chu KU, Qi K, et al. Pathologic features associated with nonsentinel lymph node metastases in patients with metastatic breast carcinoma in a sentinel lymph node. Cancer 2000;89:574–81.

[84] Hwang D, Krishamurthy S, Hunt KK, et al. Clinicopathologic factors predicting involvement of nonsentinel axillary nodes in women with breast cancer. Ann Surg Oncol 2003;10:248–53.

[85] Barranger E, Coutant C, Flahault A, et al. An axilla scoring system to predict non-sentinel lymph node status in breast cancer patients with sentinel lymph node involvement. Breast Cancer Res Treat 2005;91:113–9.

[86] Alran S, De Rycke YD, Fourchotte V, et al. Validation and limitations of the use of a breast cancer nomogram predicting the likelihood of non-sentinel node involvement after a positive sentinel node biopsy. Ann Surg Oncol 2007;14:2195–201.

[87] Parks J, Fey JV, Naik AN, et al. A declining rate of axillary dissection in sentinel lymph node-positive breast cancer patients is associated with the use of a multivariate nomogram. Ann Surg 2007;245:462–8.

[88] Rutgers EJ, Meijnen P, Bonnefoi H. European Organization for Research and Treatment of Cancer: Clinical trials update of the European Organization for Research and Treatment of Cancer Breast Cancer Group. Breast Cancer Res 2004;6:165–9.

[89] Samoilova E, Davis JT, Hinson J, et al. Lymph node involvement: which breast cancer patients may benefit from less aggressive axillary dissection? Ann Surg Oncol 2007;14:2221–7.

[90] Cronin-Fenton DP, Ries LA, Clegg LX, et al. Rising incidence rates of breast carcinoma with micrometastatic lymph node involvement. J Natl Cancer Inst 2007;99:1044–9.

[91] International (Ludwig) Breast Cancer Study Group. Prognostic importance of occult axillary lymph node micrometastases from breast cancers. Lancet 1990;335:1565–8.

[92] Dowlatshahi K, Fan M, Snider HC, et al. Lymph node micrometastases from breast carcinoma: reviewing the dilemma. Cancer 1997;80:1188–97.

[93] Tan LK, Giri D, Panageas K, et al. Occult micrometastases in axillary lymph nodes of breast cancer patients are significant: a retrospective study with long-term follow-up (abstract). Proc Am Soc Clin Oncol 2002;21:37.

[94] Colleoni M, Rotmensz N, Peruzzotti G, et al. Size of breast cancer metastases in axillary lymph nodes: clinical relevance of minimal lymph node involvement. J Clin Oncol 2005; 23:1379–89.

[95] National Cancer Institute, US National Institute of Health clinical trials. International Breast Cancer Study Group (IBCSG). Galiberti V Trial 23-01. Phase III randomized study of surgical resection with or without axillary lymph node dissection in women with a clinically node-negative breast cancer with a sentinel micrometastasis. Available at: http://www.cancer.gov/clinical trials/IBCSG 23-01, 2004. Accessed December 1, 2007.

[96] White RL Jr, Wilke LG. Update on the NSABP and ACOSOG breast cancer sentinel node trials. Am Surg 2004;70:420–4.

[97] Leonard GD, Swain SM. Ductal carcinoma in situ, complexities and challenges. J Natl Cancer Inst 2004;96:906–20.

[98] van Deurzen CHM, Hobbelink MGG, van Hillegersberg R, et al. Is there an indication for sentinel node biopsy in patients with ductal carcinoma in situ of the breast? A review. Eur J Cancer 2007;43:993–1001.

[99] Zavagno G, Carcoforo P, Marconato R, et al. Role of axillary sentinel lymph node biopsy in patients with pure ductal carcinoma in situ of the breast. BMC Cancer 2005;5:28.

[100] Veronesi P, Intra M, Vento AR, et al. Sentinel lymph node biopsy for localized ductal carcinoma in situ? Breast 2005;14:520–2.

[101] Cody SH. Sentinel lymph node biopsy for DCIS: are we approaching consensus? Ann Surg Oncol 2007;12:2179–81.

[102] Moore KH, Sweeney KJ, Wilson ME, et al. Outcomes for women with ductal carcinoma in-situ and a positive sentinel node: a multi institutional audit. Ann Surg Oncol 2007;14: 2911–7.

[103] Broekhuizen LN, Wijsman JH, Peterse JL, et al. The incidence and significance of micrometastases in lymph nodes of patients with ductal carcinoma in situ and T1a carcinoma of the breast. Eur J Surg Oncol 2006;32:502–6.

[104] Klauber-DeMore N, Tan LK, Liberman L, et al. Sentinel lymph node biopsy: is it indicated in patients with high-risk ductal carcinoma-in-situ and ductal carcinoma-in-situ with microinvasion? Ann Surg Oncol 2000;7:636–42.

[105] Jimenez RE, Visscher DW. Clinicopathologic analysis of microscopically invasive breast carcinoma. Hum Pathol 1998;29:1412–9.

[106] Zavotsky J, Hansen N, Brennan MB, et al. Lymph node metastasis from ductal carcinoma in situ with microinvasion. Cancer 1999;85:2439–43.

[107] Intra M, Zurrida S, Maffini F, et al. Sentinel lymph node metastases in microinvasive breast cancer. Ann Surg Oncol 2003;10:1160–5.

[108] Zavagno G, Belardinelli V, Marconato R, et al. Sentinel lymph node metastasis from mammary ductal carcinoma in situ with microinvasion. Breast 2007;16:146–51.

[109] Fortunato L, Santoni M, Drago S, et al. Sentinel lymph node biopsy in women with pT1a or "micro-invasive" breast cancer. The Breast, in press.

[110] SI Wong, Chao C, Edwards MJ, et al. Accuracy of sentinel lymph node biopsy for patients with T2 and T3 breast cancer. Am Surg 2001;67:522–6.

[111] Coombs N, Chen W, Taylor R, et al. A decision tool for predicting sentinel node accuracy from breast tumor size and grade. Breast J 2007;13:593–8.

[112] Bedrosian I, Reynolds C, Mick R, et al. Accuracy of sentinel lymph node biopsy in patients with large primary breast tumors. Cancer 2000;88:2540–5.

[113] Olson JA, Fey J, Winaver J, et al. Sentinel lymphadenectomy accurately predicts nodal status in T2 breast cancer. J Am Coll Surg 2000;191:593–9.

[114] Chung MH, Ye W, Giuliano AE. Role of sentinel lymph node dissection in the management of large (> 5 cm) invasive breast cancer. Ann Surg Oncol 2001;8:688–92.

[115] Lelievre L, Houvenaeghel G, Buttarelli M, et al. Value of sentinel lymph node procedure in patients with large size breast cancer. Ann Surg Oncol 2006;14:621–6.

[116] Schule J, Frisell J, Ingvar C, et al. Sentinel node biopsy for breast cancer larger than 3 cm in diameter. Br J Surg 2007;94:948–51.

[117] Schrenk P, Wayand W. Sentinel-node biopsy in axillary lymph node staging for patients with multicentric breast cancer. Lancet 2001;357:122.

[118] Fernandez K, Swanson M, Verbanac K, et al. Is sentinel lymphadenectomy accurate in multifocal and multicentric breast cancer? [abstract 29] Proceedings of the 55th Annual Cancer Symposium of the Society of Surgical Oncology. 2002. p. S9–16.

[119] Kumar R, Jana S, Heiba SI, et al. Retrospective analysis of sentinel node localization in multifocal, multicentric, palpable or non palpable breast cancer. J Nucl Med 2003;44:7–10.

[120] Tousimis E, Van Zee KJ, Fey JV, et al. The accuracy of sentinel lymph node biopsy in multicentric and multifocal invasive breast cancers. J Am Coll Surg 2003;197:529–35.

[121] Goyal A, Newcombe RG, Mansel RE. Sentinel lymph node biopsy in patients with multifocal breast cancer. Eur J Surg Oncol 2004;30:475–9.

[122] Knauer M, Konstantiniuk P, Haid A, et al. Multicentric breast cancer: a new indication for sentinel node biopsy—a multi-institutional validation study. J Clin Oncol 2006;24:3374–80.

[123] Ferrari A, Dionigi P, Rovera F, et al. Multifocality and multicentricity are not contraindications for sentinel lymph node biopsy in breast cancer surgery. World J Surg Oncol 2006;4: 79–86.

[124] Gentilini O, Trifirò G, Soteldo J, et al. Sentinel lymph node biopsy in multicentric breast cancer. The experience of the European Institute of Oncology. Ann Surg Oncol 2006;32:507–10.

[125] D'Eredita G, Giardina C, Ingravallo G, et al. Sentinel lymph node biopsy in multiple breast cancer using subareolar injection of the tracer. Breast 2007;16:316–22.

[126] Breslin TM, Cohen LF, Sahin A, et al. Sentinel lymph node biopsy is accurate after neoadjuvant chemotherapy for breast cancer. J Clin Oncol 2000;18:3480–4.

[127] Tafra L, Verbanac KM, Lannin DR. Preoperative chemotherapy and sentinel lymphadenectomy for breast cancer. Am J Surg 2001;182:312–5.

[128] Fernandez A, Cortes M, Benito E, et al. Gamma probe sentinel node localization and biopsy in breast cancer patients treated with a neoadjuvant chemotherapy scheme. Nucl Med Commun 2001;22:361–6.

[129] Julian TB, Dusi D, Wolmark N. Sentinel node biopsy after neoadjuvant chemotherapy for breast cancer. Am J Surg 2002;184:315–7.

[130] Stearns V, Ewing CA, Slack R, et al. Sentinel lymphadenectomy after neoadjuvant chemotherapy for breast cancer may reliably represent the axilla except for inflammatory breast cancer. Ann Surg Oncol 2002;9:235–42.

[131] Brady EW. Sentinel lymph node mapping following neoadjuvant chemotherapy for breast cancer. Breast J 2002;8:97–100.

[132] Schwartz GF, Meltzer AJ. Accuracy of axillary sentinel lymph node biopsy following neoadjuvant (induction) chemotherapy for carcinoma of the breast. Breast J 2003;9:374–9.

[133] Piato JR, Barros AC, Pincerato KM, et al. Sentinel lymph node biopsy in breast cancer after neoadjuvant chemotherapy. A pilot study. Eur J Surg Oncol 2003;29:118–20.

[134] Reitsamer R, Peintinger F, Rettenbacher L, et al. Sentinel lymph node biopsy in breast cancer patients after neoadjuvant chemotherapy. J Surg Oncol 2003;84:63–7.

[135] Kang SH, Kim SK, Kwon Y, et al. Decreased identification rate of sentinel lymph node after neoadjuvant chemotherapy. World J Surg 2004;28:1019–24.

[136] Lang JE, Esserman LJ, Ewing CA, et al. Accuracy of sentinel lymphadenectomy after neoadjuvant chemotherapy: effect of clinical node status at presentation. J Am Coll Surg 2004;199:856–62.

[137] Shimazu K, Tamaki Y, Taguchi T, et al. Sentinel lymph node biopsy using periareolar injection of radiocolloid for patients with neoadjuvant chemotherapy-treated breast carcinoma. Cancer 2004;100:2555–61.

[138] Balch GC, Mithani SK, Richards KR, et al. Lymphatic mapping and sentinel lymphadenectomy after preoperative therapy for stage II and III breast cancer. Ann Surg Oncol 2003;10:616–21.

[139] Aihara T, Munakata S, Morino H, et al. Feasibility of sentinel node biopsy for breast cancer after neoadjuvant endocrine therapy: a pilot study. J Surg Oncol 2004;85:77–81.

[140] Mamounas EP, Brown A, Anderson S, et al. Sentinel node biopsy after neoadjuvant chemotherapy in breast cancer: results from National Surgical Adjuvant Breast and Bowel Project Protocol B-27. J Clin Oncol 2005;23:2694–702, Erratum in: J Clin Oncol. 2005;23: 4808.

[141] Tausch C, Konstantiniuk P, Kugler F, et al. Sentinel lymph node biopsy after preoperative chemotherapy for breast cancer: findings from the Austrian Sentinel Node Study Group. Ann Surg Oncol 2006 May 24 (Epub ahead of print).

[142] Shen J, Gilcrease MZ, Babiera GV, et al. Feasibility and accuracy of sentinel lymph node biopsy after preoperative chemotherapy in breast cancer patients with documented axillary metastases. Cancer 2007;109:1255–63.

[143] Newman EA, Sabel MS, Nees AV, et al. Sentinel lymph node biopsy performed after neoadjuvant chemotherapy is accurate in patients with documented node-positive breast cancer at presentation. Ann Surg Oncol 2007;14:2946–52.

[144] Kinoshita T. Sentinel lymph node biopsy is feasible for breast cancer patients after neoadjuvant chemotherapy. Breast Cancer 2007;14:10–5.

[145] Xing Y, Foy M, Cox DD, et al. Meta-analysis of sentinel lymph node biopsy after preoperative chemotherapy in patients with breast cancer. Br J Surg 2006;93:539–46.

[146] Fisher B, Anderson S, Bryant J, et al. Twenty-year follow-up of a randomized trial comparing total mastectomy, lumpectomy, and lumpectomy plus irradiation for the treatment of invasive breast cancer. N Engl J Med 2002;347:1233–41.

[147] Veronesi U, Marubini E, Del Vecchio M, et al. Local recurrences and distant metastases after conservative breast cancer treatments: partly independent events. J Natl Cancer Inst 1995;87:19–27.

[148] Roumen RMH, Kuijy GP, Liem LH. Lymphatic mapping and sentinel node harvesting in patients with recurrent breast cancer. Eur J Surg Oncol 2006;32:1076–81.

[149] Sood A, Youssef IM, Heiba SI, et al. Alternative lymphatic pathway after previous axillary node dissection in recurrent/primary breast cancer. Clin Nucl Med 2004;29:698–702.

[150] Agarwal A, Heron DE, Sumkin J, et al. Contralateral uptake and metastases in sentinel lymph node mapping for recurrent breast cancer. J Surg Oncol 2005;92:4–8.

[151] Newman EA, Cimmino VM, Sabel MS, et al. Lymphatic mapping and sentinel lymph node biopsy for patients with local recurrence after breast-conservation therapy. Ann Surg Oncol 2006;13:52–7.

[152] Taback B, Nguyen P, Hansen N, et al. Sentinel lymph node biopsy for local recurrence of breast cancer after breast-conserving therapy. Ann Surg Oncol 2006;13:1099–104.

[153] Intra M, Trifiro G, Galimberti V, et al. Second axillary sentinel node biopsy for ipsilateral breast tumour recurrence. Br J Surg 2007;94:1216–9.

[154] Port ER, Garcia-Etienne CA, Park J, et al. Reoperative sentinel lymph node biopsy: a new frontier in the management of ipsilateral breast tumor recurrence. Ann Surg Oncol 2007;14:2209–14.

[155] Barone JL, Feldman SM, Estabrook A, et al. Reoperative sentinel lymph node biopsy in patients with locally recurrent breast cancer. Am J Surg 2007;194:491–3.

[156] Axelsson CK, Jønsson PE. Sentinel lymph node biopsy in operations for recurrent breast cancer. Eur J Surg Oncol 2007 Oct 26 (Epub ahead of print).

[157] Nori J, Vanzi E, Bazzocchi M, et al. Role of axillary ultrasound in the selection of breast cancer patients for sentinel node biopsy. Am J Surg 2007;193:16–20.

[158] Bonnema J, van Geel AN, van Ooijen B, et al. Ultrasound-guided aspiration biopsy for detection of nonpalpable axillary node metastases in breast cancer patients: new diagnostic method. World J Surg 1997;21:270–4.

[159] Kanter AY, van Eijck CH, van Geel AN, et al. Multicentre study of ultrasonographically guided axillary node biopsy in patients with breast cancer. Br J Surg 1999;86:1459–62.

[160] Sato K, Tamaki K, Tsuda H, et al. Utility of axillary ultrasound examination to select breast cancer patients suited of optimal sentinel node biopsy. Am J Surg 2004;187:679–83.

[161] Deurloo EE, Tanis PJ, Gilhujis KGA, et al. Reduction in the number of sentinel lymph node procedures by pre-operative ultrasonography of the axilla in breast cancer. Eur J Cancer 2003;39:1068–73.

[162] Kuenen-Boumeester V, Menke-Pluymers M, de Kanter AY, et al. Ultrasound-guided fine needle aspiration cytology of axillary lymph nodes in breast cancer. A pre-operative staging procedure. Eur J Cancer 2003;39:170–4.

[163] Veronesi U, Marubini E, Mariani L, et al. The dissection of internal mammary nodes does not improve the survival of breast cancer patients. 30-year results of a randomized trial. Eur J Cancer 1999;35:1320–5.

[164] Estourgie SH, Nieweg OE, Valdes Olmos RA, et al. Lymphatic drainage patterns from the breast. Ann Surg 2004;239:232–7.

[165] Turner-Warwick RT. The lymphatics of the breast. Br J Surg 1959;46:574–82.

[166] Park C, Sied P, Morita E, et al. Internal mammary sentinel lymph node mapping for invasive breast cancer: implications for staging and treatment. Breast J 2005;11:29–33.

[167] Paganelli G, Galimberti V, Trifirò G, et al. Internal mammary node lymphoscintigraphy and biopsy in breast cancer. Q J Nucl Med 2002;46:138–44.

[168] Galimberti V, Veronesi P, Arnone P, et al. Stage migration after biopsy of internal mammary chain lymph nodes in breast cancer patients. Ann Surg Oncol 2002;9:924–8.

[169] Farrus B, Vidal-Sicart S, Velasco M, et al. Incidence of internal mammary node metastases after a sentinel lymph node technique in breast cancer and its implication in the radiotherapy plan. Int J Radiat Oncol Biol Phys 2004;60:715–21.

[170] Carcoforo P, Sortini D, Feggi L, et al. Clinical and therapeutic importance of sentinel node biopsy of the internal mammary chain in patients with breast cancer: a single-center study with long-term follow-up. Ann Surg Oncol 2006;13:1338–43.

ELSEVIER
SAUNDERS

Surg Oncol Clin N Am
17 (2008) 701–708

SURGICAL
ONCOLOGY CLINICS
OF NORTH AMERICA

Index

Note: Page numbers of article titles are in **boldface** type.

A

Ablation, local, for curative hepatic resection of bilobar colorectal metastases, 558–560

Adenocarcinoma, pancreatic, treatment of, European perspective on, **569–586**

Adhesion, cell, in prognosis of gastric carcinoma, 474

Adjuvant therapy, for pancreatic adenocarcinoma, 577
systemic, for melanoma, 640–643
chemotherapy, nonspecific immune stimulants, and vaccines, 640–641
interferon-alpha, 641–643
need for predictive factors, 643

Anatomic resection, and parenchymal preservation in liver resection for hepatocellular carcinoma, 617–618

Apoptosis, in prognosis of gastric carcinoma, 473–474

Autoantibodies, as predictive factors in adjuvant therapy for melanoma, 643

B

Biliary drainage, preoperative, in pancreatic adenocarcinoma, 571–572

Bilobar distribution, of colorectal liver metastases, prognostic value of, 554

Biopsy, sentinel lymph node, in breast cancer, **673–699**

Bleeding, prevention of, in liver resection for hepatocellular carcinoma, 618–622

Breast cancer, sentinel lymph node biopsy in, **673–699**
enhanced pathology, 679–682
false-negative rate, 676
identification of sentinel node and type of injection, 675–676
intraoperative examination, 677–679
morbidity, 676–677
predicting involvement of non-sentinel lymph nodes, 682–683
prognostic significance of micrometastases, 683–684
role in special circumstances, 684–691
ductal carcinoma in situ, 684–685
for multicentric disease, 686–687
internal mammary sentinel lymph node biopsy, 690–691
neoadjuvant chemotherapy, 687–688
preoperative identification of node involvement by ultrasound, 689–690
repeat, for recurrent breast cancer, 688–689
tumor diameter, 685–686

C

Cell adhesion, in prognosis of gastric carcinoma, 474

Cell cycle, in prognosis of gastric carcinoma, 473–474

Chemoradiotherapy, for advanced cancer of esophagus and gastroesophageal junction, definitive, 496–498
induction, 492–495
tumor response to, in rectal cancer, 545–546

Chemotherapy, as adjuvant therapy for melanoma, 640–641
for rectal cancer, 543–544
for soft-tissue sarcoma, 658–661
adjuvant, 658
chemoradiation, 659–660